One Health

People, Animals, and
the Environment

One Health

People, Animals, and the Environment

EDITED BY

Ronald M. Atlas

University of Louisville, Louisville, KY 40292

and

Stanley Maloy

San Diego State University, San Diego, CA 92182

ASM
PRESS

Washington, DC

Library of Congress Cataloging-in-Publication Data

One health: people, animals, and the environment / edited by Ronald M. Atlas, University of Louisville, Louisville, KY, and Stanley Maloy, San Diego State University, San Diego, CA.
   volumes cm
Includes index.
   ISBN 978-1-55581-842-5 (print) -- ISBN 978-1-55581-843-2 (electronic) 1. Zoonoses.
2. Human-animal relationships. 3. Human ecology. 4. Communicable diseases in animals.
5. Public health. 6. Environmental health. 7. Animal health. I. Atlas, Ronald M., 1946- editor of compilation. II. Maloy, Stanley R., editor of compilation.
   RA639.O53 2014
   362.19695'9--dc23

                              2013044586

doi:10.1128/9781555818432

Printed in the United States of America

10 9 8 7 6 5 4 3 2
Address editorial correspondence to: ASM Press, 1752 N St., N.W., Washington, DC 20036-2904, USA.
Send orders to: ASM Press, P.O. Box 605, Herndon, VA 20172, USA.
Phone: 800-546-2416; 703-661-1593. Fax: 703-661-1501.
E-mail: books@asmusa.org
Online: http://www.asmscience.org

CONTENTS

One Health: What Is It and Why Is It Important?

Zoonotic and Environmental Drivers of Emerging Infectious Diseases

One Health and Antibiotic Resistance

Disease Surveillance

Making One Health a Reality

CONTRIBUTORS

Kyle Adair • Centre for Immunity, Infection & Evolution, and Ashworth Laboratories, University of Edinburgh, Edinburgh EH9 3JT, United Kingdom

Salvador Almagro-Moreno • Department of Microbiology and Immunology, Geisel School of Medicine at Dartmouth, Hanover, NH 03755

Ronald M. Atlas • Department of Biology, University of Louisville, Louisville, KY 40292-0001

Hazel A. Barton • Department of Biology, University of Akron, Akron, OH 44325-3809

Liam Brierley • Centre for Immunity, Infection & Evolution, and Ashworth Laboratories, University of Edinburgh, Edinburgh EH9 3JT, United Kingdom

Edmundo Calva • Departamento de Microbiología Molecular, Instituto de Biotecnología, Universidad Nacional Autónoma de México, Cuernavaca, Morelos 62210, Mexico

Veronica Casas • Center for Microbial Sciences, San Diego State University, San Diego, CA 92182

David W. Chapman • Department of Organizational Leadership, Policy, and Development, University of Minnesota-Twin Cities, Minneapolis, MN 55455

Edward E. Clark • Wildlife Center of Virginia, Waynesboro, VA 22980

Peter Daszak • EcoHealth Alliance, New York, NY 10001

Julian Davies • Department of Microbiology and Immunology, Life Science Centre, University of British Columbia, Vancouver, BC V6T 1Z3, Canada

John Deen • Department of Veterinary Population Medicine, University of Minnesota College of Veterinary Medicine, St. Paul, MN 55108

Matthew Dixon • The Centre on Global Health Security, Chatham House, The Royal Institute of International Affairs, London SW1Y 4LE, United Kingdom

Bernadette Dunham • Center for Veterinary Medicine, U.S. Food and Drug Administration, Rockville, MD 20855

Julie C. Ellis • Tufts University, Cummings School of Veterinary Medicine, North Grafton, MA 01536

Macdonald W. Farnham • Department of Veterinary Population Medicine, University of Minnesota College of Veterinary Medicine, St. Paul, MN 55108

John R. Fischer • Southeastern Cooperative Wildlife Disease Study, College of Veterinary Medicine, University of Georgia, Athens, GA 30602

Richard French • University of New Hampshire, New Hampshire Veterinary Diagnostic Laboratory, Durham, NH 03824

Carolyn Garcia • School of Nursing, University of Minnesota-Twin Cities, Minneapolis, MN 55455

Colin M. Gillin • Wildlife Health and Population Lab, Oregon Department of Fish and Wildlife, Corvallis, OR 97330

Duncan Hannant • Department of Applied Immunology, School of Veterinary Medicine and Science, University of Nottingham Sutton Bonington Campus, Nottingham LE12 5RD, United Kingdom

David L. Heymann • The Centre on Global Health Security, Chatham House, The Royal Institute of International Affairs, London SW1Y 4LE, United Kingdom, and Department of Infectious Disease Epidemiology, London School of Hygiene and Tropical Medicine, London WC1E 7HT, United Kingdom

Megan K. Hines • Wildlife Data Integration Network, Department of Surgical Sciences, University of Wisconsin School of Veterinary Medicine, Madison, WI 53706

Parviez R. Hosseini • EcoHealth Alliance, New York, NY 10001

William D. Hueston • Department of Veterinary Population Medicine, University of Minnesota College of Veterinary Medicine, St. Paul, MN 55108

Martyn Jeggo • Geelong Centre for Emerging Infectious Diseases, Deakin University, Waurn Ponds Campus, Geelong, Victoria VIC 3220, Australia

Jeremy C. Jones • Department of Infectious Diseases, Division of Virology, St. Jude Children's Research Hospital, Memphis, TN 38105

William B. Karesh • EcoHealth Alliance, New York, NY 10001

Lonnie J. King • College of Veterinary Medicine, Ohio State University, Columbus, OH 43210

Zeynep A. Koçer • Department of Infectious Diseases, Division of Virology, St. Jude Children's Research Hospital, Memphis, TN 38105

Richard Kock • Department of Pathology & Infectious Diseases, The Royal Veterinary College, North Mymms, Hatfield, Hertfordshire AL9 7TA, United Kingdom

Meggan E. Kraft • Department of Veterinary Population Medicine, University of Minnesota College of Veterinary Medicine, St. Paul, MN 55108

Annie Li • City University of Hong Kong, Department of Biology and Chemistry, Kowloon Tong, Kowloon, Hong Kong

Elizabeth H. Loh • EcoHealth Alliance, New York, NY 10001

John S. Mackenzie • Curtin University, Perth, Western Australia WA 6012, Australia, and Burnet Institute, Melbourne, Victoria VIC 3004, Australia

Lawrence C. Madoff • ProMED-mail, University of Massachusetts Medical School, Massachusetts Department of Public Health, Jamaica Plain, MA 02130

Michael Mahero • Department of Veterinary Population Medicine, University of Minnesota College of Veterinary Medicine, St. Paul, MN 55108

Stanley Maloy • Center for Microbial Sciences, San Diego State University, San Diego, CA 92182-1010

Cris Marsh • Wildlife Data Integration Network, Department of Surgical Sciences, University of Wisconsin School of Veterinary Medicine, Madison, WI 53706

Patrick P. Martin • New York State Department of Environmental Conservation Wildlife Health Unit, Albany, NY 12233-4752

Robert G. McLean • Division of Biology, Kansas State University, Manhattan, KS 66506

Tracey S. McNamara • Western University of Health Sciences, Pomona, CA 91766

Dave McRuer   •   Wildlife Center of Virginia, Waynesboro, VA 22980

G. Medina-Vogel   •   Facultad de Ecología y Recursos Naturales, Universidad Andrés Bello, República 440, Santiago, Chile

Stephen S. Morse   •   Department of Epidemiology, Mailman School of Public Health, Columbia University, New York, NY 10032

Lawrence Mugisha   •   Department of Wildlife and Resource Management, Makerere University College of Veterinary Medicine, Animal Resources and Biosecurity, Kampala, Uganda

Kris A. Murray   •   EcoHealth Alliance, New York, NY 10001

Louis H. Nel   •   Department of Microbiology and Plant Pathology, Faculty of Natural and Agricultural Sciences, University of Pretoria, Pretoria, 0001, South Africa

Felicia B. Nutter   •   Department of Biomedical Sciences, Cummings School of Veterinary Medicine, Tufts University, North Grafton, MA 01536

Serge Nzietchueng   •   Department of Veterinary Population Medicine, University of Minnesota College of Veterinary Medicine, St. Paul, MN 55108

Debra Olson   •   School of Public Health, University of Minnesota-Twin Cities, Minneapolis, MN 55455

Albert D. M. E. Osterhaus   •   Department of Viroscience, Erasmus Medical Centre, 3000 CA Rotterdam, The Netherlands, and Artemis Research Institute for Wildlife Health in Europe, 3584 CK Utrecht, The Netherlands

Amy Pekol   •   Department of Organizational Leadership, Policy, and Development, University of Minnesota-Twin Cities, Minneapolis, MN 55455

Katharine M. Pelican   •   Department of Veterinary Population Medicine, University of Minnesota College of Veterinary Medicine, St. Paul, MN 55108

Leslie A. Reperant   •   Department of Viroscience, Erasmus Medical Centre, 3000 CA Rotterdam, The Netherlands

Hannah T. Reynolds   •   Department of Biology, University of Akron, Akron, OH 44325-3809

Cheryl Robertson   •   School of Nursing, University of Minnesota-Twin Cities, Minneapolis, MN 55455

Melinda K. Rostal   •   EcoHealth Alliance, New York, NY 10001

Carol Rubin   •   National Center for Emerging and Zoonotic Infectious Diseases, Centers for Disease Control and Prevention, Atlanta, GA 30333

Innocent B. Rwego   •   Department of Veterinary Population Medicine, University of Minnesota College of Veterinary Medicine, St. Paul, MN 55108, and Department of Biological Sciences, Makerere University, Kampala, Uganda

Emi K. Saito   •   National Surveillance Unit, Centers for Epidemiology and Animal Health, USDA APHIS Veterinary Services, Fort Collins, CO 80526

Krysten L. Schuler   •   Animal Health Diagnostic Center, Ithaca, NY 14850

William F. Siemer   •   Human Dimensions Research Unit, Department of Natural Resources, Cornell University, Ithaca, NY 14853

Claudia Silva   •   Departamento de Microbiología Molecular, Instituto de Biotecnología, Universidad Nacional Autónoma de México, Cuernavaca, Morelos 62210, Mexico

Kurt Sladky   •   Wildlife Data Integration Network, Department of Surgical Sciences, University of Wisconsin School of Veterinary Medicine, Madison, WI 53706

Jonathan Sleeman   •   National Wildlife Health Center, U.S. Geological Survey, Madison, WI 53711

Victoria Szewczyk   •   Wildlife Data Integration Network, Department of Surgical Sciences, University of Wisconsin School of Veterinary Medicine, Madison, WI 53706

Ronald K. Taylor   •   Department of Microbiology and Immunology, Geisel School of Medicine at Dartmouth, Hanover, NH 03755

Dominic A. Travis   •   Department of Veterinary Population Medicine, University of Minnesota College of Veterinary Medicine, St. Paul, MN 55108

Robert G. Webster   •   Department of Infectious Diseases, Division of Virology, St. Jude Children's Research Hospital, Memphis, TN 38105

Peregrine L. Wolff   •   Nevada Department of Wildlife, Reno, NV 89512

Mark E. J. Woolhouse   •   Centre for Immunity, Infection & Evolution, University of Edinburgh, Ashworth Laboratories, Edinburgh EH9 3JT, United Kingdom

Lisa Yon   •   School of Veterinary Medicine and Science, University of Nottingham Sutton Bonington Campus, Nottingham LE12 5RD, United Kingdom, and Twycross Zoo-East Midland Zoological Society, Twycross CV9 3PX, United Kingdom

Carlos Zambrana-Torrelio   •   EcoHealth Alliance, New York, NY 10001

PREFACE

One Health, the emerging discipline that brings together human, animal, and environmental health, is critical for the future control of infectious diseases. Over the past 30 years, new infectious diseases have been arising at an unprecedented frequency. Many diseases such as *Escherichia coli* O157:H7 infection, Lyme disease, hantavirus pulmonary syndrome, Nipah virus disease, and severe acute respiratory syndrome (SARS) were unknown before 1982. Other diseases that seemed to be dying out are now reemerging, including rabies and food-borne diseases. Some diseases like West Nile fever have leaped across oceans and spread across continents. Antibiotic resistance is increasing at an alarming rate. Where are the new diseases coming from? Why is the incidence of these diseases increasing? What can we do to respond to these health threats that seemingly arise suddenly? The answers to these questions lie in the One Health approach for achieving harmonized strategies for disease detection and prevention.

The vast majority of emerging infectious diseases in humans are zoonoses. The factors responsible for many of these diseases in humans often share common themes: environmental disruption by humans, exposure of microbes to a different niche that selects for new virulence traits and facilitates transmission to animals, and genetic changes that permit subsequent transmission to humans. In retrospect, this sequence is not surprising. Microbial evolution occurs rapidly. The increase in the human population has prompted the encroachment of humans into new environments, disrupting the ecology of these habitats and bringing humans and domestic animals into contact with wildlife. Exposure to wildlife facilitates the transmission of new diseases that were previously contained within localized niches.

This process is not unidirectional. Devastating infectious diseases in animals often result from human disruption of habitat. Examples include toxoplasmosis in marine mammals, leptospirosis in river otters, white-nose bat syndrome, and many other diseases that impact threatened species and reduce biodiversity.

Furthermore, as clearly demonstrated by the international spread of SARS and influenza and the impact of chytridiomycosis on amphibian populations worldwide, the emergence and re-emergence of infectious diseases are global problems. Extensive international travel and trade networks make it possible for pathogens to move from anywhere in the world to dense population centers within days.

This interdependence between human health, animal health, and environmental health underpins the concept of "One Health." Solutions to the growing problems with infectious disease demand collaboration between experts in many disciplines, including human medicine, animal medicine, and environmental sciences. However, there remain many barriers to implementation of an interdisciplinary One Health approach. Education of physicians, veterinarians, and environmental scientists is typically done as a focused discipline with little emphasis on the other domains. Most funding sources are directed specifically at human medicine, animal medicine, or environmental science, rather than the interfaces among these domains. Further, there is often ineffective communication between governmental agencies responsible for each of these domains within and between countries. Now, however, driven by the tremendous health and economic impact of infectious disease, the barriers are beginning to break down.

One Health is a paradigm shift in how we respond to the threat of emerging infectious diseases. The traditional approach has been to identify a sick person or animal, identify the pathogen, and apply a therapy to reduce the symptoms of disease. In contrast, the One Health approach focuses on surveillance of the environment, animals, and humans to predict an outbreak of disease *before* it happens, then to bring together environmental scientists, animal experts, and human physicians to develop upstream interventions that prevent the transmission of disease. This approach was not feasible before the development of computational approaches to analyze the large, complex data sets required to compile information from around the globe, evaluate the data, and pinpoint potential problems. In addition to reports from physicians and veterinarians, the data-gathering required for effective surveillance also includes social networking tools and new rapid laboratory approaches for DNA sequence analysis. Thus, although the close relationship between the environment, animals, and humans has been recognized for ages, the One Health initiative provides practical solutions that have broad implications. Interestingly, the greatest acceptance of One Health is seen in the developing world, where it is having significant impacts on control of infectious diseases.

This book presents core concepts, compelling evidence, successful applications, and the remaining challenges of One Health approaches to thwarting the threat of emerging infectious disease. The scientific insights described are timeless, and the potential solutions are timely. The One Health approach is simply too important to ignore.

Ronald M. Atlas and Stanley Maloy
November 2013

One Health: What Is It and Why Is It Important?

One Health: People, Animals, and the Environment
Edited by Ronald M. Atlas and Stanley Maloy
© 2014 American Society for Microbiology, Washington, DC
doi:10.1128/microbiolspec.OH-0012-2012

Chapter 1

Combating the Triple Threat: The Need for a One Health Approach

Lonnie J. King[1]

INTRODUCTION

We live in a world that is rapidly changing, complex, and progressively more interconnected. The convergence of people, animals, and their products embedded in a threatened environment has resulted in an unprecedented 21st-century mixing bowl. This convergence has created a new dynamic, one in which the health of three domains—animals, people, and the environment—is now profoundly and inextricably linked and elaborately woven together.

One way to think about this interconnectivity is to picture the domains of people, animals, and the environment as a group of interconnected circles (Fig. 1) that push and pull on one another and create profound forces through their interactions. The interaction of these forces is similar to the dynamics of Newton's third law of motion, which simply states that for every action there is an equal and opposite reaction. Thus, our actions and interventions in any of the three domains have an impact on the other domains. In today's world, these forces have mostly resulted in negative impacts on the health of all three. In addition, with the growing global populations of people and animals, human-animal interfaces are accelerating, expanding, and becoming increasingly consequential. The ultimate result is a threat to the health and well-being of people, animals, and the environment, where problems in one domain are causing greater challenges and problems in the others and have created the biological equivalent of the third law of motion.

To effectively address the connected and changing health challenges of today and tomorrow, we must alter our mindset and consider health through more of an ecological, holistic, and systems-based approach. There is a growing acceptance and revival of the concept of "One Health" to better understand and more appropriately address our contemporary challenges and the threats to the health of people, animals, and the environment. The essence of One Health is a collaborative, integrated, and multidisciplinary approach to improve health in all three domains rather than restrict our views and interventions to any single domain.

---

[1]College of Veterinary Medicine, Ohio State University, Columbus, OH 43210.

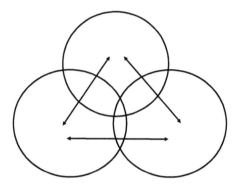

Ecosystem Health

Animal Health   Human Health

Figure 1. The domains and forces of One Health.
doi:10.1128/microbiolspec.OH-0012-2012.f1

BACKGROUND

While noninfectious diseases, chronic diseases, and environmental degradation are of growing importance to our health, central to the concept of One Health is understanding and controlling the infectious diseases that have helped shape the course of human history. The conditions that promote and favor the emergence and reemergence of infectious diseases are well established and have become even more entrenched as the 21st century evolves. These conditions were identified and described by an Institute of Medicine report in 2003 that referred to a new convergence model and factors producing a "perfect microbial storm" (1).

The perfect microbial storm has been created due to the following factors: adaptation of microbes; global travel, trade, and transportation; host susceptibility; climate change; economic development and land use; human demographics and behavior; poverty; social inequity; breakdown of public and animal health infrastructures; and war and the intent to do harm (1). Most of these factors are anthropogenic and have produced a new milieu and ingredients for a global mixing bowl, in which microbes have greater opportunities to establish new niches, cross species lines, be transported globally, become resistant, and very quickly create new exposures and challenges in the populations of people and animals and in the environment. Microbes can be transported directly among hosts, indirectly through food and water, or through vectors such as mosquitoes and ticks, and they may survive as environmental contaminants or microbial populations where they are maintained in nature outside of living hosts.

The result has been the creation of a new era of emerging and reemerging diseases that has been characterized especially by new zoonotic diseases. Over the last 3 decades, approximately 75% of new emerging human diseases have been zoonotic and many have come from and/or through wildlife (2). These diseases are also being found in new geographic locations. For example, in 2003 just in the United States, West Nile virus, monkeypox, and severe acute respiratory syndrome (SARS) infections were all found concurrently, and none of these diseases had ever previously been found in the Western Hemisphere.

The factors that created the perfect microbial storm are still in place and have largely been unabated. Thus, the era of emerging infections and new zoonoses is likely to continue. In a recent foresight study, scientists predicted that there will be two to four new emerging diseases every year. The highest probability for emergence will be associated with RNA viruses, especially those found at the human-animal interface (3). We are reminded that the current HIV/AIDS epidemic, which has resulted in more than 40 million human cases worldwide, had its origin in a chimpanzee retrovirus that jumped species and then adapted itself to human-to-human transmission. Exotic animals and bush meat are now popular and represent significant products in global trade and new threats to both human and animal health.

Our complex and interrelated global health threats are, unfortunately, also caused by complex and interrelated issues and problems, and thus lack simple solutions. The concept of "wicked problems" comes from the world of business but also aptly describes our health threats. Wicked problems are characterized by complexity, uniqueness, enigma, the lack of simple solutions, and the failure of past solutions to address them, and they are often symptomatic of other problems. Wickedness does not refer to the difficulty of the problem, but rather to its inability to be solved by standard approaches used in the past (4). For example, in the future the prevention of many diseases such as food-borne illnesses will come from new strategies and interventions focused on the animal or environmental domains emphasizing prevention, as opposed to the narrow focus of the past, which targeted people suffering from such illnesses and thus limited the response to the human domain.

The former director of the World Health Organization, Gro Harlem Brundtland, once said, "In a modern world, bacteria and viruses travel almost as fast as money. With globalization a single microbial sea washes over all human kind. There are no health sanctuaries" (address to Davos World Economic Forum, January 29, 2001). That sea also washes over all other species, and the microbial world has new opportunities for transmission, new niches and species to infect, and new geographical sites in which to become established. Thus we are, indeed, part of one large, interconnected, global village, where one country's problem can be another country's problem in a matter of hours.

HUMAN DOMAIN

The world population currently has a growth rate of 1.2% per year, and the next century will represent a period of exponential growth. The global population now exceeds 7 billion people and is estimated to increase to over 9 billion by the middle of this century. It is estimated that 90% of the global population growth will take place in the developing world and the world's fastest growth will actually take place in periurban settings that are now a part of almost all large cities in developing countries (5). Today almost 1 billion people inhabit these sites. Global slums are creating unprecedented conditions where new emerging and reemerging diseases are highly probable outcomes. There is further concern that developing countries lack the public and animal health infrastructures needed to quickly detect an emerging health threat or to effectively respond to or control such threats. In an interconnected world, this reality makes the entire world riskier and more vulnerable.

At the same time, we are now witnessing an era characterized by the phenomenal relocation, migration, and movement of people worldwide. The global economy is a key driver causing people to shift from rural settings to urban centers. Furthermore, new diasporas are being created as populations relocate globally due to the changing economy and job availability, and large populations of refugees are being created due to social and political unrest. In addition to this unique human relocation phenomenon, people are also traveling more. Today more than 1 billion people cross international borders each year. Not only are people on the move, but animals, vectors, food, and other commerce are also on the move and microbes are given unprecedented opportunities to migrate rapidly.

The world is literally in motion and on the move. Geographers refer to the world as "collapsed space." Our global travel, trade, commerce, and human movements have literally merged space, resulting in the acceleration and increase in interactions of people, animals, and animal products with potential exposure to microbes capable of crossing species lines. To add further to this risk, people are invading new territories and changing habitats and a substantial part of the world's surface has been inexorably altered, threatening the environment and its sustainability.

Finally, there are growing segments of our human population that have acquired vulnerabilities to certain diseases. In the United States, and indeed worldwide, there is an increase in the global cohort of people classified as seniors. In the United States, the baby boomers are approaching retirement and may represent a large population that could collectively experience a potential reduced immunity with age. We now have growing populations of immunocompromised individuals, including cancer patients, organ transplant patients, and HIV/AIDS patients, who are part of a growing cohort with greater susceptibility to infectious diseases.

One of the key factors determining health is poverty. Poor health is both a cause of and a result of poverty. Often people are trapped in poverty for a lifetime, and their health and quality of life are also reduced and threatened over an entire lifetime. While poverty takes many tolls, one of the most tragic has been its inexorable link with infectious diseases.

Approximately 1 billion people live on less than $2 a day. Worldwide, almost two-thirds of the rural poor and one-third of the urban poor depend on livestock to provide them with essential household income and a source of food and nutrients (6). Poor livestock keepers are found especially in Southeast Asia, Africa, and India. This large global population is threatened by zoonotic diseases because of their close proximity to livestock and dependence on animal products. Zoonotic diseases carry a double impact. They add substantially to disease morbidity, mortality, and loss of productivity of livestock and poultry themselves but may also produce illnesses in their keepers. A recent study by the International Livestock Research Institute highlighted a strong association among poverty, hunger, livestock keeping, and zoonoses (20). Globally, the top 13 zoonotic diseases are responsible for 2.4 billion cases of illness and 2.2 million human deaths per year. Examples of these zoonoses include gastrointestinal parasites, leptospirosis, cysticercosis, bovine tuberculosis, rabies, brucellosis, toxoplasmosis, and Q fever (6). Livestock and poultry production is rapidly increasing in the developing world, where the demand for protein from animal sources is rapidly expanding and the production of livestock and poultry holds the promise of a path out of poverty.

A One Health perspective is essential to reducing the huge economic, social, and health impact of zoonoses in developing countries. These diseases often involve wildlife as well as domestic animals, and almost all of these zoonoses are amenable to agriculture-based interventions, which gives further credence to One Health strategies.

ANIMAL DOMAIN

As the world's human population grows significantly, animal populations are also increasing rapidly. The growth in companion animals and recreational animals such as horses is also on the rise. Exotic animal pets are popular, and the illegal export and movement of these animals is a growing problem both because of human exposure to potentially new zoonotic agents and because of the emergence of novel diseases in new animal species. HIV/AIDS, malaria, and tuberculosis represent the major infectious diseases today. However, all three are likely to have had their origin in animal populations and subsequently adapted and become capable of person-to-person transmission.

A major global trend today is the substantial growth and expansion of food animal populations due to the growing demand for protein from animal sources in human diets. There were more than 24 billion food animals produced last year to help feed more than 7 billion people (6). The Food and Agriculture Organization of the United Nations describes a new agricultural revolution and predicts that there will be a demand for a 50% increase in animal proteins over the next 1 to 2 decades. This remarkable agricultural revolution is based on the relative increase in wealth in many developing countries and the subsequent change in diets toward more animal products (7).

In addition to the need to produce an unprecedented number of food animals, this livestock revolution is driving profound changes in how livestock and poultry are produced, where they are produced, and the environmental consequences of this phenomenon. While literally billions of food animals will need to be produced using more integrated, larger, and specialized production systems, they will be reared and produced to a progressively greater extent in the developing countries of the world. As part of this phenomenon, there will be an expansion of grazing lands and more grain crops will need to be produced to feed these animals. Major issues including environmental sustainability, nutrient management, and an enlarging carbon footprint are growing and emergent challenges.

GLOBAL FOOD SYSTEMS

Inherent in the concept of the great convergence is the creation of an immense and widely distributed global food system. In 2011, U.S. producers and ranchers alone produced almost 93 billion pounds of meat. Food imports and exports represent one of the world's largest trade and commercial markets. Currently the United States imports approximately 15% of its food; however, some products like shrimp and other seafood, fruits, and vegetables are imported to a much higher degree (8). Global food systems are remarkable but also add to the risk of transporting microbes. Microbes can move worldwide faster than their incubation periods, and the threat to both human and animal health is increasing, with food and water as potential vehicles for the dissemination of pathogens.

As in people, animal diseases are also emerging and reemerging. Global agricultural businesses are increasingly concerned about the exposure, vulnerabilities, and biosecurity of their supply chains, products, and animals. Diseases such as influenza, foot-and-mouth disease, bovine spongiform encephalopathy, and African swine fever have emerged and produced major outbreaks with huge economic losses as well as other consequences, including morbidity and mortality of animals; loss of products; costs of control and recovery; loss of global markets; disruptions of supply chains; loss of protein sources; landscape and environmental damages; loss of income and jobs; detrimental impacts on the economic and social well-being and health of rural communities; and potential public health costs, especially for zoonotic diseases. There are further concerns regarding the loss of wildlife populations and biodiversity, animal suffering, human psychological costs, and potential loss of the public's confidence. Recent experiences in the United Kingdom dealing with epidemics of bovine spongiform encephalopathy and foot-and-mouth disease have given us a new appreciation of the consequences of trying to address devastating diseases of livestock and poultry. In addition to the horrific losses to the animal populations themselves, these epidemics altered people's lives and left deep and long-term social, economic, and psychological scars in many individuals and communities. Furthermore, the SARS epidemic, which originated and was amplified by animals in special live-animal markets, resulted in serious losses to tourism, financial markets, and numerous ancillary businesses. Thus, the incursions of such diseases today have much greater consequences than they did previously and go much further and deeper than just the impact on agricultural communities. Looking though a One Health prism is essential to view and truly understand the driving forces and impacts of these diseases but also to offer insights into the use of new interventions and prevention schemes.

Because of the economic and psychological consequences of incursions of exotic diseases in large populations of animals, another concern and vulnerability has emerged: the intentional introduction of pathogens by bioterrorists. Of the current list of select agents, 80% are zoonotic and could be found in animal populations before human cases are found. Certainly there is a growing need to incorporate animal and environmental surveillance as part of a national One Health preparedness and surveillance plan.

Food Safety

The animal health and public health domains are even more connected today through our food systems and form an important interface with growing concerns. The CDC now estimates that there are approximately 48 million food-borne illnesses in the United States every year, resulting in 128,000 hospitalizations and 3,000 deaths annually (9). Although we lack similar global data, a rough extrapolation suggests that there could be as many as 1 billion such illnesses worldwide each year. Without question, the burden of food-borne disease represents a huge health care cost. A number of food-borne diseases such as norovirus and hepatitis are transmitted directly from person to person with food as a common vehicle; however, many food-borne illnesses are zoonotic and are transmitted across domains.

CDC studies have also demonstrated changing patterns of attribution. Plant-derived foods such as leafy greens, tomatoes, and sprouts have been implicated in more and more food-borne disease outbreaks. In the recent past, transmission has been linked to peanut butter, pizza, spinach, ice cream, cookie dough, pet food, melons, mangoes, peppers, and carrot juice. There is also concern about the concept of "stealth" vehicles in transmission. There are numerous food ingredients that are often mixed in with foods, such as spices, that can be vehicles for transmission but are often not considered in outbreak investigations (10).

In addition to the traditional food-borne pathogens such as *Escherichia coli* and *Salmonella*, *Campylobacter*, and *Listeria* spp., new outbreaks often reveal new agents. The FoodNet System, which analyzes outbreaks, has revealed adenoviruses, sapoviruses, picobirnaviruses, and Saffold virus as potential pathogens. To further complicate our understanding of the safety of our food, transmission vehicles can change when microbes are given new opportunities. For example, the Nipah virus, first found as a zoonotic disease outbreak in Malaysia that killed pigs and people associated with them, has recently been found as a contaminant in date palm sap, a food source in Bangladesh. *Pteropus* fruit bats are the asymptomatic carriers. *Trypanosoma cruzi* is the parasite that causes Chagas disease and is usually transmitted to people via reduviid insects, yet it has recently been found in sugar cane juice in Brazil. There is a remarkable spectrum of foods and pathogens involved in food-borne illnesses and this is an ever-changing dynamic. Produce is of growing importance as a vehicle for food-borne pathogens, yet animal reservoirs are often the origin of these infections. One Health gives us the proper lens to view and better understand this linkage and, more importantly, to develop new insights for changing our interventions and prevention strategies. In many instances, ill people are the endpoint of a complicated epidemiological cycle and serve as indicator hosts; however, if we continue to focus exclusively on food-borne illness by responding to human outbreaks and just conducting retrospective analyses, we will miss the true sites of origin of these diseases and we will forgo critical prevention strategies in other domains. To a certain extent, ill people serve as sentinels of a larger ecological problem and, as such, may not be the best focal point for our interventions. One Health is a mindset that is proactive and preventive; it helps to shift our attention "upstream" to the ecological, animal, and environmental sources responsible for these illnesses and, therefore, helps us to identify the most effective points for the initiation of food safety actions.

ENVIRONMENTAL DOMAIN

Our environment has continued to undergo changes, mostly to the detriment of our various ecosystems. The threat to the health of our environment is largely anthropogenic. While we are concerned about the sustainability of the environment itself, we also understand more clearly that diseases, too, are often a result of environmental disruption and changes.

The increasing incidence of Lyme disease is very much the result of human changes to the environment, especially on the East Coast of the United States. Forests have been reduced and fragmented and development has chased off predators; thus, an expanding population of deer and white-footed mice helped preserve both *Ixodes* ticks and the *Borrelia* organism. The disease consistently spills over into human populations colocated in these new ecological sites. When ecosystems are disrupted along with our natural biodiversity, we often remove the protective effects of multiple species (11).

Some scientists have referred to today's era as part of Earth's sixth mass extinction, with unprecedented loss of plant and animal species largely due to disruptive human activities (12). As a consequence, there is heightened concern that the protective and buffering effect of biodiversity is being lost and microbes could enter directly into people without first infecting other species that are no longer available as hosts.

Habitat disruption and alteration of land use also affect vector populations. An additional concern is climate change and the potential of changing the geographic range of disease vectors. There are more than 3,000 species of mosquitoes, some of which are very efficient and effective disease transmitters. Historians estimate that mosquitoes may be responsible for half the deaths in human history (13). Malaria, yellow fever, and recently a serious dengue epidemic are vector-borne diseases. The animal disease bluetongue, discovered recently and now found across much of Europe, may be a consequence of the expansion of the *Culicoides* (biting midge) vector due to warmer temperatures. In addition, Schmallenberg virus, an emerging disease affecting domestic ruminants in Europe, is a newly found orthobunyavirus and likely transmitted by *Culicoides* vectors. These vectors seemingly have established new geographic niches, possibly due to warmer temperatures. Rift Valley fever has caused both animal and human epidemics in Africa after flooding rains have greatly increased the population of mosquitoes. Cholera, caused by *Vibrio cholerae*, may be associated with typhoons that flood Bangladeshi lowlands and produce a favorable environment for plankton growth and subsequent larger numbers of vibrio organisms that live off the plankton and then infect people. An epidemic outbreak of cholera in Haiti that followed a devastating earthquake appears to have been introduced into the water supplies by an infected aid worker from Asia.

Recent events have demonstrated that fungi are becoming greater global threats to agriculture, forests, and wild animals than was previously understood. Countless amphibians have been killed; some species have become extinct; and some food crops such as wheat, rice, and soybeans have all experienced serious fungal infections. One-third of the world's amphibian population is globally threatened or extinct due to an epidemic of fungal infections (14).

Increased global trade and travel, changing agricultural practices, and perhaps global warming are responsible for the increase in fungal infections and their geographic shift. Two major animal crises—the profound decline in amphibian species and a disease outbreak in North American bats—have given us new cause for concern. *Batrachochytrium dendrobatidis* is a fungus whose spores survive in streams and ponds and is responsible for a tragic loss of biodiversity in Central and North America and Australia. Bat white-nose syndrome is caused by *Geomyces destructans* and has killed approximately 6 million bats in the United States (19). These fungi can persist in the environment and live outside their hosts for years. In addition, cryptococcal meningitis (*Cryptococcus neoformans*) is estimated to cause 1 million human infections annually, especially in immunocompromised populations. *Cryptococcus gattii*, which has spread into western Canada and the northwestern United States from Australasia, is a fungus that has infected people, domestic animals, marine mammals, and forests. This fungus has shifted in both its geographic location and ecologic niche. Scientists have been able to identify only a small percentage of the global fungal species. They are clearly part of the 21st-century convergence of people and animals in a changing environment. There is further speculation that fungi may adapt very well to globalization and now represent another emerging triple threat to health.

Nature supports many of our human endeavors. Forests help filter our water, bees and birds help pollinate our crops, and our many diverse animal species help serve as filters and buffers for infectious microbes, thus protecting people from exposure to potential pathogens. As we experience warmer temperatures across the globe, there is concern that the ranges and life cycles of vectors may change significantly and alter the exposure of humans to vector-borne and waterborne diseases. Our understanding of these dynamics gives us a new appreciation of the term "ecology of disease." Thus, if our natural world breaks down, our human and animal health can be negatively affected, often in ways we have never experienced.

CONSEQUENCES OF THIS UNPRECEDENTED CONVERGENCE

There is no question that we live in a world that has become riskier and is on a trajectory to become even more so as our space collapses and more and more people and animals converge and exist in ecosystems that are changing and are not sustainable.

As a consequence, microbes, as they have done for eons, are taking advantage—they adapt; move globally; cross species lines; become resistant to antimicrobials; have increasing numbers of hosts, vectors, and products from which to choose; and are able to target populations with greater vulnerabilities. As our microbial swarms gain a greater advantage and influence, their scope, scale, and impact also increase and there is an undeniable and direct correlation to an increased threat to our health.

An added concern is that in many countries, infrastructures to support both human and animal health are not commensurate with the increasing levels of threat. There is a concern that current economic conditions have reduced funds and investment in public and animal health safety nets and that there has been an erosion of some key systems supporting surveillance and rapid detection and response capacities. Finally, there is also a new appreciation that outbreaks of disease go beyond health costs and may lead to significant losses in travel, commerce, supply chains, and potentially public trust and confidence.

A CALL FOR A NEW MODEL TO CONFRONT THIS CHALLENGE

Our growing interconnectedness and the "wicked" nature of our problems have created not only more complex challenges but also the need to rethink and recreate new solutions and strategies to address the triple threat to our health. Inherent in this contemporary condition is the fact that old solutions no longer work as well and new solutions haven't been invented or effectively incorporated.

One Health is a concept that embraces disease ecology. The holistic understanding of ecology and our connectedness gives us new insights into the control and prevention of disease and improvement of our health. However, this mindset is almost counter to our training in medicine, especially clinical medicine, where we seek definitive diagnoses, try to establish an immediate cause-and-effect relationship, and determine and implement the best treatment. Medicine and science have resulted in phenomenal breakthroughs but have also created a bias toward reductionism as we have made new molecular and genomic discoveries. In part, this bias has led us away from holistic and ecological studies and away from a fuller appreciation of the complexities and dynamics of disease processes, especially for zoonoses. One Health gives us a better balance between reductionism and ecological approaches and leads to more effective medical interventions.

One Health is the collaborative effort of multiple disciplines working locally, nationally, and globally to attain optimal health for people, animals, and our environment (15). It is a paradigm that recognizes the interconnectedness of people, animals, and the environment and emphasizes disease prevention. The scale and complexity of health threats demand that scientists, researchers, and others move beyond the confines of their own disciplines, professions, and mindsets and explore new organizational models of team science; a One Health concept embodies this declaration. The scope of One Health is impressive, broad, and growing. Much of the recent focus of One Health has been limited to emerging infectious diseases, yet the concept clearly embraces environmental and ecosystem health, social sciences, ecology, noninfectious and chronic diseases, wildlife, land use, antimicrobial resistance, biodiversity, and much more.

While these components are appreciated within our understanding of the broad dimensions of health, they also add to the complexity of One Health and the difficulty in implementing strategies, building effective coalitions, and mobilizing scientific communities that embrace One Health. Although there may be different definitions of One Health, there is broad consensus that a new framework for preventing infectious diseases is essential rather than the alternative of constantly responding reactively to these diseases.

The World Health Organization defines health as not merely the absence of disease but rather as a state of well-being and wellness that encompasses physical, mental, and spiritual health, resulting in healthier, safer, happier, and more productive lives. One Health is a concept that enables us to better understand this broad definition of health and that health is based on many factors and represents an ever-changing dynamic.

The factors determining health include genetics, social circumstances, environmental conditions, behavior, and medical care. The last, medical care, represents less than 25% of the total impact of determining our health status. In the United States, we spend approximately $2 trillion on health care per year, yet a very small and disproportionate amount of this total is spent on disease prevention and health promotion, where the greatest health impact can be achieved (16). One Health stresses prevention by incorporating other factors and shifting interventions upstream, closer to the source of the problem. Armed with this knowledge, scientists, researchers, and health care workers need to form One Health teams that cross disciplines and professions to better understand and improve health.

The concepts expressed as One Health are not new, but are predicated on the discoveries of others such as Louis Pasteur in the late 19th century, and were widely accepted before the advent of specialized medicine. These concepts have "reemerged" as One Health because they place the problem of infectious disease emergence within ecosystems, a relationship championed by the late Nobel laureate Joshua Lederberg. In his essay "Infectious History," Lederberg observed that "an axiomatic starting point for progress [against emerging infectious diseases] is the simple recognition that humans, animals, plants and microbes are cohabitants of this planet. That leads to refined questions that focus on the origin and dynamics of instabilities within this context of cohabitation. These instabilities arise from two main sources loosely definable as ecological and evolutionary" (17).

Adopting a One Health approach is an example of changing paradigms, as described by philosopher of science Thomas Kuhn in his seminal work, *The Structure of Scientific Revolutions* (18). With regard to medical science and addressing emerging diseases, we have reached an era when old models don't work as well but new models have yet to be created, a time when basic assumptions must be questioned and changed.

Such changes need not be led by the scientific community. The paradigm shift to One Health may be consumer driven. Indeed, One Health should be considered in terms of its economic benefits to stakeholders, and its value judged according to evidence of its superiority to current approaches. The evidence has to be based on metrics of reduced costs, reduction or elimination of cases and deaths, and greater effectiveness.

CONCLUDING REMARKS

There is nothing on the horizon to suggest that the factors and conditions driving the "perfect microbial storm" are lessening or abating. Our world continues to be more and more connected: trade, travel, and commerce are growing; populations of people, animals, and wildlife continue to grow and the interfaces between animals and people are both accelerating and intensifying; a global food system is expanding; pollution and contamination of our environment along with habitat destruction continue unchecked; climate change may alter our exposure to vector-borne and waterborne infections; our biodiversity of plants and animals is rapidly being lost; poor health continues to be both a cause and consequence of poverty; vulnerable populations are increasing in numbers; and microbes are gaining the upper hand through their ability to establish new niches and become resistant to antimicrobial agents. The result is a triple threat to the health of people, animals, and our environment. These factors also represent the principal evidence needed to mobilize health professionals toward adapting a new One Health approach to reduce these threats. Until we address the underlying factors that lead to disease emergence and reemergence, we will just continue to try to address these problems one at a time as we have done in the past. In today's world, we must commit and refocus our efforts holistically and collaboratively. We can no longer just focus on humans and microbes but rather must shift our attention to the interplay among people, animals, and the environment—One Health.

Understanding the mechanisms that underlie newly emerging and reemerging infectious diseases is one of the most difficult scientific problems facing society today. Significant knowledge gaps exist for many studies of emerging infectious diseases. Coupled with failures in the response to the resurgence of infectious diseases, this lack of information is embedded in a simplistic view of pathogens and disconnected from a social and ecological context, and it assumes a linear response of pathogens to environmental change. In fact, the natural reservoirs and transmission rates of most emerging infectious diseases are affected primarily by environmental factors, such as seasonality or meteorological events, typically producing nonlinear results that are inherently unpredictable. A more realistic view of emerging infectious diseases requires a holistic perspective and incorporates social as well as physical, chemical, and biological dimensions of our global systems. The notion of One Health captures this depth and richness and, most importantly, the interactions of human and natural systems. Furthermore, there must be a synthesis of interdisciplinary approaches aligned with social-ecological approaches to garner an improved understanding of emerging infectious diseases, to better manage them, and to successfully address the wicked problems underlying the triple threat to health.

Citation. King LJ. 2013. Combating the triple threat: the need for a One Health approach. Microbiol Spectrum 1(1):OH-0012-2012. doi:10.1128/microbiolspec.OH-0012-2012.

REFERENCES

1. **Smolinski MS, Hamburg MA, Lederberg J (ed).** 2003. *Microbial Threats to Health: Emergence, Detection and Response*, p 19. National Academies Press, Washington, DC.
2. **Taylor LH, Latham SM, Woolhouse ME.** 2001. Risk factors for human disease emergence. *Philos Trans R Soc London B Biol Sci* **356:**983–989.
3. **Brownlie J, Peckham C, Waage J, Woolhouse M, Lyall C, Meagher L, Tait J, Baylis M, Nicoll A.** 2006. *Foresight. Infectious Diseases: Preparing for the Future. Future Threats.* Office of Science and Innovation, London, United Kingdom.
4. **Camillus JC.** 2008. Strategy as a wicked problem. *Harvard Bus Rev* **86:**99–106.
5. **FAOSTAT.** 2012. *FAO statistical database.* Food and Agriculture Organization of the United Nations, Rome, Italy. http://faostat3.fao.org/home/index.html.
6. **International Livestock Research Institute.** 2012. *Mapping of Poverty and Likely Zoonoses Hotspots. Zoonoses Project 4: Report to Department for International Development, UK*, p 4–27. International Livestock Research Institute, Nairobi, Kenya.
7. **Delgado C, Rosegrant M, Steinfeld F, Ehui S, Courbois C.** 1999. *Lifestock to 2020: the Next Food Revolution*, p 1–12. Food, Agriculture and the Environment Discussion Paper 28. International Food Policy Research Institute, Washington, DC.
8. **Florkowski WJ.** 2008. Status and projections for foods imported into the United States, p 1–7. *In* Doyle MP, Erickson MC (ed), *Imported Foods: Microbiological Issues and Challenges.* ASM Press, Washington, DC.
9. **Scallon E, Hoekstra RM, Angulo FJ, Tauxe RV, Widdowson MA, Roy SL, Jones JL, Griffin PM.** 2011. Foodborne illness acquired in the United States—major pathogens. *Emerg Infect Dis* **17:**7–15.
10. **Tauxe R.** 2008. *Roots of foodborne illness. Meeting report.* New York Academy of Sciences, New York, NY.
11. **Ostfeld RS.** 2011. *Lyme Disease: the Ecology of a Complex System*, p 113–143. Oxford University Press, New York, NY.
12. **Wake DB, Vredenburg VT.** 2008. Colloquium paper: are we in the midst of the sixth mass extinction? A view from the world of amphibians. *Proc Natl Acad Sci USA* **105**(Suppl 1)**:**11466–11473.
13. **Specter M.** 2012. The mosquito solution. *The New Yorker* (Annals of Science) July 9, 2012, 38–40.
14. **Kupferschmidt K.** 2012. Mycology. Attack of the clones. *Science* **337:**636–638.
15. **King LJ, Anderson LR, Blackmore CG, Blackwell MJ, Lautner EA, Marcus LC, Meyer TE, Monath TP, Nave JE, Ohle J, Pappaioanou M, Sobota J, Stokes WS, David RM, Glasser JH, Mahr RK.** Executive summary of the AVMA One Health Initiative Task Force report. *J Am Vet Med Assoc* **233:**259–261.
16. **Committee on Living Well with Chronic Disease: Public Health Action to Reduce Disability and Improve Functioning and Quality of Life.** 2012. *Living Well with Chronic Illness: A Call for Public Health Action.* National Academies Press, Washington, DC.
17. **Lederberg J.** 2000. Infectious history. *Science* **288:**287–293.
18. **Kuhn T.** 1996. *The Structure of Scientific Revolutions*, 3rd ed, p 3–27. University of Chicago Press, Chicago, IL. First published 1962.

19. **Reynolds HT, Barton HA.** 2013. White-nose syndrome: human activity in the emergence of an extirpating mycosis. *Microbiol Spectrum* **1**(1):OH-0008-2012. doi:10.1128/microbiolspectrum.OH-0008-2012.

20. **Grace D, Mutua F, Ochungo P, Kruska R, Jones K, Brierley L, Lapar L, Said M, Herrero M, Phuc PM, Thao NB, Akuku I, Ogutu F.** 2012. *Mapping of poverty and likely zoonoses hotspots.* International Livestock Research Institute. http://hdl.handle.net/10568/21161.

One Health: People, Animals, and the Environment
Edited by Ronald M. Atlas and Stanley Maloy
© 2014 American Society for Microbiology, Washington, DC
doi:10.1128/microbiolspec.OH-0011-2012

Chapter 2

The Value of the One Health Approach: Shifting from Emergency Response to Prevention of Zoonotic Disease Threats at Their Source

David L. Heymann[1,2] and Matthew Dixon[1]

EMERGENCY RESPONSE TO NEWLY IDENTIFIED HUMAN INFECTIONS

When an infectious disease organism from an animal breaches the species barrier to infect a human, it enters an immunologically naïve population. Depending on incompletely understood risk factors, which depend on both the organism and the infected human, there are several possible transmission pathways: (i) no further transmission, with the human an endpoint as in rabies and variant Creutzfeldt-Jakob disease; (ii) nonsustained human-to-human transmission such as presently occurs in close human contact with persons with influenza A (H5N1) and human monkeypox (1–4); (iii) sustained human-to-human transmission following initial transmission from an animal source, as observed with influenza A (H1N1) that emerged as a pandemic in 2009; and (iv) sustained transmission that leads to endemicity (Fig. 1). HIV presents the most important recent example of the latter, but the pattern of animal infections becoming endemic in humans appears to have occurred throughout history, suggesting that most, if not all, endemic infections in humans have come from animals (5, 6).

The ecosystem in which microbes, humans, and animals exist is in delicate balance. Any changes to its equilibrium can afford increased opportunities for microbes to breach the species barrier. Opportunities occur through direct human contact with livestock and wild animals and/or their waste materials in shared ecosystems (7). They also occur through human-animal contact along the food production and marketing chain (8). These opportunities are increasing because of greater levels of infringement of human populations on animal habitats through urbanization, logging, mineral extraction, and recreation; and increasing demand for animal-based foods and other shifting dietary preferences that require more intensive animal husbandry and are based on international trade.

While human behavior plays a role in the type and extent of animal contact, and therefore the risk that an infectious organism will cross the species barrier, the inherent

[1]The Centre on Global Health Security, Chatham House, The Royal Institute of International Affairs, London SW1Y 4LE, United Kingdom; [2]Department of Infectious Disease Epidemiology, London School of Hygiene and Tropical Medicine, London WC1E 7HT, United Kingdom.

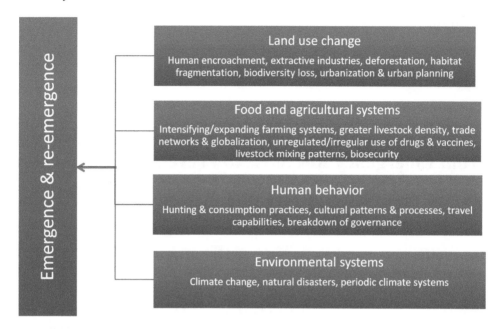

Figure 1. Potential pathways after emergence. doi:10.1128/microbiolspec.OH-0011-2012.f1

biology and genetics of the infectious organism also play a fundamental role. Some microbes are genetically unstable—the genome may be prone to mutations, replication error, reassortment, or recombination during reproduction in the animal or human host. Such alterations in the genome can change the transmission properties and increase or decrease virulence. Modification of the microbial genome can thus equip a microbe with the ability to cause illness, to transmit, and/or to survive (9). RNA viruses in particular demonstrate a strong propensity to mutate and develop into human infections that emerge from animals and are transmissible from human to human (10).

The term "emerging infection" is often used to describe newly identified zoonotic infections at the animal-human interface. Often they are first identified many years after the breach in the species barrier has occurred (11). During the past 40 years newly identified zoonotic—or emerging—infections have been identified that range from Ebola and Marburg hemorrhagic fever viruses to HIV, the paramyxoviruses (Hendra and Nipah viruses), and certain food-borne bacterial infections (e.g., verocytotoxin-producing *Escherichia coli* O157) (12, 13). Most emerging infections have been first identified in humans, before the animal source was known, and many of them reemerge when the risk factors for cross-species transmission align.

In some situations, an infection with the putative zoonotic organism is asymptomatic or causes mild human illness. At other times it causes severe human illness and there is need for an immediate and potentially emergency response in the infected human population to save lives and contain the infection through treatment and/or disease management.

The clinical response to zoonotic infections is often costly, an economic burden that can be particularly difficult in low-income countries where health budgets are already heavily restricted. Postexposure prophylaxis for rabies, for example, has been estimated (conservatively) to cost $40 in sub-Saharan Africa and $49 in Asia, a cost that equals 5.8 and 3.9%, respectively, of the annual per capita gross national income (14). But zoonotic infections can also be costly in industrialized countries. Health services utilization, work absenteeism, and direct costs for hospitalization of persons with H1N1 in Spain have been estimated at €6,236 per inpatient (15).

Following an outbreak caused by an emerging infection, an epidemiological investigation helps to assess the risk to humans—and to determine the source, and if the source is an animal, to understand whether there is continued risk of transmission to humans. A range of emergency response measures must then be implemented, including surveillance, contact tracing, isolation, social distancing, vaccination or prophylaxis (if vaccines and/or medicines are available), and in some instances culling of the animal source. The revised International Health Regulations (IHR 2005) (16) require World Health Organization (WHO) member states to rapidly assess an emerging infectious disease outbreak and notify the WHO, and through WHO the global community, if the outbreak fits the criteria established for a public health emergency of international concern and causes a risk of international spread (17).

Intensive culling of cattle after research had identified causal links between bovine spongiform encephalopathy (BSE) in cattle and variant Creutzfeldt-Jakob disease in humans, for example, was estimated to have cost the United Kingdom government $5.75 billion, including $2 billion in lost exports (18); culling of flocks of H5N1-infected chickens, coupled with inadequate compensation in Asian countries, cost an average of $210 per farmer, a high cost in a population whose average monthly income is $120 (19) (Fig. 2). If an emerging infection becomes endemic in human populations, the disease burden and cost can have a major and prolonged economic impact. The impact of AIDS in terms of lost economic output is significant, particularly in the poorest countries;

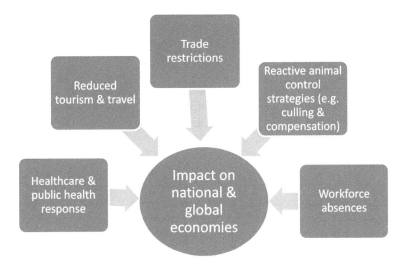

Figure 2. Economic impact of recent emerging infection events.
doi:10.1128/microbiolspec.OH-0011-2012.f2

reductions of 2 to 4% in the national gross domestic product have been calculated, for example, across a range of African countries (20).

Severe acute respiratory syndrome (SARS) was the first major emerging infection identified in the 21st century. A close examination of its origins, the outbreak and human sickness and death that it caused, the international response, and the effect it had on Asian economies provides a clear lesson of the impact of emerging infections and the reasons they must be assessed and managed with urgency to ensure a rapid and effective response.

First detected because it caused a severe atypical pneumonia, SARS soon became a burden in hospitals in the Guangdong Province of China, where many patients required respiratory support and broad-spectrum antibiotics had no effect. Hospital workers caring for these patients became infected as well, and one of them—a medical doctor who had treated patients in the Guangdong Province—traveled to Hong Kong, where he stayed in a hotel on the same floor as both Chinese and international guests. Some of these other hotel guests became infected, but it is not clearly understood how—hypotheses ranged from transmission through the hotel ventilation system to transmission in a shared closed environment such as occurs when people use the same elevator (21).

Those who became infected at the hotel were admitted to Hong Kong hospitals when they became ill or traveled to other countries, many times while still in the incubation period, to become seriously ill at their next destination. Hospitalized, they too became sources of infection of hospital workers, who in turn unintentionally infected other patients and family members.

Molecular and epidemiological investigation suggested that the infection of the index case (never identified) was a onetime event. As more information became available, it was further hypothesized that this initial infection was due to close contact with an infected animal, probably a civet cat, thought to have been a carrier of a coronavirus that mutated, either in the animal or an infected human, in such a way as to cause severe human illness (22).

The world's interconnectivity through air transport facilitated the international spread of SARS. Its electronic connections also permitted a virtual collaborative effort for surveillance, and for an emergency outbreak investigation, management, and containment: the most favorable patient management regimens and modes of transmission were rapidly identified; the causative organism was identified and characterized; international travel advisories were recommended to stop international spread; and after human-to-human transmission had been interrupted, the scientific evidence that was collected during the outbreak was used for guidelines in preparation for another outbreak should it occur (23).

SARS resulted in 8,422 probable infections and 916 (11%) deaths; in addition, the economic impact of the outbreak on gross domestic product was estimated at $30 billion to $100 billion from decreased commerce, travel, and tourism (24). Unlike HIV, the SARS coronavirus did not become endemic, and economic recovery was rapid.

Research to examine various hypotheses of transmission and to develop medicines and vaccines was active during the outbreak, but it came to a standstill during the following year when there was no recurrence of human infection and resources were then shifted to other research priorities.

SARS and other emerging infections share a common theme: infection is often first detected in human populations, in which an emergency clinical response and hypothesis-generating outbreak investigation begin before the source of infection is understood.

Initial recommendations for control are often precautionary—based on the evidence available from the current outbreak or previous outbreaks caused by similar organisms—and they can cause severe negative economic impact.

If it were possible to identify infectious organisms carried by wild and domestic animals and to predict if, when, and where they would emerge in humans, and if these animals could then be somehow removed from contact with humans or cleared of infection, human sickness and death could be prevented and economies protected.

A One Health approach to prevent human infection by enhanced detection and surveillance in both wild and domestic animals is actively being pursued, including identification of geographic areas where the greatest number of emergent infections have occurred historically (25). Such geographic localization is followed by prediction of which organisms might emerge based on an understanding of what infectious organisms are present in wild and domestic animal populations at those sites. Genetic sequencing of these infectious organisms and comparison of the sequence information to that from other known infectious organisms is then done in an attempt to discern genetic changes that could lead to emergence (26, 27).

If the One Health approach could be expanded to understand and mitigate the determinants, or factors, that align to shape the risk of animal infection and breaches in the species barrier from animals to humans, both populations could be protected from sickness and death, and economies even better protected. The current paradigm of emergency response, and that of prediction and prevention, could then be shifted even further upstream to management and mitigation of the determinants of the risks that lead to emergence, thus preventing emergence at the source (Fig. 3).

UNDERSTANDING THE DETERMINANTS OF EMERGENCE AND THEIR MITIGATION

The determinants of emergence are risk factors that align in such a manner as to modify the equilibrium among and between three species: humans, animals, and the

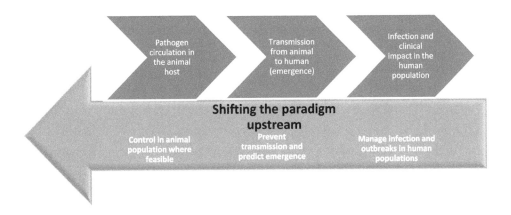

Figure 3. Shifting the paradigm from emergency response to preventing emergence at its source. doi:10.1128/microbiolspec.OH-0011-2012.f3

infectious organisms carried by those animals. The determinants cross many sectors, including human and animal health, animal husbandry, agriculture, community planning, water and sanitation, commerce, forestry, mining, food processing of animals, trade, and agriculture. Specific determinants must be identified in each instance of an emergence, understood, and then mitigated to prevent the same alignment and emergence in the future.

It is because of the cross-sectoral origin of these determinants that a One Health approach—defined as a collaborative effort of multiple disciplines to attain optimal health for people, animals, and the environment (28)—is of value. Figure 4 shows how this One Health approach builds on analyses of previous emergence events to (i) identify

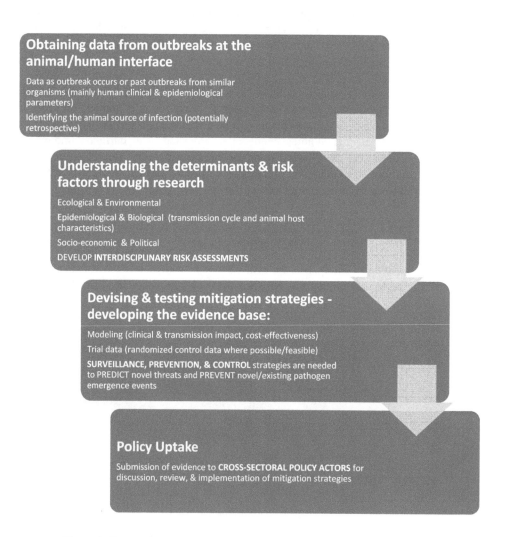

Figure 4. Flow chart showing steps for transforming evidence at the animal-human interface into policy. doi:10.1128/microbiolspec.OH-0011-2012.f4

the determinants that have aligned in past or current emergence events in such a manner as to facilitate or permit emergence; (ii) engage partners and stakeholders outside of the traditional medical community to ensure that these determinants are understood; and (iii) with these partners and stakeholders, propose and implement strategies that will mitigate and decrease the negative impact of emergence events in the short term and contribute to prevention of emergence in the future.

Such a One Health approach over time could be used to change the existing paradigm of detection and emergency response to prevention, or to a decrease in the frequency of emergence, by mitigation of the determinants that have the potential to cause emergence. Mitigation requires observation and analysis of events that occur, or have occurred in the past, to identify the various government and other sectors involved and to develop the sector-specific strategies and policies that will prevent their occurrence. These strategies must then be put in place across all sectors involved through cross-sector—One Health—collaboration.

In the case of SARS, there was a flurry of field research activity in the Guangdong Province during and just after the outbreak, but over time funding decreased and research slowed. Among the research that was completed was a study of workers in some of the province's wet markets that suggested that up to 22% (12/55) had antibody evidence of a coronavirus infection related to the SARS coronavirus, but that none had a history of severe respiratory symptoms such as were occurring in persons with SARS (29). Further field research might have helped better elucidate the risk factors for emergence, but it was not conducted, and the epidemiology remains unclear.

Determinants of emergence, in addition to working in a wet market, as suggested by the completed study, might also include hunting wild animals, killing and/or butchering/ preparing wild animal meat for consumption in a restaurant, or living in a household that buys live or recently killed wild game meat from a wet market.

Even though evidence is available from just one epidemiological study of SARS, a series of actions outside the human and animal health sectors could be useful in preventing a future outbreak of another emerging pathogen in the Guangdong Province. These include education of all those who come into contact with wild game (and domestic animals) about how to protect themselves against infection; regulation with enforcement of wet markets and eating establishments that does not drive these activities underground, but rather ensures safe animal handling; and regulation and enforcement of trade between hunters and markets and between markets and those who purchase. Other activities might be research to determine whether any wild animals could be raised commercially under conditions that prevent their infection and risk to humans, or further downstream, more effective education of health workers about infection control. This latter activity would ensure that if other actions such as those above failed to prevent emergence, amplification of transmission of emergent organisms could be prevented.

There are numerous other situations in which emergence occurs, and numerous reports in the medical literature that fully or partially analyze these events. People living and working in small rural farming communities carved out of tropical rain forests, savannas, mountains, and deserts often come in close proximity to wild animals, or to domestic animals they tend that in turn are in close proximity to wild animals. Exposures range from direct contact with wildlife and domestic animals to indirect contact through water, garden products, or other ecosystems in the environment that have been contaminated by animal waste materials. A 2004 serological survey demonstrated that 1% of inhabitants in rural villages who had reported exposure to primates presented with antibodies to simian foamy virus (30). Hantavirus outbreaks have occurred in rural American Indian communities when humans have become infected by inhaling dust particles contaminated by the urine of rats, and have occurred in other areas—recently in a national park in the United States—where humans and the waste products of rodents came in close contact (31). Human monkeypox—caused by an orthopoxvirus carried by rodents in tropical rain forests of sub-Saharan Africa—occasionally causes infection in hunters and others living in small rural communities who come in contact with forest animals they have killed or butchered (32).

In larger urban communities, human contact with animals may be limited to domestic pets, a few farm animals in close proximity to households, or rodents and other animals that have adapted to the environment and come in contact with humans or other animals as they range (e.g., cows and chickens in parts of Asia) or browse (e.g., urban foxes and rodents). The continued high rate of contact between humans and animals in both smaller backyard and larger market systems within these networks permits constant human exposure to and infection with the virus. Children and adults in Asia are thought to have been infected with the H5N1 influenza A virus by contact with living chickens in backyards, and adults have been shown to become infected at some point during the process of raising or slaughtering/butchering chickens (33). A recent multisource outbreak of human monkeypox in the United States was associated with the importation of exotic animals for pets from West Africa, which served as a reservoir for infection of other animals in pet shops that then infected the children with whom they came in contact (34).

With increasing population density, particularly where rural-urban migration is a common trend, a breakdown in environmental sanitation/waste disposal from burgeoning population demands can create ecological niches for sustained transmission of animal pathogens through the environment, water, or food contaminated by animal waste (35). Major outbreaks of giardiasis—caused by an intestinal parasite that has a reservoir in livestock and wild animals—have occurred in the state of Wisconsin and in St. Petersburg (Russia), linked to contamination of drinking water systems (36).

Civil disturbance, destruction of community infrastructure, and resultant migration of human populations can likewise alter the interaction of humans and animals and lead to emergence. Lassa fever outbreaks in refugee camps following civil war in western Africa, for example, forced displaced human populations to migrate in mass numbers and relocate to camps with extremely poor housing and living conditions, an environment where the natural host for the Lassa fever virus, the rodent *Mastomys natalensis*, can thrive (37).

Determinants of emergence in these settings are poor or inadequate urban planning, lack of understanding by populations about risks associated with animal contact, failure to adopt and adhere to safe farming practices, and failure to maintain sanitation and water infrastructure. A One Health approach must work across all these sectors, assisting communities to develop a safer living environment through urban planning, developing and maintaining robust water and sanitation infrastructure, controlling rodent and other animal populations in near-proximity urban areas, ensuring safe animal husbandry, and providing understanding of risks through community-based education.

In addition to workers who have contact with domestic animals, other occupations are risk factors for human infection from wild animals. The 1998 Nipah virus outbreak in Malaysia was attributed to initial transmission of the virus at the livestock-wildlife interface (from bats to pigs, which served as the amplifying host) and then to pig farmers and slaughterhouse workers (38). In Malaysia, the Nipah virus is thought to have been transmitted to humans who collected or drank palm wine that was contaminated with guano of Nipah-infected bats (39).

Outbreaks of Ebola hemorrhagic fever have also been linked to occupation: the index case of the Ebola outbreak in the Democratic Republic of the Congo is thought to have been a local inhabitant whose occupation was preparing charcoal in the tropical rain forest (40) and who was exposed to an Ebola-infected animal or to the guano of the bat reservoir.

The origin of HIV emergence has been linked to both hunting and butchering of chimpanzees for consumption (41); the SARS infectious organism (coronavirus) spread to humans in China through either close contact with wild animals in wet markets or preparation of wild animals for consumption; and recurrent outbreaks of Ebola hemorrhagic fever are linked to ongoing hunting and butchering of nonhuman primates (42).

Extractive industries such as logging and mining open previously uninhabited parts of forests or other terrain to human settlement. Moving humans for work purposes to such naïve ecosystems increases the opportunity for their exposure, and that of their domestic animals, to infections present in the wildlife population (30). Though reports of outbreaks associated with the extractive industries have not yet been published, such events are thought to be of real but low potential. Such events are likely to have high impact, and it is known that habitat modification and fragmentation after deforestation or other extraction procedures can affect both animals and the vectors that transmit infections, as described for yellow fever or plague from wild animals to humans (43).

Determinants of emergence related to occupation include hunting and working in areas where either wild or domestic animals can transmit infection. Some of the determinants involve wild animals—contact with animals or indirectly with the vectors that carry infection from animals to humans such as mosquitoes. In addition to community education about occupational risks of infection, industry must be encouraged or legally required to ensure that workers are protected and safe from wild animal exposure whether they work in the slaughterhouse, mining, or forestry industry, and special attention must be paid to regulation of markets that sell wild animals and prevention of those that are clandestine.

Climate change may also be a factor in emergence of human infection. Rainfall associated with El Niño-Southern Oscillation in East Africa, for example, has contributed to frequent outbreaks of Rift Valley fever as a result of flooding that increases breeding sites of the mosquito vector (44). The frequency of *Leptospira* transmission from rodents to humans has been shown to increase following heavy rains and flooding in Latin America, Bangladesh, and India (45). Lassa fever has also emerged after severe drought in Sierra Leone, when rodents carrying the virus were forced to move closer to humans so that they could survive on agricultural products in cultivated fields or storage facilities, contaminating human food supplies (46).

Determinants related to climate change require (i) more robust civil engineering projects to prevent flooding and to channel water for irrigation, (ii) better rodent and wild animal control, and (iii) continued participation globally in the negotiation of the United Nations Framework Convention on Climate Change (47).

The 20th and 21st centuries have seen shifting dynamics across food and agricultural production systems, from rapidly intensifying systems throughout Southeast Asia to the rise of periurban farming practices in developing countries and the globalization of production and supply. Growing demand for animal-based food in many developing countries has led to more complex food chains. An increase in the numbers of animals has been followed by rapid expansion of both food and live-animal processing and trade networks, enabling food safety hazards and infectious organisms to travel with ease.

The emergence of Rift Valley fever in the Arabian Peninsula has been linked to the illegal importation of cattle from eastern Africa, where outbreaks are frequent (48). H5N1 influenza is endemic in poultry stock within a number of Southeast Asian countries where a multitude of live-animal trade networks exist. The rapid expansion of poultry production has led to increases in other food-borne zoonoses, particularly from eggs and egg products, which account for approximately 15% of food-borne infectious disease outbreaks across Europe (49). Changes in wide-scale, industrial processing of meat and animal by-products have been shown to also have the potential to lead to major large-scale zoonotic outbreaks. BSE emerged in cattle in the United Kingdom in the late 1980s, a result of reduction in the chemical solvent and temperature used for the rendering process for bone meal, ultimately enabling the infectious organism (a prion) to transfer back to livestock through feed made from bone meal (50). Outbreaks of *E. coli* O157 have consistently been shown to originate from meat and meat products, resulting in serious illness and death (51).

Overuse of antibiotics in livestock animals is thought to have led to an increase in antimicrobial-resistant bacteria in animals. This has been a primary consequence of extensive, often unregulated use of antibiotics for "growth promotion" in animal feed (52). Introducing antibiotics into the microbial gut flora of livestock animals alters evolutionary pressures on the microbes present, often increasing selection toward antibiotic resistance.

There is still much debate within the scientific community as to the contribution of antibiotics in farming systems to the rise of antibiotic resistance, and the implications for emerging antibiotic resistance in human populations are even less well understood. But there is general consensus that farming systems are likely to contribute to the flow of antibiotic-resistant microbes in the wider ecosystem and in humans by runoff into water used or consumed by humans, especially in economically poor settings where farming communities exist alongside densely populated human environments with poor sanitation/sewage systems (53, 54).

The interaction between animals and the environment also plays an important role in other infections. Fecal contamination by feral swine, for example, is thought to have led to *E. coli* O157:H7 transmission to crops and resultant human outbreaks of hemolytic-uremic syndrome in both Europe and North America (55).

Though hunting and trade in wild animals may be negligible in terms of food products for consumption, they have been implicated in the emergence of highly significant infectious diseases such as a point source Ebola outbreak in the tropical rain forest of Gabon among a group of men who had killed and butchered a chimpanzee for food in the mid-1990s (56).

Determinants of infectious organisms in the food chain include breaches in personal protection during animal husbandry and slaughter, in quality control during food processing, and during storage and shipment. Other determinants include overuse of antibiotics and runoff from animal farms to water and the environment. Most of these breaches are accidental—and some are caused by attempts to economize to maximize profit.

Prevention of infectious disease emergence through the food chain and agricultural system must include intervention at each of the various steps along the pathway from the farm to the fork. If infectious organisms pass through the food chain and enter foods, their impact can be minimized at the final intervention point, where animal-derived foods can be prepared carefully in the factory, restaurant, and household either by cooking or other means to remove or mitigate the risk of infection. They could be controlled earlier— during the period animals are being raised, during slaughter, and during transport. Each known cause of emergence must be assessed for risk, and those that are considered risks must be mitigated. Mitigation plans must take into account the risks of wild animal exposure from land use and farming and must plan and implement strategies that mitigate risks of exposure that occur from activities such as deforestation and a reduction in biodiversity. They must also take into account human behavior and ensure that populations most at risk clearly understand the measures required to reduce high-risk behavior.

TURNING EVIDENCE INTO POLICY THROUGH A ONE HEALTH APPROACH

A great amount of scientific knowledge about the risk factors or determinants of emergence at the animal-human interface is already available from previous investigations and risk assessments of emergent events. More knowledge can be obtained from in-depth study of each new emergence event as it occurs. Research must also take into account human behavior and determine whether populations most at risk understand the measures that might be required to reduce or protect from high risk (57).

Translation of this knowledge into policy can help shift the paradigm from detection, assessment, and response further upstream to prevention of emerging infections at the source, thus better protecting animal and human health and protecting economies.

But many of these proposed evidence-based policies will encounter political barriers, especially when commercial benefits are at stake. The differences between the goals of the animal and human health sectors must be clearly understood. Agriculture is for profit —whether it is raising cattle for milk, poultry for eggs and meat, or pigs for meat and meat products. The mitigation strategies that are most easily accepted are therefore those that are shown to be cost-effective and have no negative impact on profit. For policy options that do not appear to be cost-effective, it is more difficult to achieve acceptance by all sectors of costly mitigation strategies, and enforceable legislation may be the only way they can be addressed. But it is clear that those preventive interventions that are cost-effective for the animal industry (and associated sectors such as trade, commerce, and the environment) will have a better chance of being accepted than others that could decrease profit, and barriers among the different sectors must be broken down by using clear and easy-to-understand evidence of the cost-effectiveness of a variety of risk mitigation strategies. Through cooperative efforts at the animal-human interface using a One Health approach, emergence events in the future can be decreased, and lives and economies saved.

At the same time, stronger and joint surveillance and risk assessment are required at the animal-human interface to serve as a safety net for those emergence events that occur despite any mitigation policies that are in place. Monitoring of both livestock and wildlife animal populations is fundamental to identifying and assessing these emerging threats at an early stage and taking appropriate action. The United Kingdom fulfills this need through its Human Infections and Risk Surveillance group, which conducts monthly horizon scanning to identify emerging and potentially zoonotic infections that may pose a threat to the nation's public health. Other countries have adopted joint animal-human surveillance and risk assessment activities as well, and this One Health perspective in surveillance—integrating animal and human surveillance with human activities (particularly in human populations at greatest risk)—will likely yield a cost-effective and sustainable approach to monitoring the flow of pathogens at the human-animal-environment interface (58). A recent World Bank report (59) concluded that there is significant merit in integrating surveillance activities that cover emerging zoonosis threats (which attract considerable funding) with persistent and endemic zoonotic disease monitoring.

In summary, it not enough to identify and understand the determinants that cause emergence of an infection at the animal-human interface if mitigation of these determinants is to lead to successful prevention of emergence. Various evidence-based mitigation strategies must be proposed, their cost-effectiveness assessed and understood, and scenarios developed that clearly provide the information needed by those responsible for the policies across sectors that deal with issues including animal and human health, trade, education, and urban planning. Working together to prevent infections at the human-animal interface requires a true One Health approach.

Citation. Heymann DL, Dixon M. 2013. The value of the One Health approach: shifting from emergency response to prevention of zoonotic disease threats at their source. Microbiol Spectrum 1(1):OH-0011-2012. doi:10.1128/microbiolspec.OH-0011-2012.

REFERENCES

1. **Yousaf MZ, Qasim M, Zia S, Khan MR, Ashfaq UA, Khan S.** 2012. Rabies molecular virology, diagnosis, prevention and treatment. *Virol J* **9:**50. doi:10.1186/1743-422X-9-50.
2. **Trevitt CR, Singh PN.** 2003. Variant Creutzfeldt-Jakob disease: pathology, epidemiology, and public health implications. *Am J Clin Nutr* **78:**651–656.
3. **Liu J, Xiao H, Lei F, Zhu Q, Qin K, Zhang XW, Zhang XL, Zhao D, Wang G, Feng Y, Ma J, Liu W, Wang J, Gao GF.** 2005. Highly pathogenic H5N1 influenza virus infection in migratory birds. *Science* **309:**1206. doi:10.1126/science.1115273.
4. **Ellis CK, Carroll DS, Lash RR, Peterson AT, Damon IK, Malekani J, Formenty P.** 2012. Ecology and geography of human monkeypox case occurrences across Africa. *J Wildl Dis* **48:**335–347.
5. **Smith GJ, Vijaykrishna D, Bahl J, Lycett SJ, Worobey M, Pybus OG, Ma SK, Cheung CL, Raghwani J, Bhatt S, Peiris JS, Guan Y, Rambaut A.** 2009. Origins and evolutionary genomics of the 2009 swine-origin H1N1 influenza A epidemic. *Nature* **459:**1122–1125.
6. **Holmes EC.** 2001. On the origin and evolution of the human immunodeficiency virus (HIV). *Biol Rev Camb Philos Soc* **76:**239–254.
7. **Bengis RG, Leighton FA, Fischer JR, Artois M, Mörner T, Tate CM.** 2004. The role of wildlife in emerging and re-emerging zoonoses. *Rev Sci Tech* **23:**497–511.

8. **Delgado C, Rosegrant M, Steinfeld H, Ehui S, Courbois C.** 1999. *Livestock to 2020: the Next Food Revolution.* Food, Agriculture, and the Environment Discussion Paper 28. International Food Policy Research Institute, Washington DC.

9. **Lloyd-Smith JO, George D, Pepin KM, Pitzer VE, Pulliam JR, Dobson AP, Hudson PJ, Grenfell BT.** 2009. Epidemic dynamics at the human-animal interface. *Science* **326:**1362–1367.

10. **Taylor LH, Latham SM, Woolhouse ME.** 2001. Risk factors for human disease emergence. *Philos Trans R Soc Lond B Biol Sci* **356:**983–989.

11. **Wolfe ND.** 2010. The transition from pandemic response to pandemic prevention, p 33–35. *In* Institute on Science for Global Policy (ed), *Emerging and Persistent Infectious Diseases: Focus on Surveillance.* Institute on Science for Global Policy, Washington, DC.

12. **Kruse H, Kirkemo AM, Handeland K.** 2004. Wildlife as source of zoonotic infections. *Emerg Inf Dis* **10:**2067–2072.

13. **Thorns CJ.** 2000. Bacterial food-borne zoonoses. *Rev Sci Tech* **19:**226–239.

14. **World Health Organization.** 2005. *Control of neglected zoonotic disease: challenges and the way forward.* World Health Organization, Geneva, Switzerland. http://www.who.int/zoonoses/Consultation_Sept05_en.pdf (last accessed January 17, 2013).

15. **Galante M, Garin O, Sicuri E, Cots F, García-Altés A, Ferrer M, Dominguez A, Alonso J.** 2012. Health services utilization, work absenteeism and costs of pandemic influenza A (H1N1) 2009 in Spain: a multicenter-longitudinal study. *PLoS One* **7:**e31696. doi:10.1371/journal.pone.0031696.

16. **World Health Organization.** 2005. *International Health Regulations (2005)*, 2nd ed. World Health Organization, Geneva, Switzerland. http://whqlibdoc.who.int/publications/2008/9789241580410_eng.pdf (last accessed January 18, 2013).

17. **Rodier G, Greenspan AL, Hughes JM, Heymann DL.** 2007. Global public health security. *Emerg Infect Dis* **13:**1447–1452.

18. **Marsh Inc.** 2008. *The Economic and Social Impact of Emerging Infectious Disease: Mitigation through Detection, Research, and Response.* http://www.healthcare.philips.com/main/shared/assets/documents/bioshield/ecoandsocialimpactofemerginginfectiousdisease_111208.pdf (last accessed June 5, 2013).

19. **Hancock J, Cho G.** 2008. *Assessment of likely impacts of avian influenza on rural poverty reduction in Asia: responses, impacts and recommendations for IFAD strategy.* IFAD occasional papers no. 6. International Fund for Agricultural Development, Rome, Italy. http://www.ifad.org/operations/projects/regions/pi/paper/6.pdf (last accessed June 5, 2013).

20. **Dixon S, McDonald S, Roberts J.** 2002. The impact of HIV and AIDS on Africa's economic development. *BMJ* **324:**232–234.

21. **Chan-Yeung M, Xu RH.** 2003. SARS: epidemiology. *Respirology* **8**(Suppl)**:**S9–S14.

22. **Wang LF, Eaton BT.** 2007. Bats, civets and the emergence of SARS. *Curr Top Microbiol Immunol* **315:**325–344.

23. **World Health Organization, Department of Communicable Disease Surveillance and Response.** 2004. *WHO SARS Risk Assessment and Preparedness Framework.* World Health Organization, Geneva, Switzerland. http://www.who.int/csr/resources/publications/CDS_CSR_ARO_2004_2.pdf (last accessed January 17, 2013).

24. **Keogh-Brown MR, Smith RD.** 2008. The economic impact of SARS: how does the reality match the predictions? *Health Policy* **88:**110–120.

25. **International Livestock Research Institute.** 2012. *Mapping of Poverty and Likely Zoonoses Hotspots. Zoonoses Project 4: Report to Department for International Development, UK.* International Livestock Research Institute, Nairobi, Kenya. http://cgspace.cgiar.org/bitstream/handle/10568/21161/ZooMap_July2012_final.pdf (last accessed June 5, 2013).

26. **Biek R, Real LA.** 2010. The landscape genetics of infectious disease emergence and spread. *Mol Ecol* **19:**3515–3531.

27. **Barclay E.** 2008. Predicting the next pandemic. *Lancet* **372:**1025–1026.

28. **American Veterinary Medical Association.** 2008. *One Health: a New Professional Imperative.* Final report of One Health Initiative Task Force. American Veterinary Medical Association, Schaumburg, IL. https://www.avma.org/KB/Resources/Reports/Documents/onehealth_final.pdf (last accessed June 5, 2013).

29. **Parry J.** 2003. Asymptomatic animal traders prove positive for SARS virus. *BMJ* **327:**582. doi:10.1136/bmj.327.7415.582-a.

30. **Wolfe ND, Dunavan CP, Diamond J.** 2007. Origins of major human infectious diseases. *Nature* **447:**279–283.

31. **World Health Organization.** 2012. Outbreak news. Hantavirus pulmonary syndrome, Yosemite National Park, United States of America. *Wkly Epidemiol Rec* **87:**345–346.

32. **Reynolds MG, Carroll DS, Karem KL.** 2012. Factors affecting the likelihood of monkeypox's emergence and spread in the post-smallpox era. *Curr Opin Virol* **2:**335–343.

33. **Coker RJ, Hunter BM, Rudge JW, Liverani M, Hanvoravongchai P.** 2011. Emerging infectious diseases in southeast Asia: regional challenges to control. *Lancet* **377:**599–609.

34. **Sejvar JJ, Chowdary Y, Schomogyi M, Stevens J, Patel J, Karem K, Fischer M, Kuehnert MJ, Zaki SR, Paddock CD, Guarner J, Shieh WJ, Patton JL, Bernard N, Li Y, Olson VA, Kline RL, Loparev VN, Schmid DS, Beard B, Regnery RR, Damon IK.** 2004. Human monkeypox infection: a family cluster in the midwestern United States. *J Infect Dis* **190:**1833–1840.

35. **Smolinski MS, Hamburg MA, Lederberg J (ed).** 2003. *Microbial Threats to Health: Emergence, Detection, and Response.* National Academies Press, Washington, DC.

36. **Addiss DG, Davis JP, Roberts JM, Mast EE.** 1992. Epidemiology of giardiasis in Wisconsin: increasing incidence of reported cases and unexplained seasonal trends. *Am J Trop Med Hyg* **47:**13–19.

37. **Lalis A, Leblois R, Lecompte E, Denys C, ter Meulen J, Wirth T.** 2012. The impact of human conflict on the genetics of *Mastomys natalensis* and Lassa virus in West Africa. *PLoS One* **7:**e37068. doi:10.1371/journal.pone.0037068.

38. **Luby SP, Gurley ES, Hossain MJ.** 2009. Transmission of human infection with Nipah virus. *Clin Infect Dis* **49:**1743–1748.

39. **Keesing F, Belden LK, Daszak P, Dobson A, Harvell CD, Holt RD, Hudson P, Jolles A, Jones KE, Mitchell CE, Myers SS, Bogich T, Ostfeld RS.** 2010. Impacts of biodiversity on the emergence and transmission of infectious diseases. *Nature* **468:**647–652.

40. **Groseth A, Feldmann H, Strong JE.** 2007. The ecology of Ebola virus. *Trends Microbiol* **15:**408–416.

41. **LeBreton M, Prosser AT, Tamoufel U, Sateren W, Mpoudi-Nigole E, Diffol JL, Burke DS, Wolfe ND.** 2006. Patterns of bushmeat hunting and perceptions of disease risk among central African communities. *Anim Conserv* **9:**357–363.

42. **Rizkalla C, Blanco-Silva F, Gruver S.** 2007. Modeling the impact of Ebola and bushmeat hunting on western lowland gorillas. *Ecohealth* **4:**151–155.

43. **Pongsiri MJ, Roman J, Ezenwa VO, Goldberg TL, Koren HS, Newbold SC, Ostfeld RS, Pattanaykak SK, Salkeld DJ.** 2009. Biodiversity loss affects global disease ecology. *Bioscience* **59:**945–954.

44. **Anyamba A, Chretien JP, Small J, Tucker CJ, Formenty PB, Richardson JH, Britch SC, Schnabel DC, Erickson RL, Linthicum KJ.** 2009. Prediction of a Rift Valley fever outbreak. *Proc Natl Acad Sci USA* **106:**955–959.

45. **Lau CL, Smythe LD, Craig SB, Weinstein P.** 2010. Climate change, flooding, urbanisation and leptospirosis: fuelling the fire? *Trans R Soc Trop Med Hyg* **104:**631–638.

46. **Ogbu O, Ajuluchukwu E, Uneke CJ.** 2007. Lassa fever in West African sub-region: an overview. *J Vector Borne Dis* **44:**1–11.

47. **de Boer Y.** 2012. *An international climate treaty: is it worth fighting for? (meeting transcript).* Chatham House, London, United Kingdom. http://www.chathamhouse.org/sites/default/files/public/Meetings/Meeting%20Transcripts/280212deboer.pdf (last accessed January 20, 2013).

48. **Balkhy HH, Memish ZA.** 2003. Rift Valley fever: an uninvited zoonosis in the Arabian peninsula. *Int J Antimicrob Agents* **21:**153–157.

49. **European Food Safety Authority.** 2009. Special measures to reduce the risk for consumers through *Salmonella* in table eggs—e.g. cooling of table eggs. Scientific Opinion of the Panel on Biological Hazards. *EFSA J* **957:**1–29.

50. **Prusiner SB.** 1997. Prion diseases and the BSE crisis. *Science* **278:**245–251.

51. **Soon JM, Chadd SA, Baines RN.** 2011. *Escherichia coli* O157:H7 in beef cattle: on farm contamination and pre-slaughter control methods. *Anim Health Res Rev* **12:**197–211.

52. **Barton MD.** 2000. Antibiotic use in animal feed and its impact on human health. *Nutr Res Rev* **13:**279–299.

53. **Segura PA, François M, Gagnon C, Sauve S.** 2009. Review of the occurrence of anti-infectives in contaminated wastewaters and natural and drinking waters. *Environ Health Perspect* **117:**675–684.

54. **Abraham WR.** 2011. Megacities as sources for pathogenic bacteria in rivers and their fate downstream. *Int J Microbiol* **2011:**798292. doi:10.1155/2011/798292.

55. **Jay MT, Cooley M, Carychao D, Wiscomb GW, Sweitzer RA, Crawford-Miksza L, Farrar JA, Lau DK, O'Connell J, Millington A, Asmundson RV, Atwill ER, Mandrell RE.** 2007. *Escherichia coli* O157: H7 in feral swine near spinach fields and cattle, central California coast. *Emerg Infect Dis* **13**:1908–1911.

56. **Khan AS, Tshioko FK, Heymann DL, Le Guenno B, Nabeth P, Kerstiëns B, Fleerackers Y, Kilmarx PH, Rodier GR, Nkuku O, Rollin PE, Sanchez A, Zaki SR, Swanepoel R, Tomori O, Nichol ST, Peters CJ, Muyembe-Tamfum JJ, Ksiazek TG.** 1999. The reemergence of Ebola hemorrhagic fever, Democratic Republic of the Congo, 1995. *J Infect Dis* **179**(Suppl 1):S76–S86.

57. **Cascio A, Bosilkovski M, Rodriguez-Morales AJ, Pappas G.** 2011. The socio-ecology of zoonotic infections. *Clin Microbiol Infect* **17**:336–342.

58. **The FAO-OIE-WHO Collaboration.** 2010. *Sharing responsibilities and coordinating global activities to address health risks at the animal-human-ecosystems interfaces (A Tripartite Concept Note).* http://www.who.int/foodsafety/zoonoses/final_concept_note_Hanoi.pdf (last accessed January 20, 2013).

59. **World Bank.** 2010. *People, Pathogens, and Our Planet: Volume One—Towards a One Health Approach for Controlling Zoonotic Diseases.* World Bank, Washington, DC. https://openknowledge.worldbank.org/handle/10986/2844 (last accessed June 5, 2013).

One Health: People, Animals, and the Environment
Edited by Ronald M. Atlas and Stanley Maloy
© 2014 American Society for Microbiology, Washington, DC
doi:10.1128/microbiolspec.OH-0013-2012

Chapter 3

The Human-Animal Interface

Leslie A. Reperant[1] and Albert D. M. E. Osterhaus[1,2]

INTRODUCTION

The human-animal interface is as ancient as the first bipedal steps taken by humans. It has grown and expanded with the human species' prehistoric and historical development to reach the unprecedented scope of current times. Several facets define the human-animal interface, guiding the scope and range of human interactions with animal species. These facets have continued to evolve and expand since their emergence, promoting disease emergence. Placing the human-animal interface in its historical perspective allows us to realize its versatile and dynamic nature. Changes in the scope and range of domestication, agriculture, urbanization, colonization, trade, and industrialization have been accompanied by evolving risks for cross-species transmission of pathogens. Because these risks are unlikely to decrease, improving our technologies to identify and monitor pathogenic threats lurking at the human-animal interface should be a priority.

The human-animal interface is a defining feature of the One Health concept. It is a continuum of contacts and interactions between humans, animals, their products, and their environment, and represents the medium allowing cross-species transmission of zoonotic and emerging human and animal pathogens. The human-animal interface is characterized by a number of attributes that have been acquired throughout the evolutionary history of the human species and the development of mankind (1). The main attributes of the human-animal interface include the evolutionary pathogen heritage of the human species as well as human demographics and behaviors associated with the human inventions of domestication, agriculture and food production, urbanization, worldwide migration, colonization and trade, and industrialization and globalization (Fig. 1). These attributes have not ceased to evolve as mankind has grown and expanded, reaching unprecedented scope in parallel with the unabated growth of human impact on the environment. As such, the human-animal interface represents an ever-growing driver of the emergence of infectious diseases in humans and, perhaps less well recognized, in animal species associated with humans and in wildlife.

In humans, emerging zoonotic infectious diseases can be divided into those caused by pathogens that repeatedly cross the species barrier and result in sporadic cases of

[1]Department of Viroscience, Erasmus Medical Centre, 3000 CA Rotterdam, The Netherlands; [2]Artemis Research Institute for Wildlife Health in Europe, 3584 CK Utrecht, The Netherlands.

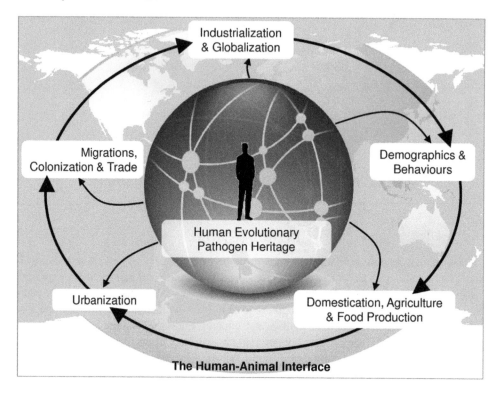

Figure 1. Schematic of the human-animal interface. The different facets of the human-animal interface include the evolutionary pathogen heritage of the human species and human demographics and behaviors associated with domestication, agriculture and food production, urbanization, worldwide migration, colonization and trade, and industrialization and globalization. These facets interact and expand as mankind continues to develop. doi:10.1128/microbiolspec.OH-0013-2012.f1

infection without further spread in the new host species; those caused by pathogens that cross the species barrier and spread in limited fashion in the new host species; and those caused by pathogens that after crossing the species barrier eventually adapt and spread efficiently in the new host species, resulting in epidemics or even pandemics. Recently developed data have demonstrated that only a few mutations may be sufficient to allow pathogens to acquire efficient transmissibility in a new host species (2–4). The main attributes of the human-animal interface favor both the cross-species transmission of zoonotic pathogens and the emergence, evolution, and eventual establishment of efficiently transmitted novel pathogens in humans. In animals associated with humans, such as domestic, feral, and commensal animals, and in wildlife, emerging infectious diseases also can be divided into these three categories; however, those of the last category are most often identified and reported, due to their potential greater impact. In this article, we will review the characteristics of the main attributes of the human-animal interface and their impact on the cross-species transmission and emergence of pathogens in humans and animals.

EVOLUTIONARY PATHOGEN HERITAGE OF THE HUMAN SPECIES

The evolutionary pathogen heritage of the human species is often forgotten when considering the human-animal interface, although it represents its most primordial attribute (1). It characterizes the scope and range of the interface that existed between the human species and its ancestral predecessors. It puts forth the diversity of pathogens that the human species inherited following vertical transmission and cospeciation upon human evolutionary debut (Fig. 2). Thus, a number of strict human pathogens or remnants thereof that exist today, from DNA and RNA viruses (e.g., herpesviruses, endogenous retroviruses) to mycobacteria (e.g., species of the *Mycobacterium tuberculosis* complex), protozoans (e.g., *Plasmodium* spp. and *Trypanosoma* spp.), and ectoparasites (e.g., *Pediculus* lice), are the result of ancestral cross-species transmission of zoonotic pathogens at the birth of the *Homo* genus, some 2.5 million years ago, and of further cospeciation ever since (5–9). Other pathogens and parasites, such as human T-lymphotropic viruses (HTLVs), enteroviruses, various hepatitis viruses, *Helicobacter pylori*, and *Taenia* spp., were acquired by species of the *Homo* genus following horizontal cross-species transmission before the rise of the modern human species (5, 10, 11). These pathogens most likely emerged as a result of predation on prey animal species, including other primates. As these pathogens further adapted and became

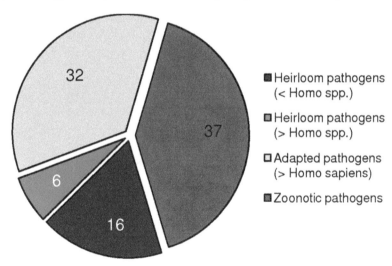

Figure 2. Ancestral origins of human pathogens. Most pathogens capable of infecting the human species have originated from animal pathogens that crossed the species barrier, in particular across the domesticated human-animal interface. Human viruses belonging to 32 different genera have their ancestral origins in animal precursors and have adapted to efficiently transmit among humans (light pink), while viruses belonging to 37 different genera are zoonotic pathogens with no or limited ability to transmit among humans (dark pink). The remaining pathogens are heirloom pathogens that cospeciated with the human species. Of these, viruses belonging to 16 different genera were vertically transmitted from hominin ancestral species at the emergence of the *Homo* genus (dark blue), while viruses belonging to 6 different genera were vertically transmitted from related *Homo* spp. to the modern human *Homo sapiens* at the time of its emergence (light blue). doi:10.1128/microbiolspec.OH-0013-2012.f2

established in *Homo* spp., they also cospeciated and were transmitted vertically to the modern human species, *Homo sapiens*, about 200,000 years ago. Patterns of cospeciation of these so-called heirloom pathogens and their hosts were highlighted by phylogenetic analyses (5). These analyses revealed pathogen phylogenies that closely mirrored those of their host species, with times of divergence of pathogen species coinciding with those of their respective hosts (12, 13).

Although the evolutionary pathogen heritage of the human species principally defines the prehistoric human-animal interface of >200,000 years ago, understanding its range and scope highlights the diversity of pathogens that the human species was susceptible to at the time of its emergence. Phylogenetic tools and the current genomic era increasingly provide the means to address this diversity and demonstrate that a wide range of pathogens had already crossed the unique human-animal interface of those times. Most of the pathogens that have infected the human species since its evolutionary debut have in common a relatively strict species specificity, tend to cause persistent or chronic infections typically of relatively low pathogenicity in immune-competent individuals, and are transmitted among humans mainly following intimate encounters like mucosal, skin, and blood- or other body fluid-borne contacts (1). These pathogens have cospeciated with the human species, while in parallel, sister pathogen species have cospeciated with other primates and often with most other species of the animal realm. Studying this particular attribute of the human-animal interface may thus improve our understanding of the mechanisms behind some pathogens' limited host range, strict species specificity, and relative inability to currently cross the species barrier.

The particulars of the pathogens inherited upon the emergence and early evolution of the human species and the relative rarity of acute or virulent infections then are in sharp contrast with current times. Epidemiological theory demonstrates that the size of host communities is essential for the evolution and maintenance of more acute and/or more virulent pathogens that induce solid immunity (14, 15). It is therefore likely that the social behavior and demographics of the early human species, in particular of hunter-gatherers, precluded the establishment of such more acute or more virulent pathogens. Therefore, classically acute pathogens, such as measles virus and smallpox virus, were unlikely to emerge at those times. This highlights the importance of the behavioral and demographic changes defining the prehistoric and historical development of the human species in further shaping the modern human-animal interface as we know it today.

DOMESTICATION AND AGRICULTURE

After hunter-gatherers migrated out of the African homeland and dispersed around the globe, significant behavioral innovations took place remarkably simultaneously in several regions of the world (16). About 12,000 years ago, previously highly mobile human groups settled in what would be seen as the world's first villages and domesticated valuable wild plant and animal species for food and feed production. While ancient evidence for these behavioral innovations was first excavated from the soil of the Fertile Crescent, similarly dated evidence has been brought to light in Mesopotamia, China, South America, and the eastern part of North America. The novel farming economies swiftly spread globally from these homelands of agriculture to replace most hunter-gatherer economies around the world.

The behavioral innovations associated with the birth of domestication and agriculture during the so-called Neolithic revolution initiated increasingly close contacts and interactions between animal species and humans, drastically altering the prehistoric human-animal interface (16). Before the Neolithic revolution, interactions between humans and animals were mainly those of predator-prey systems (1). The Neolithic revolution led to animal husbandry and care and associated activities for the production of food. It resulted in a major historical transition characterized by massive emergence of novel human and domestic animal pathogens, as revealed by phylogenetic analyses. Thus, mumps virus, smallpox virus, *Corynebacterium diphtheriae*, and *Bordetella pertussis* emerged in humans soon after the birth of domestication and agriculture, although their animal hosts of origin cannot be identified with certainty (17). Similarly, strains of caliciviruses, rotaviruses, and other pathogens transmitted via environmental reservoirs, such as certain strains of *Salmonella* spp., emerged and spread among cattle, swine, and humans soon after the birth of domestication (1, 5, 18). While it is difficult to trace their exact cross-species transmission history, they have spread recurrently from livestock to humans and vice versa since then. Interestingly, *Taenia* spp. and possibly *Mycobacterium bovis* of cattle also emerged around the time of domestication and have their ancestral origins in the pathogens of humans acquired thousands of years earlier by *Homo* spp. living on the African savannah (10, 19).

The exchange of pathogens between domestic animals and humans, resulting in the emergence of novel pathogens in novel host species, has not ceased since the birth of domestication and agriculture. Domestication and agriculture drive domestic species in close contact not only with humans but also with one another, and favor the evolution and establishment of commensal animal species, such as rats and mice. They result in the mixing of a diverse range of animal species and ideal conditions for the cross-species transmission of pathogens. For example, it has been suggested that feline leukemia viruses emerged following the cross-species transmission of rodent retroviruses and further adaptation of these pathogens to domestic cats (20). Recently canine hepatitis C virus was identified in domestic dogs and estimated to have emerged 500 to 1,000 years ago (21). It is closely related to the human hepatitis C virus, known to infect humans since prehistoric times. It is therefore tempting to speculate that cross-species transmission of hepatitis C-like virus from humans to domestic dogs occurred sometime during the Middle Ages (1). Another recently discovered virus, the human metapneumovirus, closely related to the avian metapneumovirus, is thought to have emerged about 150,000 to 200,000 years ago presumably following poultry-to-human transmission (22). It adapted to the human species and spread globally in the human population, so that today, most individuals ≥5 years of age have been infected at least once by this pathogen. Likewise, the recently discovered human bocavirus is proven to be a recombinant parvovirus of cattle and canine host origins, and infects most children before 5 years of age, suggesting that it has been established in the human population for some time (23, 24). Influenza viruses may have emerged as early as the 5th century B.C. or before, as reports of suggestive epidemics can be found in the Hippocratic Corpus. However, it is typically accepted that influenza pandemics occurred recurrently in human populations at least from the 16th century A.D. onward, and their origins can be found in animal viruses that crossed to the human species, most probably after passage in domestic animals, such as swine or poultry (25, 26). Feline panleukopenia virus has been known as a pathogen of domestic cats since the beginning of the last century, and recognized as a naturally occurring pathogen in wild carnivores, such as mink, foxes, and raccoons, since the 1940s. In the late 1970s, canine parvovirus emerged in domestic dogs following cross-species transmission of feline panleukopenia virus and adaptation to its novel host (26). It rapidly spread worldwide and now represents a major pathogen of domestic dogs. These examples certainly highlight the continued cross-species transmission of pathogens between and among animal species and humans at the domestic human-animal interface, followed by adaptation to the newly "colonized" species.

The cross-species transmission of zoonotic and nonzoonotic pathogens between animals and humans and among animal species associated with humans further intensified as the diversity of pet, food, and commensal animal species expanded to the unprecedented levels of current times. Exotic pet species, such as reptiles and rodents, are the source of a plethora of pathogens for humans, from ubiquitous ones such as *Salmonella* spp. to foes that have challenged mankind since medieval times and exotic pathogens such as *Yersinia pestis* and monkeypox virus (27). Remarkably, cross-species transmission of many of these pathogens occurs both from animals to humans as well as between animal species, illustrating the scope of the domestic human-animal interface. Likewise, the unequaled development of bush meat consumption in many developing countries to meet the pressing demand for food by rapidly growing human populations has expanded the range of food animal species in the recent past to unparalleled numbers (28). Animal species used for bush meat have been incriminated in spectacular cross-species transmissions of a number of new zoonotic pathogens, including HIV, Ebola viruses, bat lyssaviruses, and recently discovered coronaviruses, i.e., severe acute respiratory syndrome coronavirus (SARS-CoV) and hCoV-EMC (29, 30). As previously, many of these pathogens cross the species barrier not only from animals to humans but also among animal species. Lastly, the continued encroachment of mankind into natural habitats, in association with the expansion of agriculture, creates novel environmental conditions favoring a wide range of new commensal species that thrive in anthropogenic environments due to behavioral flexibility and adaptability. In the recent past, these species, newly associated with humans, such as fruit bats in Asia and Oceania and New World rodents, have been the sources of whole new groups of zoonotic pathogens, from henipaviruses to New World hantaviruses (31–33). Rodents and bats are mammals belonging to the orders *Rodentia* and *Chiroptera*, respectively, which together represent 60% of all mammalian species. While a few species of rodents have had a long association with humans and their shared pathogens, the wide diversity of rodent as well as bat species makes them an undoubtedly important reservoir pool for zoonotic pathogens in the future. Bats in particular are increasingly recognized as maintenance hosts for a plethora of pathogens typically found to be highly virulent in other mammals, such as rabies and other lyssaviruses, filoviruses, and coronaviruses.

Both commensal and wildlife species used for bush meat create an efficient link between the domestic human-animal interface and wildlife, favoring the cross-species transmission of wildlife pathogens from host species not directly associated with humans. Although evidence for this is largely lacking, some pathogens that emerged soon after the birth of domestication and agriculture may have originated from wildlife reservoirs or commensals. Smallpox virus, for example, is closely related to gerbilpox viruses, and may have crossed to humans from a rodent host (5). *Y. pestis* may have evolved from an ancestral strain of *Yersinia pseudotuberculosis* infecting rodents, possibly in relation to the birth of domestication and associated demographic and behavioral changes in commensals (34). It may have further evolved into different populations, associated with different rodent species and/or geographic areas, and at the origin of the historical plague pandemics in humans. The role of commensal or bush meat species as relays in the cross-species transmission of pathogens of wildlife is well illustrated in historical and more recent times. Major scourges of ancient and medieval history were associated with commensals, such as typhus and plague. *Y. pestis* at the origin of the Black Death was carried by black rats that accompanied humans along the Silk Road, before causing one of the most devastating historical plague pandemics (35). More recently, bush meat species infected with Ebola viruses in Africa or SARS-CoV in Southeast Asia were but relay species in the cross-species transmission of these bat viruses to humans (28). Likewise, domestic swine and horses were relay species in the cross-species transmission of fruit bat henipaviruses (Nipah virus in Malaysia and Hendra virus in Australia, respectively) to humans (31, 36). The destruction of natural habitats and encroachment of agriculture created altered conditions for fruit bats, which colonized cultured and farmed environments, eventually infecting domestic animals and humans with these novel pathogens. In a way, agriculture and farming practices, in combination with the destruction of natural habitats, led to the colonization of anthropogenic environments by fruit bats and turned them into novel commensal species. Similarly, in South America, the recent encroachment of agriculture into natural habitats led to the colonization of cultures by a variety of rodent species, not unlike the ancient colonization of anthropogenic environments by commensal rodent species of the Old World, resulting in multiple cross-species transmissions of new bunya- and arenaviruses to humans (32, 33).

Although the number of new zoonotic pathogens emerging in the human species following cross-species transmission from domestic, commensal, or wild animals appears to be on the rise, it may be worthwhile to determine whether advances in laboratory technologies and awareness do not significantly account for these exploding numbers. In fact, since its prehistoric kickoff, the domestic human-animal interface has created melting-pot conditions for both host and pathogen species, spurring the cross-species transmission of pathogens (1). It is nevertheless beyond doubt that the trends in cross-species transmissions of animal pathogens to humans and among animal species associated with humans will not subside in the future. Beyond bringing animal species and humans in close contact, domestication and agriculture also initiated food and feed production, allowing population sizes of the human, domestic, and commensal species to boom up to this day. In addition, the unprecedented globalized distribution of food and feed products facilitates the emergence and spread of novel pathogens of humans and animals alike. These demographic changes further fueled cross-species transmissions of pathogens, their emergence, and eventually their long-term maintenance in growing populations.

FOOD PRODUCTION, POPULATION GROWTH, AND HUMAN URBANIZATION

The birth of domestication and agriculture some 12,000 years ago initiated food and feed production that have allowed the massive population growth of the human species and associated animal species to this day (16). As populations grew, humans congregated in villages of expanding size, leading to the start of urbanization. Babylon in Mesopotamia was one of the first cities to reach 200,000 inhabitants during ancient history. As early cities developed, they retained the characteristics of villages, with domestic and food production animal species kept in close proximity to humans. As such, these cities hosted dense populations of humans and of domestic and commensal animals, fueling the cross-species transmission of pathogens, and eventually favoring their long-term maintenance in novel host species. It led to the birth of crowd diseases that have plagued humans and associated animal species ever since. As cities expanded and developed into the major population centers of current times, they grew to host ever larger and denser populations of humans and associated animals, providing fertile soil for the sustained spread of pathogens. In this light, it is interesting to note that more and more mammalian, avian, and other wildlife as well as feral species are being linked with newly emerging habitats associated with human urbanization (37).

Epidemiological theory demonstrates that pathogens causing acute immunizing infections require a critical community size to be maintained in the host population, below which these pathogens are unable to persist (14, 15). Measles virus, for example, confers strong lifelong immunity and is known to require a community of 200,000 to 500,000 individuals to persist in the human population and recur as cyclic epidemics. Similarly, smallpox virus, *B. pertussis*, and other acute pathogens that emerged in humans soon after the birth of domestication and agriculture required critical community sizes to spread and persist, which were met by the growing human population. The invention of food production following the birth of domestication and agriculture gradually set the stage for the evolution of these pathogens to cause acute, virulent, and highly immunizing infections. Growing populations during the last stages of prehistory likely sustained these pathogens in the making, leading to the full-blown crowd diseases of ancient history and following the rise of urbanization. Thus, the oldest putative physical evidence of smallpox is seen as pustules on the mummified skin of Pharaoh Ramses V (20th Dynasty, 12th century B.C.) (Fig. 3) (38). Later, the report of devastating epidemics in the Hippocratic Corpus convincingly demonstrates the common occurrence of acute infections that swept through human populations by the 5th century B.C.

The demographic changes of the last ages of prehistoric and ancient history, as seen in humans following the invention of food production and accompanied by the rise of urbanization, also affected domestic animal species. These changes likely favored the establishment and maintenance of pathogens, and possibly the evolution of more-acute or -virulent pathogens in these species. It further illustrates the influence of the urban human-animal interface on disease emergence in animal populations associated with humans. Crowd diseases of domestic animals, such as rinderpest in cattle, peste des petits ruminants in sheep and goats, and canine distemper in domestic dogs, which are caused by morbilliviruses closely related to measles virus, likely emerged and evolved as the domestic animal populations grew denser to feed growing populations of humans congregating in villages and cities. An illustrative example is that of *Bordetella bronchiseptica*, a common upper respiratory tract pathogen of a wide range of wild and domestic animals. A *B. bronchiseptica*-like ancestor was likely the precursor of *B. pertussis*, which causes whooping cough in humans (14). While the latter causes acute infections in humans, the former typically causes chronic and mild infections in animal species. As seen previously, sufficiently large human communities were required for the

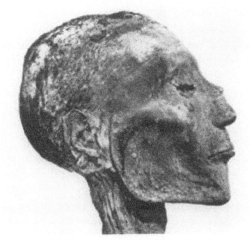

Source: World Health Organization

Figure 3. Evidence of smallpox infection of Pharaoh Ramses V. Poxlike lesions reminiscent of smallpox pustules can be seen on the head of the 3,000-year-old mummy. Source: World Health Organization.
doi:10.1128/microbiolspec.OH-0013-2012.f3

evolution of *B. pertussis* toward an acute form in humans (14). Remarkably, certain strains of *B. bronchoseptica* cause more acute and/or more virulent infections in swine and dogs, and may have evolved as a result of large population sizes and densities of these domestic animals, not unlike *B. pertussis* in humans.

Urbanization is associated not only with dramatic demographic changes in human and animal populations but also with major behavioral changes, further contributing to the emergence and spread of pathogens in humans and associated animal species. In fact, the settlement of humans in the first villages during prehistory was associated with poorer health compared with that of mobile hunter-gatherers, due to unbalanced diet, more sedentary life habits, and crowded conditions favoring pathogen transmission (39). In its debut, historical urbanization was likewise associated with poor sanitary conditions and crowding. Medieval diseases, such as typhus and bubonic plague, were often associated with commensal host species, in particular rodents, flourishing in cities rich in granaries and deficient in waste treatment (40). The account of the Plague of Athens of 430 B.C. by Thucydides illustrates well the spread of typhoid fever by the fecal pathogen *Salmonella enterica* through a crowded and unsanitary city (41). Remarkably, Thucydides reported the spread of the disease not only in humans but also in animals, suggesting that the pathogen may not have been a strictly human pathogen at that time. As such, urbanization provided ideal conditions for the sustained spread of pathogens and recurring epidemics, from the buildup of sufficiently large host populations to the mixing of humans and animal hosts to the lack of hygiene. Most interestingly, changes in behavior, improvement of hygiene, and the birth of modern medicine are direct responses to the surge of diseases associated with urbanization and the development of the human society (1). Centuries later, it is believed that urbanization and associated human behavioral changes similarly were determinant factors in the efficient spread of a modern scourge of the human species, HIV. Phylogenetic analyses revealed that HIV-1, responsible for the majority of the AIDS pandemic worldwide, had crossed the species barrier from chimpanzees to humans multiple times and decades before the efficient spread of the pathogen in the human population starting in the 1980s (42). Urban migration, poverty, social inequality, sexual promiscuity, and shared use of needles, all of which affected developing cities in Africa at that time, as well as war-related sociocultural changes are thought to be decisive behavioral drivers that allowed for the eventual adaptation of HIV and its efficient transmission in the human population (43).

Behavioral changes affected not only humans migrating to cities but also commensals and other urban-dwelling animal species. In recent times, the prevalence of a number of pathogens, including zoonotic pathogens, has been shown to be greater in wild animal populations residing in urbanized and anthropogenic environments than in those residing in more rural or natural habitats (37). Higher transmission rates of these pathogens are often associated with both higher densities of host populations and behavioral changes, such as the use of human resources for food or shelter. For example, the prevalence of raccoon zoonotic roundworm *Baylisascaris procyonis* is reported to be higher in urbanized environments. Both an increase in parasite species richness and an increase in *B. procyonis* prevalence in raccoons are associated with crowding and the use of aggregated food resources by urban populations. Other examples of disease emergence in wildlife at the urban human-animal interface include *Borrelia burgdorferi* in white-footed mice, chronic wasting disease in mule deer, and West Nile virus in songbirds in North American urbanized areas. Behavioral flexibility and adaptation to anthropogenic environments largely contribute to these species' flourishing populations in urban and residential habitats, and also favor pathogen invasion (37).

In addition to hosting growing populations of urban-dwelling animal species, expanding urbanization also presses the demand for food production and has led to increasing demands for bush meat in many parts of the developing world, in particular Asia and Africa (28). This has two major consequences that inflate the scope of the urban human-animal interface. First, urbanization and associated pressure for food lead to greater encroachment into natural habitats, via the development of road networks and expansion of anthropogenic areas. Habitat encroachment, deforestation, and habitat fragmentation can result in increased contacts between wildlife and humans, spurring the cross-species transmission of pathogens in both directions. Major examples include the cross-species transmissions of a number of pathogens from primates to humans, including retroviruses and filoviruses (28). Second, bush meat species hunted in natural habitats are brought back to cities and urbanized areas for trade and consumption. Live-animal markets have flourished in most Asian and African cities, favoring the introduction of new pathogens in these densely populated areas. Both domestic and wild animals are present in these so-called wet markets, which have facilitated the emergence of a number of zoonotic pathogens, including influenza viruses and SARS-CoV. Shortly after the cross-species transmission of the latter from wild animals kept alive at wet markets to humans, it adapted to efficiently transmit between humans (29). It hit a dense population that would sustain its transmission, first locally and eventually around the globe. As urbanization continues to expand in developing countries, the toll that bush meat hunting is taking on wildlife populations will increase and represents a major risk lurking at the urban human-animal interface (28).

The rise of urbanization in the last ages of prehistory and into ancient history went hand in glove with the initiation of trade and associated movements of humans and animals between cities and eventually across entire regions and continents. As illustrated by the spread of SARS-CoV (29), trade and movements of humans, animals, and goods are major factors completing the modern human-animal interface. Yet domestication, agriculture, food production and urbanization, worldwide migrations, colonization, and trade and their impact on disease emergence have ancient origins.

HUMAN WORLDWIDE MIGRATION, COLONIZATION, AND TRADE

Human migrations around the globe date to prehistoric times, when groups of hunter-gatherers journeyed out of Africa to colonize the rest of the world, following coastlines or the migration of megafauna (44). Phylogeographic analyses dramatically illustrate the global spread of ancient human pathogens along prehistoric migration routes. For example, phylogeographic analyses of papillomaviruses, polyomaviruses, HTLV, *H. pylori*, and human-associated lice provide remarkable insights into ancient human migrations (5, 45). The chronic infections caused by these pathogens allowed their spread over large distances, despite the relatively slow colonization rate by prehistoric humans. In addition to dispersing pathogens along migration routes, peripatetic prehistoric humans also acquired novel pathogens as they colonized new areas. HTLV-1 strains, for example, were acquired following simian-to-human transmission of primate T-lymphotropic viruses in Asia. Phylogenetic analyses also revealed that HTLV-1 strains were transmitted from humans to other primates, and vice versa, on several occasions (46, 47). While HTLV-2 emerged in Africa about 400,000 years ago, HTLV-1 strains were introduced back to Africa upon prehistoric migrations. The large-scale dispersion of pathogens by humans thus started early in the development of the human species and gradually accelerated as the means to travel and trade progressed.

The historical colonization of new worlds during ancient history, the Middle Ages, and early modern history is associated with spectacular examples of sweeping epidemic waves caused by emerging pathogens in both colonist and resident populations. Invasions of populations by such major diseases are well described in biblical texts. During medieval times, the spread of diseases often was associated with war or conquest. The Justinian plague of the 6th to 8th century A.D. may have been caused by the *Y. pestis* bacillus, originating from the African continent. Its emergence may have been associated with the conquest led by Justinian I of most of the Mediterranean coast, including that of North Africa (35). The spread of this pathogen in humans throughout Europe and North Africa during the following centuries certainly contributed to the fall of the Byzantine Empire. The second plague pandemic, of the 14th century A.D., also was associated with war and conquest. Before the introduction of the Black Death into Sicily and Europe via trade, *Y. pestis* was used by the Mongol army to besiege the Crimean city of Caffa (48). In 1346, the Mongol army catapulted corpses infected with plague beyond the city walls, making use of a devastating biological weapon. The dawn of modern history witnessed colonization and conquest reaching more distant continents. Upon the discovery and early development of the Americas, most pathogens causing crowd diseases in the Old World, such as smallpox and measles viruses, were introduced in immunologically naïve indigenous populations, sometimes even intentionally (49, 50). These introductions resulted in virgin-soil epidemics, which decimated entire populations. In contrast, in Africa, colonists were themselves ravaged by tropical pathogens, such as *Plasmodium* spp., causing malaria, and yellow fever virus (49). These exotic diseases are thought to have hampered the institutional development of the African continent and may have strongly influenced the slave trade (51). Indeed, the influence of infectious diseases is considered primordial and likely shaped the course of early modern human history. In late modern and contemporary history, wars have continued to play a major role in the global spread of infectious diseases, from typhus and typhoid fever to the 1918 influenza pandemic and the spread of HIV-2 (25, 43).

The colonization of new worlds has lately been replaced by worldwide travel practices, for business or tourism, and comes with highly similar risks of spreading infectious diseases to unexposed populations or new geographic areas. Travelers in foreign countries may become exposed to pathogens they have never before encountered, and may within an exceptionally short period of time spread them around the globe. These travel practices have been at the origin of a plethora of reports of emerging pathogens within the past decades. These range from isolated cases of exotic diseases, such as bat lyssavirus, filovirus, or human HCoV-EMC infections (30, 52, 53), to the global spread of novel pathogens, such as that of HIV and lately of SARS-CoV, which spread to 26 countries within a few months before being brought under control through concerted public health efforts (29). The scope of current travel practices and their impact on the global spread of pathogens that emerged at the human-animal interface is most convincingly illustrated by the recent influenza pandemic of 2009 and the recurrent spread of seasonal influenza viruses around the world. Within weeks after its initial emergence in Mexico, probably following swine-to-human cross-species transmission, the 2009 pandemic influenza virus spread globally via human-to-human transmission on major air-travel routes (54). A strong correlation was found between the geographic distribution of imported cases of infection with this new influenza virus at the start of the pandemic and the international destinations of travelers from Mexico. Likewise, the global spread of seasonal influenza viruses every year follows highly consistent patterns of emergence in Southeast Asia and global migration via travel and trade connections between this region and the rest of the world (55).

Since ancient history, the development of trade and human travel between growing cities has also been an efficient driver favoring the continued circulation of pathogens in human and associated animal populations, and the spread of synchronous waves of disease across the landscape. It acted in synergy with the growing size of host populations, reaching levels sufficient for long-term maintenance of crowd diseases. On a broad geographic scale, *Y. pestis* at the origin of the devastating Black Death epidemic in Europe had been introduced into Sicily via trade routes in the Mediterranean Sea (35). The bacteria had been picked up by black rats in Asia and spread both to conquering armies and to merchants traveling the Silk Road. After entry into Europe, waves of the bubonic plague pandemic ravaged the continent within a few years. On a more restricted geographic scale, measles reports of the 20th century in the United Kingdom have provided invaluable insights into the waves of measles epidemics that sweep through the human population, from large cities hosting large enough communities to maintain the virus toward smaller and more rural communities (56). These waves of disease created remarkable dynamics of synchronous pulses of disease outbreaks radiating from large cities, kept in synchrony via trade and commuting movements of humans, into more rural areas. Likewise, seasonal influenza viruses were shown to be spread via commuting movements such as workflows in the continental United States, further highlighting the driving force of even short-distance movements of humans on the spread of infectious pathogens (57).

Movements of people are accompanied by movements of animal species, and the global spread of zoonotic and nonzoonotic pathogens of animals is an important consequence of this facet of the human-animal interface (27). As for humans, trade and movements of animals have characterized populations associated with humans for millennia. It has been suggested that the distinctively low genetic diversity of some parasites, such as *Trichinella spiralis*, in domestic animal species compared to that in wild counterpart species is a result of early trade and translocation of domestic animals by prehistoric and/or ancient farmers (58). Likewise, the worldwide distribution of a phylogenetic group of closely related Seoul virus variants may point to global dispersion of the pathogen via human-associated migration of Norway rats (*Rattus norvegicus*) (59, 60). The global spread of animal pathogens is well documented during more recent human history and has become of major concern. The introduction of rinderpest virus into Africa during the 19th century resulted in virgin-soil epidemics with high mortality burdens in local cattle breeds and wild ungulates, decimating entire populations (61). Although the virus was not zoonotic, it severely affected human populations dependent on cattle and was responsible for large-scale famines in many African countries. In Europe, the spread of highly infectious pathogens, such as foot-and-mouth disease virus, rinderpest virus, and the anthrax bacillus, resulted in bans of animal movements during epidemics as regulatory measures as early as the 18th century (62). It demonstrates the early recognition of the role this facet of the human-animal interface played in disease emergence and spread.

In current times, animal species subject to travel and trade have become more and more insidious Trojan horses for the introduction of zoonotic pathogens worldwide, in part due to increasing diversity and heavier volume of traded species. Insect vectors are perhaps among the most overlooked animal species that can be dispersed globally via human activities. The global distribution of the Asia tiger mosquito *Aedes albopictus*, an important vector of dengue virus, is associated with the trade of tires, containing water infested with mosquito eggs, via rapid air and sea transport (63). Although the means of introduction of another flavivirus, West Nile virus, into North America remains unsolved, infected *Culex* mosquitoes trapped in airplanes remain a possibility, alongside the importation of infected birds (64). SARS-CoV was introduced in the human population as a result of the trade of bush meat species in Asia (29). Remarkably, it rapidly adapted and acquired efficient transmissibility in humans, gaining the means for sustained transmission first locally and then around the globe. A major recent introduction of monkeypox virus outside its African native range was a result of the trade of exotic rodent pet species from Africa to North America (65). It resulted in >80 human cases of zoonotic infection. Less exotic zoonotic viruses, such as rabies virus, recurrently threaten to affect animal and human populations alike in disease-free countries, due to the illegal trade of domestic cats, dogs, and other carnivores from countries where the diseases are endemic (27). Likewise, major pathogens of livestock, including foot-and-mouth disease virus, may invade disease-free populations and spread like wildfire following accidental or illegal introductions. In 2001, illegal introduction of meat waste originating from Asia, where foot-and-mouth disease is endemic, resulted in a major epidemic of the disease in the

United Kingdom and soon after in other European countries (66). In the United Kingdom alone, the economic consequences of the outbreak amounted to >6 million pounds (67). Last but not least, trade may influence disease emergence not only in humans and associated animal species but also in wildlife, including in relatively pristine environments (68). Trade has been suggested as a plausible cause for the spread of the fungus *Batrachochytrium dendrobatidis*, which causes amphibian chytridiomycosis worldwide (69), as well as for the spread of the fungus *Geomyces destructans*, which causes bat white-nose syndrome in North America (70). Both diseases have been associated with massive wildlife population collapses.

The increasing diversity and heavier volume of traded animal species have been accompanied and fueled by the industrialization and globalization of the food industry in more recent history. This represents one of the most recent facets of the human-animal interface in the present globalized world.

INDUSTRIALIZATION AND GLOBALIZATION

The industrial revolution marks a historical transition in late modern history, spanning the 19th and beginning of the 20th century, and initiating the globalization that characterizes current times. The industrialization of food production was prompted by the unabated growth of the human population and resulted in massive population growth of associated animal species. This unique attribute of the modern human-animal interface is its youngest facet and has brought challenges never faced before.

The industrial revolution not only resulted in massive population growth of animal species associated with humans, including domestic, commensal, and traded species, amplifying the risks at the domestic and urban human-animal interface, but it also resulted in dramatic changes in animal husbandry, in particular farming intensification. This has led to massive encroachment of natural habitats by agriculture and farmed populations, expanding the interface between domestic animals and wildlife. It also has resulted in complex disease dynamics in domestic animals and wildlife, worsening control options in domestic animal populations (71). For example, *M. bovis* and *Brucella* spp. are zoonotic pathogens that may circulate heavily in wildlife populations, typically after initial cross-species transmission from domestic animals. These pathogens, when present in wildlife, are difficult to eradicate from livestock, as is the case in some parts of Europe and in the United States. The emergence of Nipah virus in Asia is directly linked to the encroachment of natural habitats by agriculture and pig farming (31, 36). The combination of fruit tree plantations with pig farming created favorable conditions for the cross-species transmission of this fruit bat pathogen to pigs and humans. Similarly, the combination of agriculture and fish, poultry, and pig farming in China, which is increasingly encroaching on natural water bird habitats, likely favors the circulation of influenza viruses between domestic animals and wild water birds (72, 73).

The industrialization of food production also has led to the emergence and evolution of increasing diversity in known as well as novel animal pathogens, which may rapidly disseminate worldwide via globalized trade. The origin of the high diversity of foot-and-mouth disease virus strains circulating in Eurasia has been traced to a radiation and rapid expansion event that occurred during the 19th century, coinciding with the industrial revolution (74). The emergence of human metapneumovirus from an avian metapneumovirus ancestor some 150 to 200 years ago likewise coincides with the industrialization of the poultry industry (22). The massive expansion of strain diversity of influenza viruses in swine and poultry in the recent past also correlates with the increase in the industrial populations of swine and poultry worldwide (Fig. 4) (75). In combination with intercontinental trade, complex strain dynamics and reassortments have ensued, creating an increasing pool of potentially zoonotic influenza viruses in these animal populations. The circulation of influenza viruses in dense populations of poultry further allowed the emergence of highly virulent strains, called highly pathogenic avian influenza viruses, severely altering the epidemiology of the viruses. In particular, some strains of highly pathogenic avian influenza viruses may infect humans directly from bird hosts and cause often fatal respiratory and extrarespiratory disease. Similarly, changes in husbandry practices leading to dense and large populations of animals in industrial farms kept at maximal production efficiency have resulted in the emergence of new forms of prions in cattle, causing bovine spongiform encephalopathy in cattle, a new variant of Creutzfeldt-Jakob disease in humans, and a similar disease in domestic animals like cats (76). Changes in the treatment of cattle offals in the United Kingdom in the 1980s were implemented to increase production efficiency of meat and bone meal, used as a

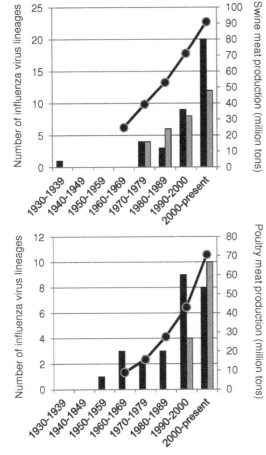

Figure 4. Diversity of avian and swine influenza viruses. The annual productions of swine and poultry meat have dramatically increased since the 1960s (upper and lower panel, connected dots). Concurrently, the number of new influenza virus lineages in swine (upper panel, black bars) and the number of outbreaks of highly pathogenic avian influenza in poultry (lower panel, black bars) have increased similarly since the discovery of the virus in pigs in the 1930s and in poultry in the 1950s. These increases in viral diversity have been accompanied by an increase in the number of swine and avian influenza virus subtypes or lineages that have caused infection in humans (upper and lower panels, gray bars). Modified from reference 75. doi:10.1128/microbiolspec.OH-0013-2012.f4

protein-rich ruminant feed supplement. These changes resulted in insufficient treatment for the destruction of nondegradable host proteins such as prions. The trade of contaminated meat and bone meal spread these new pathogens across and beyond Europe, causing an epidemic in cattle and humans. Because of the long incubation period, and in spite of all the successful but draconic intervention measures taken, cases of disease have been appearing for decades following the emergence of the pathogens and continue to appear today. Industrialization as such has created favorable conditions for the evolution and emergence of previously unmet pathogens. It is likely that these pathogens may not persist without industrial populations of domestic animals, highlighting the unique challenges brought by the industrial facet of the human-animal interface today.

Another consequence of the industrial revolution is certainly the routine use of antimicrobials in the human as well as in domestic animal populations, and the associated rise of antimicrobial resistance at the human-animal interface (77). Antimicrobial resistance initially appeared in hospitals, where most antibiotics were used, soon after their introduction. Bacterial strains resistant to multiple drugs arose in the late 1950s. Antimicrobial resistance in pathogens of animals were reported at about this time, and followed the use of antimicrobials in food production animals initiated in the 1950s for therapeutic as well as subtherapeutic and growth efficiency purposes. Although the impact of antimicrobial resistance in animal populations on human health is under debate, it is considered a significant problem that may cause heavier health burdens in the future (see reference 80).

Lastly, and among the greatest challenges of current times, industrialization likely has had a major impact on and may continue to affect global climate in the future (78). Changes in climatic conditions may further favor disease emergence at the human-animal interface, by favoring certain host-pathogen systems strongly associated with environmental conditions. Global warming thus may expand or modify migratory patterns of aquatic mammals and birds, as well as the geographic range of insect vectors of zoonotic pathogens currently considered as exotic, such as *Plasmodium* spp., Chikungunya virus, Rift Valley fever virus, Crimean-Congo hemorrhagic fever virus, dengue viruses, and yellow fever virus. Although correlating changes in the geographic distribution of vector-borne pathogens with climate change remains a challenge, the expansion of the range of tick-borne encephalitis virus in Europe and of *B. burgdorferi*, the agent of Lyme disease, in Europe and North America calls for future research (79).

CONCLUDING REMARKS

The human-animal interface is a continuously evolving entity that has affected the human species since its first bipedal steps on the earth's surface. Its attributes have not ceased to evolve and expand as mankind has developed throughout history. Understanding its evolving nature and expanding scope is a determinant for humans' race against infectious pathogens lurking across this interface. As it will continue to allow the emergence of new pathogens in humans and associated animals, developing improved tools and technologies to screen and combat pathogens before they cross the human-animal interface and adapt to spread efficiently in new hosts must be considered a priority. In recent history, two pathogens have been brought to extinction, namely, smallpox and rinderpest viruses. However, combating pathogens at the human-animal interface likely represents an advantageous head start in our battle against infectious diseases. New pathogens of humans that have their origins in animals can become major human scourges within decades, as most recently demonstrated by the human metapneumovirus and HIV. In contrast, concerted public health efforts and medical research allowed the arising SARS-CoV pandemic to be nipped in the bud as soon as the pathogen started to spread around the globe. This is a unique chapter in human history, highlighting that successes can be achieved at the forefront of combating pathogen emergence.

Citation. Reperant LA, Osterhaus ADME. 2013. The human-animal interface. Microbiol Spectrum 1(1): OH-0013-2012. doi:10.1128/microbiolspec.OH-0013-2012.

REFERENCES

1. **Reperant LA, Cornaglia G, Osterhaus AD.** 2012. The importance of understanding the human-animal interface: from early hominins to global citizens. *Curr Top Microbiol Immunol* [Epub ahead of print.] doi:10.1007/82_2012_269.
2. **Herfst S, Schrauwen EJ, Linster M, Chutinimitkul S, de Wit E, Munster VJ, Sorrell EM, Bestebroer TM, Burke DF, Smith DJ, Rimmelzwaan GF, Osterhaus AD, Fouchier RA.** 2012. Airborne transmission of influenza A/H5N1 virus between ferrets. *Science* **336:**1534–1541.
3. **Imai M, Watanabe T, Hatta M, Das SC, Ozawa M, Shinya K, Zhong G, Hanson A, Katsura H, Watanabe S, Li C, Kawakami E, Yamada S, Kiso M, Suzuki Y, Maher EA, Neumann G, Kawaoka Y.** 2012. Experimental adaptation of an influenza H5 HA confers respiratory droplet transmission to a reassortant H5 HA/H1N1 virus in ferrets. *Nature* **486:**420–428.
4. **Russell CA, Fonville JM, Brown AE, Burke DF, Smith DL, James SL, Herfst S, van Boheemen S, Linster M, Schrauwen EJ, Katzelnick L, Mosterin A, Kuiken T, Maher E, Neumann G, Osterhaus AD, Kawaoka Y, Fouchier RA, Smith DJ.** 2012. The potential for respiratory droplet-transmissible A/H5N1 influenza virus to evolve in a mammalian host. *Science* **336:**1541–1547.
5. **Van Blerkom LM.** 2003. Role of viruses in human evolution. *Am J Phys Anthropol* **122**(Suppl 37): 14–46.
6. **Gagneux S.** 2012. Host-pathogen coevolution in human tuberculosis. *Philos Trans R Soc Lond B Biol Sci* **367:**850–859.
7. **Ollomo B, Durand P, Prugnolle F, Douzery E, Arnathau C, Nkoghe D, Leroy E, Renaud F.** 2009. A new malaria agent in African hominids. *PLoS Pathog* **5:**e1000446.
8. **Stevens JR, Gibson W.** 1999. The molecular evolution of trypanosomes. *Parasitol Today* **15:**432–437.
9. **Weiss RA.** 2009. Apes, lice and prehistory. *J Biol* **8:**20.
10. **Hoberg EP, Alkire NL, de Queiroz A, Jones A.** 2001. Out of Africa: origins of the *Taenia* tapeworms in humans. *Proc Biol Sci* **268:**781–787.
11. **Linz B, Balloux F, Moodley Y, Manica A, Liu H, Roumagnac P, Falush D, Stamer C, Prugnolle F, van der Merwe SW, Yamaoka Y, Graham DY, Perez-Trallero E, Wadstrom T, Suerbaum S, Achtman M.** 2007. An African origin for the intimate association between humans and *Helicobacter pylori*. *Nature* **445:** 915–918.
12. **McGeoch DJ, Dolan A, Ralph AC.** 2000. Toward a comprehensive phylogeny for mammalian and avian herpesviruses. *J Virol* **74:**10401–10406.
13. **McGeoch DJ, Rixon FJ, Davison AJ.** 2006. Topics in herpesvirus genomics and evolution. *Virus Res* **117:** 90–104.
14. **King AA, Shrestha S, Harvill ET, Bjornstad ON.** 2009. Evolution of acute infections and the invasion-persistence trade-off. *Am Nat* **173:**446–455.
15. **Bartlett MJ.** 1957. Measles periodicity and community size. *J R Statist Soc A* **120:**48–70.
16. **Diamond J.** 2002. Evolution, consequences and future of plant and animal domestication. *Nature* **418:** 700–707.
17. **Wolfe ND, Dunavan CP, Diamond J.** 2007. Origins of major human infectious diseases. *Nature* **447:** 279–283.

18. **Hare R.** 1967. The antiquity of diseases caused by bacteria and viruses: a review of the problem from a bacteriologist's point of view, p 115–131. *In* Brothwell D, Sandison AT (ed), *Diseases in Antiquity*. Charles C Thomas, Publisher, Springfield, IL.

19. **Comas I, Gagneux S.** 2009. The past and future of tuberculosis research. *PLoS Pathog* **5**:e1000600.

20. **Roca AL, Pecon-Slattery J, O'Brien SJ.** 2004. Genomically intact endogenous feline leukemia viruses of recent origin. *J Virol* **78**:4370–4375.

21. **Kapoor A, Simmonds P, Gerold G, Qaisar N, Jain K, Henriquez JA, Firth C, Hirschberg DL, Rice CM, Shields S, Lipkin WI.** 2011. Characterization of a canine homolog of hepatitis C virus. *Proc Natl Acad Sci USA* **108**:11608–11613.

22. **de Graaf M, Osterhaus AD, Fouchier RA, Holmes EC.** 2008. Evolutionary dynamics of human and avian metapneumoviruses. *J Gen Virol* **89**:2933–2942.

23. **Allander T, Tammi MT, Eriksson M, Bjerkner A, Tiveljung-Lindell A, Andersson B.** 2005. Cloning of a human parvovirus by molecular screening of respiratory tract samples. *Proc Natl Acad Sci USA* **102**:12891–12896.

24. **McIntosh K.** 2006. Human bocavirus: developing evidence for pathogenicity. *J Infect Dis* **194**:1197–1199.

25. **Taubenberger JK, Morens DM.** 2006. 1918 influenza: the mother of all pandemics. *Emerg Infect Dis* **12**:15–22.

26. **Parrish CR, Kawaoka Y.** 2005. The origins of new pandemic viruses: the acquisition of new host ranges by canine parvovirus and influenza A viruses. *Annu Rev Microbiol* **59**:553–586.

27. **Chomel BB, Belotto A, Meslin FX.** 2007. Wildlife, exotic pets, and emerging zoonoses. *Emerg Infect Dis* **13**:6–11.

28. **Wolfe ND, Daszak P, Kilpatrick AM, Burke DS.** 2005. Bushmeat hunting, deforestation, and prediction of zoonoses emergence. *Emerg Infect Dis* **11**:1822–1827.

29. **Peiris JS, Yuen KY, Osterhaus AD, Stohr K.** 2003. The severe acute respiratory syndrome. *N Engl J Med* **349**:2431–2441.

30. **Zaki AM, van Boheemen S, Bestebroer TM, Osterhaus AD, Fouchier RA.** 2012. Isolation of a novel coronavirus from a man with pneumonia in Saudi Arabia. *N Engl J Med* **367**:1814–1820.

31. **Chua KB.** 2003. Nipah virus outbreak in Malaysia. *J Clin Virol* **26**:265–275.

32. **Charrel RN, de Lamballerie X.** 2003. Arenaviruses other than Lassa virus. *Antiviral Res* **57**:89–100.

33. **Zeier M, Handermann M, Bahr U, Rensch B, Muller S, Kehm R, Muranyi W, Darai G.** 2005. New ecological aspects of hantavirus infection: a change of a paradigm and a challenge of prevention—a review. *Virus Genes* **30**:157–180.

34. **Achtman M, Zurth K, Morelli G, Torrea G, Guiyoule A, Carniel E.** 1999. *Yersinia pestis*, the cause of plague, is a recently emerged clone of *Yersinia pseudotuberculosis*. *Proc Natl Acad Sci USA* **96**:14043–14048.

35. **Perry RD, Fetherston JD.** 1997. *Yersinia pestis*—etiologic agent of plague. *Clin Microbiol Rev* **10**:35–66.

36. **Field HE, Mackenzie JS, Daszak P.** 2007. Henipaviruses: emerging paramyxoviruses associated with fruit bats, p 133–159. *In* Childs JE, Mackenzie JS, Richt JA (ed), *Wildlife and Emerging Zoonotic Diseases: the Biology, Circumstances and Consequences of Cross-Species Transmission*. Springer, Berlin, Germany.

37. **Bradley CA, Altizer S.** 2007. Urbanization and the ecology of wildlife diseases. *Trends Ecol Evol* **22**:95–102.

38. **Hopkins D.** 1980. Ramses V: earliest known victim? *World Health* **5**:22 http://whqlibdoc.who.int/smallpox/WH_5_1980_p22.pdf (last accessed May 2, 2013).

39. **Larsen CS.** 2006. The agricultural revolution as environmental catastrophe: implications for health and lifestyle in the Holocene. *Quat Int* **150**:12–20.

40. **McCormick M.** 2003. Rats, communications, and plague: toward an ecological history. *J Interdiscip Hist* **34**:1–25.

41. **Papagrigorakis MJ, Yapijakis C, Synodinos PN.** 2008. Typhoid fever epidemic in ancient Athens, p 161–173. *In* Raoult D, Drancourt M (ed), *Paleomicrobiology: Past Human Infections*. Springer, Berlin, Germany.

42. **Yusim K, Peeters M, Pybus OG, Bhattacharya T, Delaporte E, Mulanga C, Muldoon M, Theiler J, Korber B.** 2001. Using human immunodeficiency virus type 1 sequences to infer historical features of the acquired immune deficiency syndrome epidemic and human immunodeficiency virus evolution. *Philos Trans R Soc Lond B Biol Sci* **356**:855–866.

43. **Heeney JL, Dalgleish AG, Weiss RA.** 2006. Origins of HIV and the evolution of resistance to AIDS. *Science* **313:**462–466.

44. **Bar-Yosef O, Belfer-Cohen A.** 2001. From Africa to Eurasia—early dispersals. *Quat Int* **75:**19–28.

45. **de Thé G.** 2007. Microbial genomes to write our history. *J Infect Dis* **196:**499–501.

46. **Slattery JP, Franchini G, Gessain A.** 1999. Genomic evolution, patterns of global dissemination, and interspecies transmission of human and simian T-cell leukemia/lymphotropic viruses. *Genome Res* **9:** 525–540.

47. **Verdonck K, Gonzalez E, Van Dooren S, Vandamme AM, Vanham G, Gotuzzo E.** 2007. Human T-lymphotropic virus 1: recent knowledge about an ancient infection. *Lancet Infect Dis* **7:**266–281.

48. **Wheelis M.** 2002. Biological warfare at the 1346 siege of Caffa. *Emerg Infect Dis* **8:**971–975.

49. **Acemoglu D, Robinson J, Johnson S.** 2003. Disease and development in historical perspective. *J Eur Econ Assoc* **1:**397–405.

50. **Diamond J.** 1999. *Guns, Germs, and Steel: the Fates of Human Societies.* W. W. Norton & Company, New York, NY.

51. **Curtin PD.** 1968. Epidemiology and the slave trade. *Polit Sci Q* **83:**190–216.

52. **Timen A, Koopmans MP, Vossen AC, van Doornum GJ, Gunther S, van den Berkmortel F, Verduin KM, Dittrich S, Emmerich P, Osterhaus AD, van Dissel JT, Coutinho RA.** 2009. Response to imported case of Marburg hemorrhagic fever, The Netherlands. *Emerg Infect Dis* **15:**1171–1175.

53. **van Thiel PP, van den Hoek JA, Eftimov F, Tepaske R, Zaaijer HJ, Spanjaard L, de Boer HE, Van Doornum GJ, Schutten M, Osterhaus AD, Kager PA.** 2007. Fatal case of human rabies (Duvenhage virus) from a bat in Kenya: The Netherlands, December 2007. *Euro Surveill* **13:**pii=8007.

54. **Khan K, Arino J, Hu W, Raposo P, Sears J, Calderon F, Heidebrecht C, Macdonald M, Liauw J, Chan A, Gardam M.** 2009. Spread of a novel influenza A (H1N1) virus via global airline transportation. *N Engl J Med* **361:**212–214.

55. **Russell CA, Jones TC, Barr IG, Cox NJ, Garten RJ, Gregory V, Gust ID, Hampson AW, Hay AJ, Hurt AC, de Jong JC, Kelso A, Klimov AI, Kageyama T, Komadina N, Lapedes AS, Lin YP, Mosterin A, Obuchi M, Odagiri T, Osterhaus AD, Rimmelzwaan GF, Shaw MW, Skepner E, Stohr K, Tashiro M, Fouchier RA, Smith DJ.** 2008. The global circulation of seasonal influenza A (H3N2) viruses. *Science* **320:**340–346.

56. **Grenfell BT, Bjornstad ON, Kappey J.** 2001. Travelling waves and spatial hierarchies in measles epidemics. *Nature* **414:**716–723.

57. **Viboud C, Bjornstad ON, Smith DL, Simonsen L, Miller MA, Grenfell BT.** 2006. Synchrony, waves, and spatial hierarchies in the spread of influenza. *Science* **312:**447–451.

58. **Rosenthal BM.** 2009. How has agriculture influenced the geography and genetics of animal parasites? *Trends Parasitol* **25:**67–70.

59. **Mills JN, Childs JE.** 1998. Ecologic studies of rodent reservoirs: their relevance for human health. *Emerg Infect Dis* **4:**529–537.

60. **Lin XD, Guo WP, Wang W, Zou Y, Hao ZY, Zhou DJ, Dong X, Qu YG, Li MH, Tian HF, Wen JF, Plyusnin A, Xu J, Zhang YZ.** 2012. Migration of Norway rats resulted in the worldwide distribution of Seoul hantavirus today. *J Virol* **86:**972–981.

61. **Normile D.** 2008. Rinderpest. Driven to extinction. *Science* **319:**1606–1609.

62. **Blancou J.** 2002. History of the control of foot and mouth disease. *Comp Immunol Microbiol Infect Dis* **25:** 283–296.

63. **Knudsen AB.** 1995. Global distribution and continuing spread of *Aedes albopictus*. *Parassitologia* **37:** 91–97.

64. **Rappole JH, Derrickson SR, Hubalek Z.** 2000. Migratory birds and spread of West Nile virus in the Western Hemisphere. *Emerg Infect Dis* **6:**319–328.

65. **Di Giulio DB, Eckburg PB.** 2004. Human monkeypox: an emerging zoonosis. *Lancet Infect Dis* **4:** 15–25.

66. **Gibbens JC, Sharpe CE, Wilesmith JW, Mansley LM, Michalopoulou E, Ryan JB, Hudson M.** 2001. Descriptive epidemiology of the 2001 foot-and-mouth disease epidemic in Great Britain: the first five months. *Vet Rec* **149:**729–743.

67. **Thompson D, Muriel P, Russell D, Osborne P, Bromley A, Rowland M, Creigh-Tyte S, Brown C.** 2002. Economic costs of the foot and mouth disease outbreak in the United Kingdom in 2001. *Rev Sci Tech* **21:**675–687.

68. **Daszak P, Cunningham AA, Hyatt AD.** 2000. Emerging infectious diseases of wildlife—threats to biodiversity and human health. *Science* **287:**443–449.

69. **Weldon C, du Preez LH, Hyatt AD, Muller R, Spears R.** 2004. Origin of the amphibian chytrid fungus. *Emerg Infect Dis* **10:**2100–2105.

70. **Frick WF, Pollock JF, Hicks AC, Langwig KE, Reynolds DS, Turner GG, Butchkoski CM, Kunz TH.** 2010. An emerging disease causes regional population collapse of a common North American bat species. *Science* **329:**679–682.

71. **Bengis RG, Kock RA, Fischer J.** 2002. Infectious animal diseases: the wildlife/livestock interface. *Rev Sci Tech* **21:**53–65.

72. **Gilbert M, Xiao X, Chaitaweesub P, Kalpravidh W, Premashthira S, Boles S, Slingenbergh J.** 2007. Avian influenza, domestic ducks and rice agriculture in Thailand. *Agric Ecosyst Environ* **119:**409–415.

73. **Scholtissek C, Naylor E.** 1988. Fish farming and influenza pandemics. *Nature* **331:**215.

74. **Tully DC, Fares MA.** 2008. The tale of a modern animal plague: tracing the evolutionary history and determining the time-scale for foot and mouth disease virus. *Virology* **382:**250–256.

75. **Reperant LA, Osterhaus AD.** 2012. Avian and animal influenza, p 31–39. *In* Van-Tam J, Sellwood C (ed), *Pandemic Influenza*, 2nd ed. CABI, Wallingford, United Kingdom.

76. **Brown P, Will RG, Bradley R, Asher DM, Detwiler L.** 2001. Bovine spongiform encephalopathy and variant Creutzfeldt-Jakob disease: background, evolution, and current concerns. *Emerg Infect Dis* **7:**6–16.

77. **Gold HS, Moellering RC, Jr.** 1996. Antimicrobial-drug resistance. *N Engl J Med* **335:**1445–1453.

78. **Patz JA, Epstein PR, Burke TA, Balbus JM.** 1996. Global climate change and emerging infectious diseases. *JAMA* **275:**217–223.

79. **Rogers DJ, Randolph SE.** 2006. Climate change and vector-borne diseases. *Adv Parasitol* **62:**345–381.

80. **Davies J.** 2013. Antibiotic resistance in and from nature. *Microbiol Spectrum* **1**(1):OH-0005-2012. doi: 10.1128/microbiolspec.OH-0005-2012.

One Health: People, Animals, and the Environment
Edited by Ronald M. Atlas and Stanley Maloy
© 2014 American Society for Microbiology, Washington, DC
doi:10.1128/microbiolspec.OH-0009-2012

Chapter 4

Ecological Approaches to Studying Zoonoses

Elizabeth H. Loh,[1] Kris A. Murray,[1] Carlos Zambrana-Torrelio,[1] Parviez R. Hosseini,[1] Melinda K. Rostal,[1] William B. Karesh,[1] and Peter Daszak[1]

INTRODUCTION

Concern over emerging infectious diseases and a better understanding of their causes have resulted in increasing recognition of the linkages among human, animal, and ecosystem health. Historically, the connection between animal and human health was understood and accepted, with the term "One Medicine" appearing in English texts as long ago as the 19th century (1, 2). However, during the early 20th century, human and veterinary medicine diverged into discrete fields with reduced overlap. At this time, infectious diseases afflicting humans and animals were rarely considered in the context of broader environmental issues (3).

The "One Medicine" concept was later revived in the 1960s by Calvin Schwabe, a veterinary epidemiologist and parasitologist (1, 2). However, this concept did not reflect all of the interactions between human and animal health that extend beyond individual clinical issues. Specifically, it did not include ecological concepts, public health, and the broader societal and environmental scopes that are now considered key to understanding infectious disease emergence (4).

It is now well recognized that human activities can promote the emergence of infectious diseases through the large-scale modification of natural environments, including habitat fragmentation, deforestation, urbanization, and the subsequent alteration of food webs. These perturbations can alter the ecological and evolutionary relationships among humans, wildlife, and the pathogens that move between them, resulting in disease emergence (4, 5). For example, the emergence of Nipah virus in Malaysia followed agricultural intensification that caused the direct overlap of mango orchards and commercial pig production. This resulted in cross-species transmission from flying foxes to intensively managed pigs, and subsequently to humans (6).

Of additional concern is the correlation among marked increase in human influence in previously undisturbed regions, increased global connectivity, and increased occurrence of emerging infectious diseases (4, 7–10). A recent study showed that approximately 60% of emerging diseases in humans originate in animals, with more than 70% of these

[1]EcoHealth Alliance, New York, NY 10001.

coming specifically from wildlife. In these data, a distinct increase in emergence events through time was also suggested, even after correcting for reporting bias (8).

Similarly, human activities can result in exposure of both human and wildlife populations to novel human pathogens, so spillover occurs routinely in both directions (11, 12). A good example of this is infection by several human pathogens in gorillas exposed by the ecotourism industry in central Africa (13). In recognition of such relationships, the original concept of One Medicine has evolved into a broader vision of One Health—a concept that encompasses the health of humans, animals, and their environment (Fig. 1).

Considering the potential complexity of these disease emergence events, interdisciplinary collaborations are critical to address health problems at the human-animal-environment interface (14). In particular, a suite of transboundary diseases that involve wildlife, domestic animals, and humans (e.g., henipaviruses, filoviruses, severe acute respiratory syndrome, and triple-reassortant H1N1) have led to increasing collaboration among disciplines. In each case, expertise from across the disciplines of ecology, human and veterinary medicine, public health, and the social sciences was required to unravel the complex epidemiology of these diseases and find effective management and surveillance solutions.

Over the last decade, the One Health approach has continued to gain momentum and has now been endorsed or adopted by various influential institutions, including the World Bank, the Food and Agriculture Organization, the Office International des Épizooties (World Organisation for Animal Health), the U.S. Departments of State and Agriculture, and the U.S. Centers for Disease Control and Prevention. In many regions of the world, the One Health approach is being used to improve capability and capacity to understand and respond to infectious disease events (15–19). This involves identifying the underlying

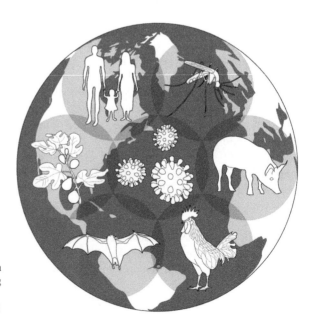

Figure 1. The One Health approach recognizes the inherent relationships among human, environmental, and animal health.
doi:10.1128/microbiolspec.OH-0009-2012.f1

drivers of disease emergence, targeting high-risk pathways and regions, and strengthening cross-sectoral collaboration in disease prevention, investigation, and response through the sharing of resources and expertise across traditionally isolated sectors (3, 20, 21).

In recent years, the rise in zoonotic emerging infectious diseases (8) has not only increased our awareness of the need for cross-sectoral collaborations but has also highlighted the disconnect between current ecological theory and biological reality (22). Theoretical ecologists have worked in this field for many years and found that ecological approaches can explain much about the dynamics of hosts and pathogens within human populations (23, 24). These approaches are now being applied practically within public health. Ecologists have also helped emphasize the role of environmental change in shaping host-pathogen interactions and infection outcomes. As the One Health movement continues to gain steam, further integration of ecological approaches into the One Health framework will be required.

In this article, we discuss the importance of ecological methods and theory to the study of zoonotic diseases by (i) discussing key ecological concepts and approaches, (ii) reviewing methods of studying wildlife diseases and their potential applications for zoonoses, and (iii) identifying future directions in the One Health movement.

ECOLOGICAL APPROACHES TO STUDYING ZOONOSES

Much of our understanding of wildlife diseases has traditionally come from detailed studies of infection at the individual level (25). Over the last 2 decades, however, researchers have increasingly applied concepts from population ecology and parasitology in natural host populations to the study of wildlife health and diseases. As a result, parasites and pathogens have been shown to regulate populations and influence population and community dynamics, host genetic diversity, and ecological and evolutionary processes (26–29). Host-pathogen interactions also have broad implications for the management of wild and captive species (30, 31). Due to their ability to cause sudden epidemics capable of rapid population declines, infectious diseases have also received considerable attention from conservation biologists (4, 32, 33).

One of the key contributions of this increased research interest in wildlife diseases is an appreciation for the role of wildlife in many livestock and human disease systems (14, 34–36). At the population level, the rate at which parasites flow from one host to another is influenced primarily by host behavior, distribution, and abundance, typically the research fodder of ecologists and wildlife biologists. Thus, a major challenge to understanding pathogen spillover from wildlife reservoirs to humans and livestock is how to link an ecological understanding of wildlife diseases with our understanding of human biology and ecology. This will involve linking data on individuals, communities, and populations of each type of host.

Host-Pathogen Ecology

Disease ecology is the study of host-pathogen interactions within the context of their environment and evolution (24). Disease caused by infectious agents can be regarded as an ecological process that involves interactions between hosts and pathogens. The spectrum of effects contributing to pathogen-induced loss of host fitness is termed virulence, and ranges from near benign to obligate mortality. Virulence depends on the properties of the pathogen as well as its host (38), both of which are often dynamic in time, are shaped by selective processes, and can be independently influenced by extrinsic factors. In this scheme, there is no functional difference between parasites and pathogens, with both causing some loss of fitness to the host, even where parasites are considered benign.

To reflect differences in their population biology, pathogens are often categorized into two broad groups of disease-inducing organisms: microparasites and macroparasites (39). Microparasites (usually viruses, bacteria, and protozoans) are characterized by their small size (often unicellular), short generation time, high reproductive rate in a host, and tendency to cause acquired immunity in surviving hosts (39, 40). Macroparasites (normally parasitic helminths and arthropods) are typically larger and have longer generation times in individual hosts or involve intermediate hosts (39, 40). Microparasites tend to cause epidemics (disease transmission events with rapidly increasing case numbers) in humans (epizootics in animals) and have the potential to cause dramatic changes in host abundance, whereas macroparasites tend to be enzootic (causing relatively stable infections through time) and generally result in more subtle population regulation. Some pathogens, such as *Batrachochytrium dendrobatidis*, the causal fungal agent of amphibian chytridiomycosis, have characteristics of both micro- and macroparasites (41), illustrating the blurry distinctions and frequent exceptions to the rules in this field.

Transmission

Transmission of disease between infected and susceptible individuals is a central process driving the dynamics of infectious diseases. Transmission is influenced by two key processes: (i) contact between hosts and infective pathogen stages (whether free living, in an infected host, or vector borne) and (ii) infection occurring upon contact. These factors depend largely on the mode of transmission (42, 43), and require information on the probability that both contact and transmission are made (25).

Theory suggests that the scaling of pathogen transmission with population size can determine whether or not a pathogen could drive host extinction. Transmission that increases with host density (linearly or nonlinearly) is termed density-dependent transmission. For example, research has shown a higher infection rate of measles in large cities compared with small villages due to significantly higher contact rates between infected and susceptible individuals in large urban centers (44). In the context of ecology, this implies that infection rate scales with host population density.

One important feature of density-dependent pathogens is that, at times, there may be a threshold density below which the pathogen cannot be sustained and the host may persist (42, 45–48). Such pathogens are more likely to regulate a population if they cause substantial mortality. One of the simplest effects of density in a host-pathogen system dominated by a single host is well typified by the effects of *Mycoplasma gallisepticum* on the local abundance of the house finch (*Carpodacus mexicanus*) in its recently invaded range. High-density areas experienced local declines in density, but areas that were newly invaded by the host experienced density increases. All areas ended up with similar densities after the *M. gallisepticum* epidemic settled into an endemic phase (49). For many pathogens that have density-dependent transmission, like influenza, high host abundance will increase transmission in a relatively straightforward fashion. However, even in multihost vector-borne disease systems (e.g., Lyme disease), host abundance and community composition have important effects on disease transmission.

In contrast, frequency-dependent pathogens infect the same number of individuals regardless of host density. For example, the transmission of West Nile virus is dependent on mosquitoes actively seeking out hosts to bite. This behavior allows the maintenance of high transmission at low population densities and may limit transmission at high population densities (21, 24, 48). Considering this, theoretically there is no threshold of susceptible host density. This is because the "force of infection"—the rate at which susceptible hosts become infected—increases with the fraction of the host population that is infectious but does not increase with overall host density. An estimation of the force of infection can be achieved by counting the number of new primary infections arising per unit time (50). The force of infection can be estimated in laboratory or field studies by examining the rate at which newborn, uninfected sentinel, or treated individuals acquire infections (42, 51). For frequency-dependent pathogens, the transmission mode may be indirect (e.g., vector borne) or nonrandom (e.g., influenced by social structure or host behavior), and thus transmission rate will be relatively invariant across a wide range of host density (42).

Contact between hosts and infective pathogen stages can be extremely difficult to measure in wildlife populations. Telemetry data are often used for animals of sufficient size to carry a transmitter to estimate contact rates, though frequently these are limited by time or error associated with radio, satellite, or geographic positioning systems. Compounding this, the majority of pathogens can infect more than one species of host (52), making it difficult to understand interspecies contact and its influence on transmission. Nevertheless, recent studies have attempted to model such multihost pathogens. For example, Craft et al. (2008) developed a modified SIR (susceptible, infectious, recovered) model with matrices to describe the dynamics of canine distemper virus within and between lion (*Panthera leo*) prides, jackal (*Canis* spp.) family groups, and spotted hyena (*Crocuta crocuta*) clans in the Serengeti. They found that differences in social structures between species can affect the size, speed, and spatial pattern of a multihost epidemic. Their results demonstrate that pathogens can expand through interspecies transmission in a geographic area in which they would normally be limited by intraspecific contact rates (53).

The capacity of a pathogen to transmit in a population is commonly quantified by the basic reproduction number, R0, which can be described mathematically. The basic reproduction number is broadly defined as the number of secondary hosts an infected host will cause, under the assumption that all hosts are equally susceptible and naïve to infection. The concept and utility of R0 is straightforward: if R0 > 1 (a parasite infecting on average more than one additional host), a pathogen can expand and persist in a population, whereas if R0 < 1 (a parasite infecting on average less than one additional host), the number of cases will diminish and a pathogen will eventually become extinct (25, 54–56). Calculating R0 is easier for human epidemics than wildlife due to generally high quality of relevant case data. However, because contact tracing is often difficult or impossible for wildlife, resulting in limited-quality, patchy data on epidemics, R0 is typically much more difficult to estimate and has limited use for managing wildlife diseases (57). In these cases, other techniques may be necessary. Examples of such techniques include capture-mark-recapture (CMR) and occupancy modeling, which are discussed further in this review.

Spatial and Temporal Structure

Recent studies have highlighted how disease transmission can also be influenced by spatial and temporal structure, dispersal patterns, and landscape heterogeneity (25, 58). For example, Koelle et al. (2009) demonstrated how spatially restricted movements result in peaks of influenza infection in humans followed by troughs (59), while similar patterns have been reported with rabies in raccoons (60). Understanding geographic and temporal variation in disease incidence has been central to improving human health globally for a number of major human diseases as well. A good example is cholera, the first disease for which organized public health surveillance and reporting was implemented. The bacterial pathogen causing cholera, *Vibrio cholerae*, is now known to be strongly associated with chitinaceous zooplankton (e.g., copepods) and shellfish, and consequently ocean currents and the events that influence them (61). This has been a key factor in unlocking the mechanisms and patterns underlying past and present cholera epidemics (62).

Disease transmission is also dependent on whether the pathogen and/or the host exhibit aggregated or random spatial distributions, as well as age-related and temporal distributions (25). Altizer et al. (2011) described the importance of temporal distribution in their study of migratory escape in monarch butterflies (*Danaus plexippus*) in eastern North America. They reported that the prevalence of the protozoan parasite *Ophryocystis elektroscirrha* increased throughout the breeding season. Prevalence was highest among adults with more intense habitat use and longer residency. They also found that butterflies that migrate the greatest distances (up to 2,500 km) have lower prevalence and a less virulent strain of the parasite than monarchs that overwinter in the same location in which they breed (58).

Land Use Change and Zoonoses

Disturbance to host-pathogen systems can have significant ramifications for disease dynamics and the impact on host populations (63). Disturbances can include the introduction of pathogens into naïve systems (e.g., along roads in newly penetrated areas), disturbance of the host's habitat (e.g., deforestation and land conversion), or bringing together species that normally have little contact (e.g., in wildlife markets), among others.

A significant number of zoonoses can be linked to large-scale land use change (5, 64, 65). Such perturbations to the environment through human-induced changes can increase human contact with wildlife species, directly affect biodiversity, and alter the ecology of hosts harboring novel diseases. This in turn may influence the relationships among human, animal, and environmental components of a disease system. Land use change may also modify vegetation structure and patterns, vector and host species behavior, distribution and abundance, and microclimates. Many of these effects may be subtle or inconspicuous and therefore difficult to elucidate. However, the effects of some of these processes have been well illustrated for several vector-borne zoonoses, including malaria and Lyme disease (5, 66). In the northeastern United States, a historical cycle of deforestation, reforestation, and habitat fragmentation has altered wildlife predator-prey populations and led to the emergence of Lyme disease (5, 66, 67). It is now suggested that loss of small-mammal predators may have cascading impacts that facilitate the emergence of zoonotic diseases, many of which rely on hosts that occupy low trophic levels (68). In tropical regions, land use changes have been linked to Chagas disease (69), yellow fever, and leishmaniasis (70). Land use changes are particularly intense in many tropical regions where primary forest is rapidly being opened up to mining, logging, plantation development, and oil and gas exploration and extraction (71, 72).

METHODS OF STUDYING WILDLIFE DISEASES: POTENTIAL APPLICATIONS FOR ZOONOSES

Diseases in wildlife populations are typically less well understood than human or livestock diseases despite an abundance of theoretical predictions and increasing appreciation for the role of wildlife in livestock and human disease systems (4, 34, 35). The difficulty of detecting epidemics and obtaining quality data from the field has encumbered the development of wildlife-specific disease research (40, 48, 73). Even during mass mortality events, detection of sick and dying wild animals is hampered by difficulties in observation and removal by scavengers, and detecting the more subtle impact of stable endemic infections is harder still (40).

Yet it is perhaps because of these challenges that useful and transferable ecological concepts have been developed that may be extended to the study of zoonotic diseases. These concepts could provide key insights into understanding pathogen emergence and dynamics in human populations, and have already yielded a range of analytical and statistical techniques and tools. These are perhaps united by the challenge of collecting well-balanced and informative data in systems where experimentation is often extremely challenging. Many of the analytical techniques that ecologists employ have been developed to minimize bias and false inference when interpreting sparse and noisy datasets. Typical ecological problems with these characteristics include understanding the behavior and movement of wildlife, estimating abundance and geographic distributions, and probing population dynamics.

Capture-Mark-Recapture (CMR)

Reliable estimates of population prevalence and infection status are essential for disease management but can be significantly biased by imperfect detection (74). In wildlife disease studies, an important, but often overlooked, problem is the extent to which detectability is dependent on disease state (75). Disease can change behavior, activity, and other physiological processes, which can lead to significant differences in the probability of sampling infected and uninfected individuals (76). In cases where infection alters detection probability, our ability to estimate a number of epidemiological parameters becomes confounded (75).

CMR is a method that has been gaining use for modeling complex disease systems and accounting for imperfect detection (75, 77, 78). CMR methods can be used to estimate numerous epidemiological parameters of potential interest, including survival and disease-induced mortality, disease-mediated detection probabilities, and transitions between disease and other states that might be useful for inferring information about transmission and recovery rates.

Where an infection reduces detection rate (e.g., by reducing activity), disease prevalence could be severely underestimated in a population and this could result in false inferences (21). For example, Faustino et al. (79) used a multistate mark-recapture model to deal with inaccuracy in disease state estimation and to estimate force of infection, recovery rates, and mortality in the wild. They found that the probability of observing a bird is dependent on its disease state (79). CMR models can also be applied to assess the broader effects of disease on the demography of a host population.

Occupancy Modeling

Like CMR, occupancy modeling has been used to deal with observation error to facilitate more reliable inferences in population and community ecology. These models have most commonly been applied to estimate what proportion of area, patches, or sample units is occupied (i.e., species present), also accounting for detectability. Occupancy is commonly used as a proxy for abundance; however, in the context of disease models, the estimated "proportion occupied" corresponds with disease prevalence in a host population. Lachish et al. (2012) used site-occupancy modeling to estimate the prevalence of malaria (*Plasmodium* spp.) in a population of wild blue tits (*Cyanistes caeruleus*) (74). They demonstrated that *Plasmodium* detection rates were strongly influenced by host pathogen load. They highlighted the utility of occupancy modeling for obtaining estimates of population prevalence under imperfect detection and illustrated that in this specific system, accounting for variation in pathogen load resulted in increased diagnostic test sensitivity (74). A general application of this approach to the study of zoonoses might involve the evaluation of multiple disease states: symptomatic versus asymptomatic. Here, the possible hierarchy of states includes an individual that is asymptomatic because it is infected (occupied), it is not infected (not occupied), or it is infected but not expressing symptoms (occupied, not detected) and therefore not detected. In contrast, a symptomatic individual must be infected (occupied).

Biogeography

Biogeography is the science of documenting and interpreting the spatial and temporal distribution of biological diversity (80, 81). The spatial distribution of species can be largely explained by evolutionary processes by which new species arise (speciation) or become extinct, or by species dynamics such as colonization (e.g., immigration). Although viruses and bacteria have important roles in ecological communities and in human health, microbial biogeography is in its infancy as a discipline (80, 82). In this section, we discuss the potential application of biogeographic theory to host-parasite interactions to help understand the factors that contribute to observed patterns, processes, and spatial and temporal dynamics of zoonotic diseases.

MacArthur and Wilson (83) proposed the idea that the number of species inhabiting a given island represents a dynamic equilibrium between immigration and extinction rates (Fig. 2). Immigration rate (defined as the rate of arrival of propagules of species not present on the island) declines from some maximum value when the island is empty, to zero when the island contains all the species in a source area or pool (e.g., other nearby islands or a continental mainland). In contrast, extinction rate (the rate of loss of insular species) increases from zero when the island is empty, to some maximum value when all

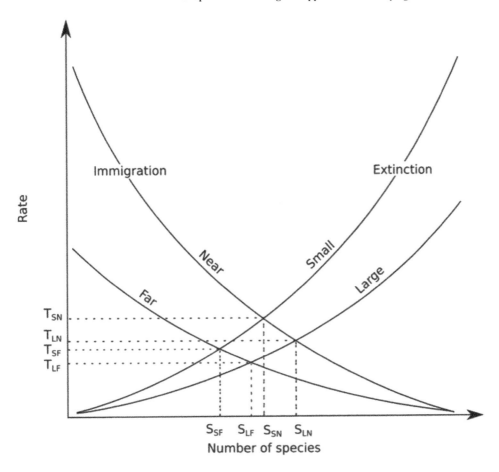

Figure 2. Dynamic equilibrium model of island biogeography. The effects of island size (small [S] and large [L]) and island isolation (near [N] and far [F]) on the number of species (S) and the rate of species turnover (T) are represented. From reference 83. doi:10.1128/microbiolspec.OH-0009-2012.f2

the species from the source area inhabit the island and are prone to extinction (Fig. 2). A stable equilibrium is reached at some species number when both the immigration and extinction rates are equal (S). Theoretically, if the system is somehow perturbed and there is a decline or increase in the species number, this value should always return to the equilibrium point.

Kuris et al. (84) proposed the idea that hosts can be viewed as islands for pathogens, in which the number of pathogen species within a given host population or in a given host species can be determined by the rate at which new pathogen species colonize the host (immigration) or by intrahost speciation and the rate at which those pathogens go extinct (85, 86). Similar to the effect of islands that are close to the source area, pathogen immigration rates may be affected by the spatial interaction of hosts. For example, host species with large distribution ranges can make contact with several other host species, increasing the probability of colonization (i.e., transmission). Likewise, extinction rates may be influenced by the host species' body size. A proposed explanation is that host species with larger body size can have more available niches and can provide more resources compared with host species with smaller body size (86). Other important factors that could influence both pathogen immigration and extinction rates are host habitat specificity, diet and social behavior, population density, and life span.

Reperant (85) employs an island biogeography approach to predict the potential drivers of emerging zoonotic and vector-borne diseases. In this model, habitat degradation and loss, fragmentation, and all human activities may modify the rates of pathogen immigration and extinction, thereby influencing host dynamics. Reperant argues that such a modified host-pathogen dynamic may explain the increase in the number of novel pathogens in human or animal populations (85). For example, the behavior of infected humans contributed to the emergence and later expansion of HIV (i.e., increasing immigration rates due to changes in human distribution) (87). Similarly, Australia's highest biosecurity risk area is in the northern region of the continent, primarily due to its proximity to, and connectivity with, neighboring countries that can act as source populations for new zoonotic and vector-borne diseases (88). Evidence for such a biogeographic process driving the assemblage of new diseases comes from an analysis showing that the vector-borne human disease assemblage of Australia is most similar to that of Papua New Guinea (when compared with all countries in the Southeast Asian region). This suggests that an informative predictor of what diseases a country will harbor is the disease assemblage of its neighbors, implicating biogeographic theory as a potential means of understanding disease distribution and spread and thereby of practical interest for coordinating management.

CONCLUDING REMARKS

Methods initially developed in the field of ecology are clearly applicable to the study of zoonoses. The majority of new emerging infectious diseases are zoonotic, and approximately 75% of these come specifically from wildlife (8); therefore, significant attention has been focused on the human-animal interface in One Health programs. The application of ecological approaches, such as CMR and occupancy modeling as well as island biogeographic theory, to disease surveillance and monitoring has great potential to inform a wide range of questions about disease effects, prevalence, and dynamics, while accounting for uncertainty induced by observation error.

We emphasize the importance of integrating a stronger ecological component into the One Health framework by discussing several examples of relevant concepts from ecology that could be applied to better understand disease dynamics and risk. Another concept that has emerged from the field of ecology is the need to shift away from random sampling over broad areas toward more systematic study designs. To achieve study objectives, a clear framework for sampling and inference will most likely result in the development of more-efficient sampling designs. Further, well-designed, systematic approaches are often more cost-efficient and provide a clearer understanding than a combination of several uncoordinated, opportunistic sampling protocols (78). Although we do not assert that the adoption of these approaches will result in a complete understanding of pathogen emergence and dynamics in human and animal populations, the continued integration of ecological approaches into One Health strategies has the potential to bring a suite of new tools into public health that have proven capable of explaining complex systems in the ecological field. This will be particularly critical over the next few decades, as we deal with increasing change in the environment, our social systems, and the dynamics of new and emerging diseases.

Acknowledgments. This work was supported by the National Science Foundation (NSF) Ecology and Evolution of Infectious Diseases program, the US Agency for International Development Emerging Pandemic Threats Program PREDICT Project, and the International Development Research Centre.

None of the authors of this manuscript has any commercial affiliations, consultancies, stock or equity interests, or patent-licensing agreements that could be considered to pose a conflict of interest regarding this manuscript.

Citation. Loh EH, Murray KA, Zambrana-Torrelio C, Hosseini PR, Rostal MK, Karesh WB, Daszak P. 2013. Ecological approaches to studying zoonoses. Microbiol Spectrum 2(1):OH-0009-2012. doi:10.1128/microbiolspec.OH-0009-2012.

REFERENCES

1. **Zinsstag J, Schelling E, Waltner-Toews D, Tanner M.** 2011. From "one medicine" to "one health" and systemic approaches to health and well-being. *Prev Vet Med* **101:**148–156.
2. **Conrad PA, Mazet JA, Clifford D, Scott C, Wilkes M.** 2009. Evolution of a transdisciplinary "One Medicine-One Health" approach to global health education at the University of California, Davis. *Prev Vet Med* **92:**268–274.
3. **Kahn LH, Kaplan B, Monath TP, Steele JH.** 2008. Teaching "One Medicine, One Health." *Am J Med* **121:**169–170.
4. **Daszak P, Cunningham A, Hyatt A.** 2000. Emerging infectious diseases of wildlife—threats to biodiversity and human health. *Science* **287:**443–449.
5. **Patz JA, Daszak P, Tabor GM, Aguirre AA, Pearl M, Epstein J, Wolfe ND, Kilpatrick AM, Foufopoulos J, Molyneux D, Bradley DJ, Members of the Working Group on Land Use Change and Disease Emergence.** 2004. Unhealthy landscapes: policy recommendations on land use change and infectious disease emergence. *Environ Health Perspect* **112:**1092–1098.
6. **Pulliam JR, Epstein JH, Dushoff J, Rahman SA, Bunning M, Jamaluddin AA, Hyatt AD, Field HE, Dobson AP, Daszak P, Henipavirus Ecology Research Group (HERG).** 2012. Agricultural intensification, priming for persistence and the emergence of Nipah virus: a lethal bat-borne zoonosis. *J R Soc Interface* **9:**89–101.
7. **Dobson A, Foufopoulos J.** 2001. Emerging infectious pathogens of wildlife. *Philos Trans R Soc Lond B Biol Sci* **356:**1001–1012.
8. **Jones KE, Patel NG, Levy MA, Storeygard A, Balk D, Gittleman JL, Daszak P.** 2008. Global trends in emerging infectious diseases. *Nature* **451:**990–993.
9. **Harvell CD, Kim K, Burkholder JM, Colwell RR, Epstein PR, Grimes DJ, Hofmann EE, Lipp EK, Osterhaus ADME, Overstreet RM, Porter JW, Smith GW, Vasta GR.** 1999. Emerging marine diseases—climate links and anthropogenic factors. *Science* **285:**1505–1510.
10. **Macdonald DW, Laurenson MK.** 2006. Infectious disease: inextricable linkages between human and ecosystem health. *Biol Conserv* **131:**143–150.
11. **Woolhouse ME, Gowtage-Sequeria S.** 2005. Host range and emerging and reemerging pathogens. *Emerg Infect Dis* **11:**1842–1847.
12. **Nunn CL, Altizer S.** 2006. *Infectious Diseases in Primates: Behavior, Ecology and Evolution.* Oxford University Press, Oxford, United Kingdom.
13. **Nizeyi JB, Innocent RB, Erume J, Kalema G, Cranfield MR, Graczyk TK.** 2001. Campylobacteriosis, salmonellosis, and shigellosis in free-ranging human-habituated mountain gorillas of Uganda. *J Wildl Dis* **37:**239–244.
14. **Daszak P, Zambrana-Torrelio C, Bogich TL, Fernandez M, Epstein JH, Murray KA, Hamilton H.** 2013. Interdisciplinary approaches to understanding disease emergence: the past, present, and future drivers of Nipah virus emergence. *Proc Natl Acad Sci USA* **110**(Suppl 1):3681–3688.

15. **Dedmon R, Briggs D, Lembo T, Cleaveland S.** 2010. One health: collaboration, recent research and developments in the global effort to eliminate rabies. *Int J Infect Dis* **14:**e159. doi:10.1016/j.ijid.2010.02.1833.

16. **Greene M.** 2010. The "One Health" initiative: using open source data for disease surveillance. *Int J Infect Dis* **14:**e162. doi:10.1016/j.ijid.2010.02.1841.

17. **Kahn RE, Clouser DF, Richt JA.** 2009. Emerging infections: a tribute to the One Medicine, One Health concept. *Zoonoses Publ Health* **56:**407–428.

18. **Mazet JA, Clifford DL, Coppolillo PB, Deolalikar AB, Erickson JD, Kazwala RR.** 2009. A "One Health" approach to address emerging zoonoses: the HALI project in Tanzania. *PLOS Med* **6:**e1000190. doi:10.1371/journal.pmed.1000190.

19. **Mullins G, Jagne J, Stone L, Konings E, Howard-Grabman L, Hartman F, Fulton M.** 2010. "One World One Health" in practice: integrating public health and veterinary curricula on emerging infectious diseases in Africa. *Int J Infect Dis* **14:**e377–e378. doi:10.1016/j.ijid.2010.02.460.

20. **Zinsstag J, Mackenzie JS, Jeggo M, Heymann DL, Patz JA, Daszak P.** 2012. Mainstreaming One Health. *EcoHealth* **9:**107–110.

21. **Murray KA, Skerratt LF, Speare R, McCallum H.** 2009. Impact and dynamics of disease in species threatened by the amphibian chytrid fungus, *Batrachochytrium dendrobatidis*. *Conserv Biol* **23:**1242–1252.

22. **Roche B, Dobson AP, Guégan JF, Rohani P.** 2012. Linking community and disease ecology: the impact of biodiversity on pathogen transmission. *Philos Trans R Soc Lond B Biol Sci* **367:**2807–2813.

23. **Grenfell BT, Bjørnstad ON, Kappey J.** 2001. Travelling waves and spatial hierarchies in measles epidemics. *Nature* **414:**716–723.

24. **Anderson RM, May RM.** 1991. *Infectious Diseases of Humans: Dynamics and Control.* Oxford University Press, Oxford, United Kingdom.

25. **Hudson P, Rizzoli A, Grenfell B, Heesterbeek H, Dobson A.** 2002. Ecology of wildlife diseases, p 1–5. *In* Hudson P, Rizzoli A, Grenfell B, Heesterbeek H, Dobson A (ed), *The Ecology of Wildlife Diseases.* Oxford University Press, Oxford, United Kingdom.

26. **Anderson RM, May RM.** 1978. Regulation and stability of host-parasite population interactions. I. Regulatory processes. *J Anim Ecol* **47:**219–247.

27. **May RM, Anderson RM.** 1978. Regulation and stability of host-parasite population interactions. II. Destabilizing processes. *J Anim Ecol* **47:**249–267.

28. **Altizer S, Dobson A, Hosseini P, Hudson P, Pascual M, Rohani P.** 2006. Seasonality and the dynamics of infectious diseases. *Ecol Lett* **9:**467–484.

29. **Crowl TA, Crist TO, Parmenter RR, Belovsky G, Lugo AE.** 2008. The spread of invasive species and infectious disease as drivers of ecosystem change. *Front Ecol Environ* **6:**238–246.

30. **Haydon DT, Laurenson MK, Sillero-Zubiri C.** 2002. Integrating epidemiology into population viability analysis: managing the risk posed by rabies and canine distemper to the Ethiopian wolf. *Conserv Biol* **16:**1372–1385.

31. **Caley P, Hone J.** 2005. Assessing the host disease status of wildlife and the implications for disease control: *Mycobacterium bovis* infection in feral ferrets. *J Appl Ecol* **42:**708–719.

32. **Smith KF, Saxdov F, Lafferty KD.** 2006. Evidence for the role of infectious disease in species extinction and endangerment. *Conserv Biol* **20:**1349–1357.

33. **Altizer S, Harvell D, Friedle E.** 2003. Rapid evolutionary dynamics and disease threats to biodiversity. *Trends Ecol Evol* **18:**589–596.

34. **Mackenzie JS, Chua KB, Daniels PW, Eaton BT, Field HE, Hall RA, Halpin K, Johansen CA, Kirkland PD, Lam SK, McMinn P, Nisbet DJ, Paru R, Pyke AT, Ritchie SA, Siba P, Smith DW, Smith GA, van den Hurk AF, Wang LF, Williams DT.** 2001. Emerging viral diseases of Southeast Asia and the Western Pacific. *Emerg Infect Dis* **7:**497–504.

35. **O'Brien SJ, Troyer JL, Roelke M, Marker L, Pecon-Slattery J.** 2006. Plagues and adaptation: lessons from the Felidae models for SARS and AIDS. *Biol Conserv* **131:**255–267.

36. **Smith KF, Acevedo-Whitehouse K, Pedersen AB.** 2009. The role of infectious diseases in biological conservation. *Anim Conserv* **12:**1–12.

37. **Reference deleted.**

38. **Ebert D, Hamilton WD.** 1996. Sex against virulence: the coevolution of parasitic diseases. *Trends Ecol Evol* **11:**A79–A82.

39. **Anderson RM.** 1979. Parasite pathogenicity and the depression of host population equilibria. *Nature* **279:** 150–152.

40. **McCallum H.** 1994. Quantifying the impact of disease on threatened species. *Pac Conserv Biol* **1:**107–117.

41. **Briggs C, Knapp RA, Vredenburg VT.** 2010. Enzootic and epizootic dynamics of the chytrid fungal pathogen of amphibians. *Proc Natl Acad Sci USA* **107:**9695–9700.

42. **McCallum H, Barlow N, Hone J.** 2001. How should pathogen transmission be modelled? *Trends Ecol Evol* **16:**295–300.

43. **Godfrey SS, Bull CM, Murray K, Gardner MG.** 2006. Transmission mode and distribution of parasites among groups of the social lizard *Egernia stokesii*. *Parasitol Res* **99:**223–230.

44. **Grenfell BT, Bolker BM.** 1998. Cities and villages: infection hierarchies in a measles metapopulation. *Ecol Lett* **1:**63–70.

45. **Begon M, Hazel SM, Telfer S, Bown K, Carslake D, Cavanagh R, Chantrey J, Jones T, Bennett M.** 2003. Rodents, cowpox virus and islands: densities, numbers and thresholds. *J Anim Ecol* **72:**343–355.

46. **Fenton A, Fairbairn JP, Norman R, Hudson PJ.** 2002. Parasite transmission: reconciling theory and reality. *J Anim Ecol* **71:**893–905.

47. **de Castro F, Bolker B.** 2005. Mechanisms of disease-induced extinction. *Ecol Lett* **8:**117–126.

48. **Lloyd-Smith JO, Cross PC, Briggs CJ, Daugherty M, Getz WM, Latto J, Sanchez MS, Smith AB, Swei A.** 2005. Should we expect population thresholds for wildlife disease? *Trends Ecol Evol* **20:**511–519.

49. **Hochachka WM, Dhondt AA.** 2000. Density-dependent decline of host abundance resulting from a new infectious disease. *Proc Natl Acad Sci USA* **97:**5303–5306.

50. **Davis S, Calvet E, Leirs H.** 2005. Fluctuating rodent populations and risk to humans from rodent-borne zoonoses. *Vector Borne Zoonotic Dis* **5:**305–314.

51. **Heisey DM, Joly DO, Messier F.** 2006. The fitting of general force-of-infection models to wildlife disease prevalence data. *Ecology* **88:**2356–2365.

52. **Woolhouse ME, Taylor LH, Haydon DT.** 2001. Population biology of multihost pathogens. *Science* **292:** 1109–1112.

53. **Craft ME, Hawthorne PL, Packer C, Dobson AP.** 2008. Dynamics of a multihost pathogen in a carnivore community. *J Anim Ecol* **77:**1257–1264.

54. **Dietz K.** 1993. The estimation of the basic reproduction number for infectious diseases. *Stat Methods Med Res* **2:**23–41.

55. **Hasibeder G, Dye C, Carpenter J.** 1992. Mathematical-modeling and theory for estimating the basic reproduction number of canine leishmaniasis. *Parasitology* **105:**43–53.

56. **Diekmann O, Heesterbeek H, Metz J.** 2000. *Mathematical Epidemiology of Infectious Diseases: Model Building, Analysis and Interpretation.* John Wiley and Sons, Chichester, United Kingdom.

57. **Hampson K, Dushoff J, Cleaveland S, Haydon DT, Kaare M, Packer C, Dobson A.** 2009. Transmission dynamics and prospects for the elimination of canine rabies. *PLoS Biol* **7:**462–471.

58. **Altizer S, Bartel R, Han BA.** 2011. Animal migration and infectious disease risk. *Science* **331:**296–302.

59. **Koelle K, Kamradt M, Pascual M.** 2009. Understanding the dynamics of rapidly evolving pathogens through modeling the tempo of antigenic change: influenza as a case study. *Epidemics* **1:**129–137.

60. **Real LA, Biek R.** 2007. Spatial dynamics and genetics of infectious diseases on heterogeneous landscapes. *J R Soc Interface* **4:**935–948.

61. **Pascual M, Rodo X, Ellner SP, Colwell R, Bouma MJ.** 2000. Cholera dynamics and El Nino-Southern Oscillation. *Science* **289:**1766–1769.

62. **Colwell RR.** 1996. Global climate and infectious disease: the cholera paradigm. *Science* **274:**2025–2031.

63. **Tompkins DM, Dunn AM, Smith MJ, Telfer S.** 2011. Wildlife diseases: from individuals to ecosystems. *J Anim Ecol* **80:**19–38.

64. **Weiss RA, McMichael AJ.** 2004. Social and environmental risk factors in the emergence of infectious diseases. *Nat Med* **10:**S70–S76.

65. **Smolinski MS, Hamburg MA, Lederberg J (ed).** 2003. *Microbial Threats to Health: Emergence, Detection, and Response.* National Academies Press, Washington, DC.

66. **LoGiudice K, Ostfeld RS, Schmidt KA, Keesing F.** 2003. The ecology of infectious disease: effects of host diversity and community composition on Lyme disease risk. *Proc Natl Acad Sci USA* **100:**567–571.

67. **Barbour AG, Fish D.** 1993. The biological and social phenomenon of Lyme disease. *Science* **260:** 1610–1616.

68. **Levi T, Kilpatrick AM, Mangel M, Wilmers CC.** 2012. Deer, predators, and the emergence of Lyme disease. *Proc Natl Acad Sci USA* **109**:10942–10947.

69. **Walsh JF, Molyneux DH, Birley MH.** 1993. Deforestation: effects on vector-borne disease. *Parasitology* **106**:S55–S75.

70. **Wilcox BA, Ellis B.** 2006. Forests and emerging infectious diseases of humans. *Unasylva* **224**:11–18.

71. **Orta-Martinez M, Finer M.** 2010. Oil frontiers and indigenous resistance in the Peruvian Amazon. *Ecol Econ* **70**:207–218.

72. **Vittor AY, Pan W, Gilman RH, Tielsch J, Glass G, Shields T, Sánchez-Lozano W, Pinedo VV, Salas-Cobos E, Flores S, Patz JA.** 2009. Linking deforestation to malaria in the Amazon: characterization of the breeding habitat of the principal malaria vector, *Anopheles darlingi. Am J Trop Med Hyg* **81**:5–12.

73. **Dhondt AA, Altizer S, Cooch EG, Davis AK, Dobson A, Driscoll MJ, Hartup BK, Hawley DM, Hochachka WM, Hosseini PR, Jennelle CS, Kollias GV, Ley DH, Swarthout EC, Sydenstricker KV.** 2005. Dynamics of a novel pathogen in an avian host: mycoplasmal conjunctivitis in house finches. *Acta Tropica* **94**:77–93.

74. **Lachish S, Gopalaswamy AM, Knowles SC, Sheldon BC.** 2012. Site-occupancy modelling as a novel framework for assessing test sensitivity and estimating wildlife disease prevalence from imperfect diagnostic tests. *Methods Ecol Evol* **3**:339–348.

75. **Jennelle CS, Cooch EG, Conroy MJ, Senar JC.** 2007. State-specific detection probabilities and disease prevalence. *Ecol Appl* **17**:154–167.

76. **Senar JC, Conroy MJ.** 2004. Multi-state analysis of the impacts of avian pox on a population of Serins (*Serinus serinus*): the importance of estimating recapture rates. *Anim Biodivers Conserv* **27**:133–146.

77. **Cooch EG, Conn PB, Ellner SP, Dobson AP, Pollock KH.** 2012. Disease dynamics in wild populations: modeling and estimation: a review. *J Ornithol* **152**:485–509.

78. **McClintock BT, Nichols JD, Bailey LL, MacKenzie DI, Kendall WL, Franklin AB.** 2010. Seeking a second opinion: uncertainty in disease ecology. *Ecol Lett* **13**:659–674.

79. **Faustino CR, Jennelle CS, Connolly V, Davis AK, Swarthout EC, Dhondt AA, Cooch EG.** 2004. *Mycoplasma gallisepticum* infection dynamics in a house finch population: seasonal variation in survival, encounter and transmission rate. *J Anim Ecol* **73**:651–669.

80. **Lomolino MV, Riddle BR, Whittaker RJ, Brown JH.** 2010. *Biogeography*, 4th ed. Sinauer Associates, Inc., Sunderland, MA.

81. **Cox CB, Moore PD.** 2010. *Biogeography: an Ecological and Evolutionary Approach*, 8th ed. John Wiley & Sons, Hoboken, NJ.

82. **Morand S, Krasnov BR (ed).** 2010. *The Biogeography of Host-Parasite Interactions*. Oxford University Press, New York, NY.

83. **MacArthur RH, Wilson EO.** 1967. *The Theory of Island Biogeography*. Princeton University Press, Princeton, NJ.

84. **Kuris AM, Blaustein AR, Alio JJ.** 1980. Hosts as islands. *Am Nat* **116**:570–586.

85. **Reperant L.** 2010. Applying the theory of island biogeography to emerging pathogens: toward predicting the sources of future emerging zoonotic and vector-borne diseases. *Vector Borne Zoonotic Dis* **10**:105–110.

86. **Poulin R.** 2004. Macroecological patterns of species richness in parasite assemblages. *Basic Appl Ecol* **5**:423–434.

87. **May RM, Gupta S, McLean AR.** 2001. Infectious disease dynamics: what characterizes a successful invader? *Philos Trans R Soc Lond B Biol Sci* **356**:901–910.

88. **Murray KA, Skerratt LF, Speare R, Ritchie S, Smout F, Hedlefs R, Lee J.** 2012. Cooling off health security hot spots: getting on top of it down under. *Environ Int* **48**:56–64.

One Health: People, Animals, and the Environment
Edited by Ronald M. Atlas and Stanley Maloy
© 2014 American Society for Microbiology, Washington, DC
doi:10.1128/microbiolspec.OH-0004-2012

Chapter 5

Emerging Infectious Diseases of Wildlife and Species Conservation

G. Medina-Vogel[1]

INTRODUCTION

Humans are rapidly transforming whole ecosystems in a number of well-documented but often poorly understood ways (1). Growing human populations and changes in land use patterns have increased contact among humans, domestic animals, and wildlife, raising the risks of transmission of numerous pathogens from animals to humans and vice versa (2, 3). Diseases are often transmitted between wild and domestic species, as well as from invasive species into resident populations (4, 5). Emergence of new infectious diseases frequently results from a change in ecology of host or pathogen (6), and when these relationships are disrupted, ecological effects may extend to many other parts of the ecosystem (7). The increase in human activities has had tremendous environmental impacts on biodiversity, including habitat loss, introduction of alien species, eradication of native species, pollution, urbanization, and anthropogenic climate change. Each of these environmental disturbances affects the ecology of infectious diseases (3).

Biodiversity is defined as the variety of life on Earth at all levels of biological organization, from genes within populations of species to species composing communities that are the biological components of ecosystems (8). Biodiversity may be related to infectious diseases at any of the following levels: the genetic variation of pathogens, vectors, and hosts; the number of species within each of these groups; the competition between species; the diversity of habitats in an ecosystem; or changes in animal behavior (9). Emerging infectious diseases of wildlife are generally related to habitat loss and fragmentation, overexploitation, introduction of invasive alien species, environmental pollution, and anthropogenic climate change (3, 10–13). There are many examples of emerging infectious diseases that have been clearly driven by direct human interventions that have altered exposure to pathogens and facilitated the transmission of disease. Moreover, the globalization of agriculture, commerce, and human travel has rapidly disseminated emerging diseases around the globe (14).

[1]Facultad de Ecología y Recursos Naturales, Universidad Andrés Bello, República 440, Santiago, Chile.

EMERGING INFECTIOUS DISEASES OF WILDLIFE

Emerging infectious diseases have been increasingly reported as a cause of death and population declines of free-living wild animals (10). In 1988, an outbreak of phocine distemper virus in the European harbor seal (*Phoca vitulina*) was stimulated by the forced southern migration of infected harp seals (*Phoca groenlandica*) due to human depletion of their food stocks by overfishing, coupled with compromised immunity caused by pollution. This outbreak killed 18,000 harbor seals throughout the North Atlantic European coasts (15–17). There are a number of examples of emerging infectious diseases of wild terrestrial and marine fauna occurring in Antarctica, as recent evidence indicates that some microorganisms may have been introduced to Antarctic wildlife as a consequence of human activity (18, 19). Disease has been recorded or suspected in several unusual mortality events of Antarctic birds, such as avian cholera caused by infection with *Pasteurella multocida* (20). The disease has also been observed on more than one occasion on sub-Antarctic Campbell Island, where *P. multocida* has been isolated from dead rockhopper penguins (*Eudyptes chrysocome*) (21), and several hundred gentoo penguin chicks (*Pygoscelis papua*) were found dead on Signy Island, Antarctica (22). In addition, bursal disease virus, a pathogen of domestic chickens, has been identified in Adélie penguins (*Pygoscelis adeliae*) (23). These data highlight the threats to penguins posed by introduced pathogens. Weimerskirch (24) demonstrated that the worldwide spread of avian cholera is probably the major cause of the decline of the large yellow-nosed albatross (*Diomedea chlororhynchos*) on Amsterdam Island as well. Another pathogenic bacterium, *Erysipelothrix*, was also implicated. Infectious diseases in Antarctica have also been recorded among other taxa. At least 1,500 crabeater seals (*Lobodon carcinophagus*) were found dead in the Crown Price Gustav Channel, Antarctic Peninsula, in 1955 (25). All affected seals had swollen necks and blood running from their mouths; on dissection their intestines were empty, their livers were pale, and pus oozed from the neck glands when incised (26). The cause was suspected to be a highly contagious virus possibly exacerbated by stress from crowding and partial starvation as a result of being trapped by ice. Abiotic factors also affect the presence, distribution, and transmission of pathogens in Antarctica, including the recent increases in temperature (27). These consequences of climate change can play an important role in disease expansion toward higher latitudes (3).

THE GEOGRAPHIC ORIGIN OF PATHOGENS

Native pathogens are those that have coexisted with their native host populations, while alien pathogens originate from different geographic regions or different populations and provide unique challenges for new hosts (28). However, distinguishing native pathogens from alien pathogens is sometimes difficult when considering disease emergence and wildlife population declines on a global scale. For example, the amphibian pathogen *Batrachochytrium dendrobatidis* is responsible for the amphibian disease chytridiomycosis (29–31). This highly pathogenic, readily transmissible emerging disease with low host specificity across an entire animal class has no precedent in modern times (32). Since the discovery of chytridiomycosis associated with declines in the amphibian populations in Australia and Central America in 1988 (29), the pathogen that causes this disease has been described in several hundred different amphibian species and has caused pandemic disease that has decimated amphibian populations (33). Nevertheless, *B. dendrobatidis* has been detected in many regions with different histories of human exposure, raising questions about whether it is native to those environments and recent changes increased its virulence or it has recently been introduced and rapidly spread around the globe.

Because of the density-dependent nature of transmission, infectious diseases had been believed to be unlikely agents of extinction (34). However, infection with the microsporidian *Steinhausia* was clearly the cause of extinction of the Polynesian tree snail, *Partula turgida* (35). Likewise, *B. dendrobatidis* has been implicated in the extinction of the golden toad (*Incilius periglenes*) in Costa Rica, as well as the sharp-snouted day frog (*Taudactylus acutirostris*) and two species of gastric-brooding frogs (*Rheobatrachus* spp.) from Australia (36, 37).

THE ROLE OF BIODIVERSITY

In addition to the direct impact of infectious disease on species diversity, the biodiversity of a habitat can influence the sensitivity of a population to infectious disease in many ways. Human alteration of the environment contributes to the loss of biodiversity and the subsequent impact of infectious disease. Several of these ecological impacts are described below.

1. *Ecological release by loss of regulation by predators and competitors.* Species extinction and the consequent reduction in biodiversity is not a random process (38, 39). In general, the "losers" are species with long life spans, large body masses, resource specialization, low reproductive rates, and other characteristics that make them much more susceptible to human activities (40). Thus, the abundance and diversity of carnivore predators may be greatly affected because they are particularly susceptible to habitat loss and fragmentation owing to their generally low population densities (38, 41, 42). This is not without consequences, as food chains contain a complex order of energy pathways that act as shock absorbers for dramatic population explosions (43). Therefore, in addition to the important role of predators in removing animals in poor health from communities (13), the reduction in top predator populations can lead to the phenomenon of ecological release of prey species that are often reservoirs of disease.

   Ecological release can also occur due to the loss of a competitor species utilizing the same food or space resource as the reservoir species (44, 45). Long-term studies have revealed the importance of interspecific competition in structuring communities of rodents in deserts; for example, an increase in the density of granivores was noted after experimentally removing larger competitors, such as the kangaroo rat, *Dipodomys* spp. (46).

2. *Ecological simplification.* A repercussion of ecological release is an increase in the abundance and geographic dispersion of generalist species,

considered as the small group of "winners" in the global loss of biodiversity (39, 47). This process, called ecological simplification, is the common denominator of current global anthropogenic change (40, 48). Generalist species have wide geographic distribution and a highly resilient ecology; further, they tend to be more competent as reservoirs or vectors compared with species with specialized niches (9, 13, 49, 50).

3. *Loss of dilution effect.* Decline in biodiversity may lead to loss of the dilution effect, considered as an ecosystem service that minimizes disease risk (11). This effect accounts for the decreased transmission of disease to a target species (e.g., Lyme disease in humans) when there is a greater number of species in the community (12). This is due to the decline in population density of reservoirs or vectors (51). In turn, there is a reduction in the frequency of encounters with these disease reservoirs or vectors (12). The result of the dilution effect is, therefore, a decrease in the prevalence of the pathogen resulting from the increase in species richness in a community (52).

THE EFFECT OF LANDSCAPE STRUCTURE

A landscape is composed of multiple habitats. The mosaic of physical and biotic conditions that define each habitat and the interfaces between habitats play an important role in the biodiversity of lakes, rivers, swamps, grasslands, forests, riparian vegetation, marine seashore, and the successional regions between them. Within this landscape there are areas with human-mediated alterations like agricultural fields, grasslands used for farm animals, controlled forests, highways, recreation areas, cities, railways, and other human contrivances that constitute a matrix surrounding the remnants of wildlife habitats. Animals living in close proximity to this man-made matrix may experience altered habitats. Some animal populations may not be able to adapt to these changes, while others effectively meld into the new landscape. The dispersal of wildlife within this landscape is restricted by the hostility of the surroundings, habitat fragmentation, and availability of animal corridors within the matrix. This results in a mosaic of habitats within the landscape, where the population abundance of a species in one habitat patch is the result of both the quality of that habitat and the hostility of the surrounding matrix (53). Wildlife populations within this landscape of fragmented habitats can have spatial structures called metapopulations, which persist as a result of the combined dynamics of extinction within a given habitat fragment and recolonization among fragments by dispersal (54). Thus, the landscape experienced by a population represents a mosaic of good and bad places for the species. Therefore, species distribution is restricted in time and space because of natural habitat discontinuity and landscape heterogeneity, and because individuals are incapable of moving through or around major barriers (55). Anthropogenic factors, consequently, can be responsible for species extinction by eliminating connecting patches or turning a surrounding habitat into a barrier (3). As a result, human-mediated habitat fragmentation may also create local populations that are completely isolated from one another (56). This concept also applies to river shores and seashores. Medina-Vogel et al. (57) and Vianna et al. (58) demonstrated that natural discontinuity of the rocky seashore patches along the coast of Chile, the main habitat of the marine otter (*Lontra felina*), is becoming fragmented as a result of the intense human activities along intervening sandy seashores and the collateral abundance of stray dogs. Within this context, domestic-wild inter-species interaction is unavoidable, with dogs acting both as predators and as vectors of diseases to marine otters (59). Thus, in terms of the importance for the ecology of infectious diseases, the habitat fragmentation process has four components: (i) reduction of the total amount of habitat in a landscape, (ii) increased distance between remaining habitat fragments, (iii) increased impact of outside factors on the remnant habitat fragments (edge effects), and (iv) changes in the species diversity within each habitat fragment (Fig. 1). The result is a significant change in the animal and plant community structure (1). For the ecology of infectious diseases, the first alteration may reduce

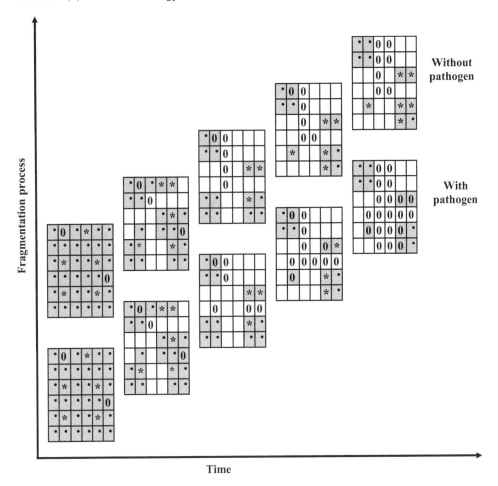

Figure 1. Effect of habitat fragmentation on three different species populations (•, *, and 0). Species 0 is less competitive against species • and *, but became a reservoir of a pathogen highly virulent for species * and less virulent for species •. By apparent competition, species 0 displaced species * and began competing for resources with species •, which was highly specialized to the disappearing habitat conditions. Empty boxes represent areas with loss of habitat. doi:10.1128/microbiolspec.OH-0004-2012.f1

the rate of contact between susceptible and infected hosts by modifying density- or frequency-dependent interactions; the second may reduce "herd immunity" of vulnerable populations by limiting exposure to pathogens; the third may facilitate the introduction of new pathogens or vectors; and the fourth may promote new species or interspecific interactions that could facilitate the transmission of disease (Fig. 1). A species which at the beginning of the process is less competitive, but acts as a host of a virulent pathogen to a second species, later can displace the second species as a result of apparent competition (60) (Fig. 1).

In western North America, prairie dog (*Cynomys* spp.) colonies vary in size and extension. Sylvatic plague caused by *Yersinia pestis* is positively correlated with the colony size (61, 62). Prairie dogs are sympatric (species found in the same area) with populations of deer mice, which are reservoir hosts for *Y. pestis* and their flea vectors. Dispersal of prairie dogs may occur more frequently in large colonies due to greater habitat suitability, thereby increasing the probability that a large colony will attract an immigrating prairie dog that is either infected or infested with infected fleas. Conversely, colony isolation, measured as the distance to the nearest plague-positive prairie dog colony, has been found to be negatively correlated with plague occurrence; even roads serve as barriers to sylvatic plague among black-tailed prairie dog colonies by affecting movement of or habitat quality for plague hosts or fleas that serve as vector for *Y. pestis* (63).

Gillespie and Chapman (64) studied parasite infection dynamics in red colobus (*Piliocolobus tephrosceles*) metapopulations inhabiting forest fragments in western Uganda. Their results demonstrate that an index of habitat degradation like stump density, as an indicator of forest extractive endeavors, significantly explained the prevalence of red colobus strongyle and rhabditoid nematode infection levels in forest fragments. In fact, they found a greater risk of infection with nematodes in the fragment with highest stump density than in the fragment with the lowest stump density. Colobus inhabiting fragments with high stump density are likely to experience a higher probability of contact with humans together with accompanying pathogens (64). This relationship between risk of disease exposure and proximity to urban areas or contact with humans has also been recorded for foxes (*Urocyon cinereoargenteus*) and bobcats (*Lynx rufus*) in urban and rural areas of California (65).

THE EFFECT OF ALIEN SPECIES

Within the context of habitat fragmentation, alien species become particularly important. Alien species are those introduced by humans deliberately or by accident into new regions. Introduction or migration of infected wild and domestic animals has been an important factor in the emergence of many epizootics. Alien species are linked to the emergence of diseases such as West Nile virus in the Americas (66), squirrel poxvirus in the United Kingdom (67), and avian malaria in Hawaii (68), among others. Furthermore, alien species can participate as vectors and reservoirs of pathogens, posing a significant threat to global biodiversity when disease is introduced into native populations (10, 69) that have not undergone selection for resistance to them (31).

Within a landscape, some animals move and live within distinctive areas, defined as their home range, and some animals territorially defend this space, thereby influencing the rate of contact with other animals as well as their own population size and density. Other animals migrate every year in a certain season following reproductive and food availability. Avoidance of competition is common in sympatric species and between native and alien species. Although competition may be avoided by sympatric species, their close proximity can provide the opportunity for transmission of pathogens (3). Infectious diseases are often maintained in a dynamic equilibrium in a population that is influenced by the landscape (70). Therefore, any environmental factor with the capability to alter the dynamic, such as the introduction of a new reservoir or hosts, may have the capacity to modify the epidemiology of pathogens (71).

THE COMBINED EFFECT—THE CASE OF *LEPTOSPIRA*

Leptospirosis is a zoonosis of global distribution. It is caused by the spirochete *Leptospira*, a pathogen with about 200 distinct serotypes (72). The severity of illness can range from an asymptomatic infection to a fatal illness involving the kidneys, liver, and other vital organs. However, there are no serotype-specific presentations of infection— each serotype may cause mild or severe disease depending on the host. Although in tropical areas incidence rates are particularly high, human cases are sporadic in Chile. Nevertheless, cases of leptospirosis in humans must be reported to the Chilean Ministry of Health. The diversity of serotypes in the population may be maintained by the reservoir hosts (73). A variety of wild and domestic animals can act as reservoir hosts for one or more serotypes and can shed the organism in their urine for months or years after being infected. This includes dogs, rats, swine, cattle, and raccoons in North America (74). Domestic as well as wild animals may come into contact with *Leptospira* by interspecies contact or by urine from farm animal reservoirs during activities such as swimming, drinking, or walking through contaminated water, soil, or mud. Humans become infected through contact of mucosal surfaces or abraded skin with contaminated soil or water or with animal urine or tissues. For example, participating in recreational activities in contaminated water increases the risk of human infection (75).

The prevalence of leptospirosis in animal populations indicates that transmission of *Leptospira* is influenced by human activities. Of 35 river otters tested for antibodies to *Leptospira interrogans*, 50% from Washington state were seropositive, but none of the 15 tested animals from Alaska were positive (76). These results correlate with levels of exposure of otters to *Toxoplasma gondii*: otters from Washington state showed high levels of exposure to *T. gondii* while otters from Alaska did not. The southern sea otter (*Enhydra lutris nereis*) population in California and the Alaskan sea otter (*E. lutris kenyoni*) population in the Aleutian Islands have also shown serological evidence of exposure to *Lepstospira* spp. (77). These results suggest that living in regions close to higher human density and its associated agricultural activities, domestic animals, and accompanying rodent populations enhance exposure of river otters to these pathogens.

An ongoing research project in southern Chile is focused on identifying viral and bacterial agents in wild and domestic animals and assessing environmental variables associated with their prevalence in different species. More than 200 samples from domestic and wild animals have been tested for *Leptospira* spp. in southern Chile. The results demonstrate a high incidence of infection: 37% in dogs, 88 to 92% in cattle, 25% in sheep, 7% in horses, 70% in swine, and 47% in wild rodents (78).

The deliberate introduction of an alien species had a major impact on transmission of *Leptospira* in wild otters in Chile. The North American mink was brought to Chile in the 1930s for the pelt industry. By the 1970s a feral population had developed from animals that had escaped from mink farms (79). The North American mink is now widely distributed throughout the Andean lacustrine and riverine habitats in Argentina and the south of Chile from 38°S latitude to Tierra del Fuego Island and adjacent archipelagos at 55°S (80–83). In rivers, lakes, and the seashore of southern Chile, the alien North American mink now coexists with the native population of southern river otters (*Lontra provocax*). This otter is one of the species that is under major conservation threats globally. It has suffered a continual reduction in habitat as a result of riparian vegetation removal, river dredging, and pollution (84–86). In contrast, mink are less sensitive to human activities and can be found near human settlements, commonly poaching poultry. Hence, populations of mink are sympatric with domestic dogs and cats and have acquired *Leptospira* infections from these interactions. In addition, mink populations are also sympatric with populations of southern river otters (80, 81, 87). Mink are semiaquatic, while otters are a more aquatic-adapted mustelid, so otters have significantly less habitat use overlap with domestic species than do mink. More than 50% of the diet of mink is wild rodents, while the diet of otters is nearly 100% aquatic macroinvertebrates and fish (80). Nevertheless, otters show the highest prevalence of *Leptospira* infections among domestic and wild species (Fig. 2). Wildlife reservoirs are those more epidemiologically tied to a population in which the pathogen can be permanently maintained and from which infestation is transmitted to the defined target population (88). The higher prevalence of *Leptospira* in river otters compared with terrestrial species provides evidence that landscape alterations by humans, invasion of domestic species, and invasion of the alien mink species exacerbated the transmission and prevalence of *Leptospira* infections in the threatened, vulnerable otter population.

CONCLUDING REMARKS

Despite evidence demonstrating the role of biodiversity depletion in the increase in zoonotic diseases, it has been suggested that the risk of emergence of infectious diseases will be higher where the biodiversity of mammals is greater, due to the assumption that each species carries an unknown number of potential pathogens (89, 90).

Three consequences of global biodiversity loss related to the emergence and increased incidence of infectious diseases are (i) ecological release, (ii) ecological simplification, and (iii) loss of the dilution effect. Thus, it is proposed that biodiversity plays a crucial role in the animals' risk of infection, and is therefore a determining factor in the emergence of new zoonotic diseases. Habitat alterations such as fragmentation, overexploitation of hosts and reservoirs, new interspecific interactions with alien species, new interspecific interactions with domestic species, pollution, and new distributions as a result of climate change are affecting biodiversity globally with unprecedented magnitude and speed. However, it seems that the factor that is of particular concern is the increase in interspecific interactions between domestic and alien species and wild species, which is bringing together hosts never before in contact. This is of special concern in natural regions including islands, national parks, and protected areas. Climate change is forcing many species into new geographic distributions, altering the animal communities in

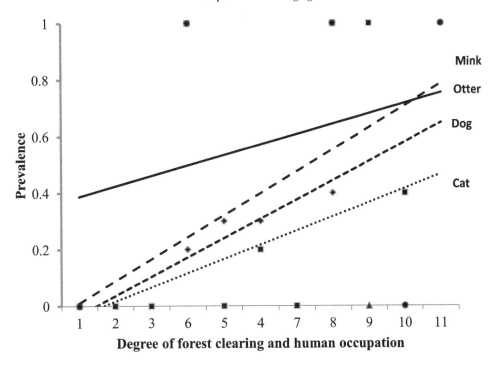

Figure 2. Relationship between the degree of landscape transformation and human presence and the prevalence of *Leptospira* spp. in animals from the lake and river districts in southern Chile. Scale representing degree of forest clearing and human occupation: 1 (essentially no alterations) to 10 (high alteration and human presence). doi:10.1128/microbiolspec.OH-0004-2012.f2

certain regions. As a result, some species will become extinct and others will expand, setting up new host-parasite, parasite-vector-host, and host-host interactions.

Biodiversity and the landscape structure play important roles in wildlife health through various mechanisms. Therefore, the "hot spots" on which to focus in monitoring emerging infectious diseases in wildlife should be located in areas with habitat loss, such as through deforestation (with special emphasis on the edges between habitat remnants and the matrix generated, and on the movement of domestic species into habitats) and where hydrological, agricultural, or aquaculture development projects are taking place. In the short term, permanent disease monitoring is needed to prevent the increase of vectors or unwanted reservoir populations and the emergence of diseases associated with trends of habitat lost and land use changes. Moreover, when defining long-term goals of maintaining the health of endangered species, disease in nearby populations of domestic and sympatric alien species should be permanently monitored.

The inclusion of studies of infectious disease in biodiversity and interspecific interactions between wildlife and domestic animals should be an important and complementary aspect to understanding human health and beyond—the health of ecosystems including humans as part of nature. As emphasized throughout the volume *One Health:*

People, Animals, and the Environment (91), most of the causative agents of emerging infectious diseases in humans are zoonotic. The advantage of focusing on biodiversity monitoring for the prevention of disease outbreaks or emergence is that even when all the necessary factors for the occurrence of illness are present (reservoir species, pathogens, intermediate or terminal hosts, and appropriate weather conditions), biodiverse communities possess the capacity to alleviate emergence events, making the biodiversity loss the ultimate determinant of the onset of illness.

Acknowledgments. Funding was provided by the Chilean Fund for Science and Technology (Fondecyt) project 1100139: "Presence of infectious diseases in wild species: the effect of alien invasive North American mink (*Neovison vison*) and the coexistence with stray dogs and cats." I also want to thank Pamela Lepe, Claudio Soto, and Lucía Alladio, students in the Ph.D. program in Conservation Medicine who assisted with reference searches.

Citation. Medina-Vogel G. 2013. Emerging infectious diseases of wildlife and species conservation. Microbiol Spectrum 1(3):OH-0004-2012. doi:10.1128/microbiolspec.OH-0004-2012.

REFERENCES

1. **Pullin AS.** 2002. *Conservation Biology*, p 345. Cambridge University Press, Cambridge, United Kingdom.
2. **Daszak P, Cunningham AA.** 2002. Emerging infectious diseases: a key role for conservation medicine, p 40–61. *In* Aguirre AA, Ostfeld RS, Tabor GM, House C, Pearl MC (ed), *Conservation Medicine: Ecological Health in Practice.* Oxford University Press, New York, NY.
3. **Medina-Vogel G.** 2010. Ecología de enfermedades infecciosas emergentes y conservación de especies silvestres. *Arch Med Vet* **42:**11–24.
4. **Garner TW, Perkins MW, Govindarajulu P, Seglie D, Walker S, Cunningham AA, Fisher MC.** 2006. The emerging amphibian pathogen *Batrachochytrium dendrobatidis* globally infects introduced populations of the North American bullfrog, *Rana catesbeiana. Biol Lett* **3:**455–459.
5. **Mañas S, Ceña JC, Ruiz-Olmo J, Palazón S, Domingo M, Wolfinbarger JB, Bloom ME.** 2001. Aleutian mink disease parvovirus in wild riparian carnivores in Spain. *J Wildl Dis* **37:**138–144.
6. **Schrag SJ, Wiener P.** 1995. Emerging infectious disease: what are the relative roles of ecology and evolution? *Trends Ecol Evol* **10:**319–324.
7. **Epstein PR.** 2002. Biodiversity, climate change, and emerging infectious diseases, p 27–39. *In* Aguirre AA, Ostfeld RS, Tabor GM, House C, Pearl MC (ed), *Conservation Medicine: Ecological Health in Practice.* Oxford University Press, New York, NY.
8. **Pimm SL, Alves MA, Chivian E, Bernstein A.** 2008. What is biodiversity?, p 3–26. *In* Chivian E, Bernstein A (ed), *Sustaining Life: How Human Health Depends on Biodiversity.* Oxford University Press, New York, NY.
9. **Molyneux DH, Ostfeld RS, Bernstein A, Chivian E.** 2008. Ecosystem disturbance, biodiversity loss, and human infectious disease, p 287–323. *In* Chivian E, Bernstein A (ed), *Sustaining Life: How Human Health Depends on Biodiversity.* Oxford University Press, New York, NY.
10. **Daszak P, Cunningham AA, Hyatt AD.** 2000. Emerging infectious diseases of wildlife—threats to biodiversity and human health. *Science* **287:**443–449.
11. **Ostfeld RS, LoGiudice K.** 2003. Community disassembly, biodiversity loss, and the erosion of an ecosystem service. *Ecology* **84:**1421–1427.
12. **Ostfeld RS.** 2009. Biodiversity loss and the rise of zoonotic pathogens. *Clin Microbiol Infect* **15**(Suppl 1): 40–43.
13. **Morand S.** 2011. Infectious diseases, biodiversity and global changes: how the biodiversity sciences may help, p 231–254. *In* López-Pujol J (ed), *The Importance of Biological Interactions in the Study of Biodiversity.* InTech, Rijeka, Croatia.
14. **Daszak P, Cunningham AA, Hyatt AD.** 2001. Anthropogenic environmental change and the emergence of infectious diseases in wildlife. *Acta Tropica* **78:**103–116.
15. **Dietz R, Ansen CT, Have P, Heide-Jørgensen MP.** 1989. Clue to seal epizootic? *Nature* **338:**627.

16. **Hall AJ, Pomeroy PP, Harwood J.** 1992. The descriptive epizootiology of phocine distemper in the UK during 1988/89. *Sci Total Environ* **115**:31–44.
17. **Heide-Jørgensen MP, Harkonen T, Dietz R, Thompson PM.** 1992. Retrospective of the 1988 European seal epizootic. *Dis Aquat Organ* **13**:37–62.
18. **Broman T, Bergström S, On SL, Palmgren H, McCafferty DJ, Sellin M, Olsen B.** 2000. Isolation and characterization of *Campylobacter jejuni* subsp. *jejuni* from macaroni penguins (*Eudyptes chrysolophus*) in the subantartic region. *Appl Environ Microbiol* **66**:449–452.
19. **Palmgren H, McCafferty D, Aspán A, Broman T, Sellin M, Wollin R, Bergström S, Olsen B.** 2000. *Salmonella* in sub-Antarctica: low heterogeneity in *Salmonella* serotypes in South Georgian seals and birds. *Epidemiol Infect* **125**:257–262.
20. **Parmelee DF, Maxson SJ, Bernstein NP.** 1979. Fowl cholera outbreak among brown skuas at Palmer Station. *Antarct J U S* **14**:168–169.
21. **de Lisle GW, Stanislawak WL, Moors PJ.** 1990. *Pasteurella multocida* infections in rockhopper penguins (*Eudyptes chrysocome*) from Campbell Island, New Zealand. *J Wildl Dis* **26**:283–285.
22. **MacDonald JW, Conroy JW.** 1971. Virus disease resembling puffinosis in the gentoo penguin *Pygoscelis papua* on Signy Island, South Orkney Islands. *Br Antarct Surv Bull* **26**:80–83.
23. **Gardner H, Kerry K, Riddle M, Brouwer S, Gleeson L.** 1997. Poultry virus infection in Antarctic penguins. *Nature* **387**:245.
24. **Weimerskirch H.** 2004. Diseases threaten Southern Ocean albatrosses. *Polar Biol* **27**:374–379.
25. **Laws RM, Taylor RJ.** 1957. A mass dying of crabeater seals, *Lobodon carcinophagus* (gray). *Proc Zool Soc Lond* **129**:315–325.
26. **Fuchs V.** 1982. *Of Ice and Men.* Anthony Nelson, London, United Kingdom.
27. **Wobeser AG.** 2006. *Essentials of Disease in Wild Animals.* Blackwell Publishing, Ames, IA.
28. **Dobson A, Foufopolus J.** 2001. Emerging infectious pathogens of wildlife. *Philos Trans R Soc Lond B Biol Sci* **356**:1001–1012.
29. **Berger L, Speare R, Daszak P, Green DE, Cunningham AA, Goggin CL, Slocombe R, Ragan MA, Hyatt AD, McDonald KR, Hines HB, Lips KR, Marantelli G, Parkes H.** 1998. Chytridiomycosis causes amphibian mortality associated with population declines in the rain forests of Australia and Central America. *Proc Natl Acad Sci USA* **95**:9031–9036.
30. **Longcore JE, Pessier AP, Nichols DK.** 1999. *Batrachochytrium dendrobatidis* gen. et sp. nov., a chytrid pathogenic to amphibians. *Mycologia* **91**:219–227.
31. **Skerratt LF, Berger L, Speare R, Cashins S, McDonald KR, Phillott AD, Hines HB, Kenyon N.** 2007. Spread of chytridiomycosis has caused the rapid global decline and extinction of frogs. *Ecohealth* **4**:125–134.
32. **Gascon C, Collins JP, Moore RD, Church DR, McKay JE, Mendelson JR III (ed).** 2007. *Amphibian Conservation Action Plan.* World Conservation Union/Species Survival Commission Amphibian Specialist Group, Gland, Switzerland and Cambridge, United Kingdom. http://www.amphibianark.org/pdf/ACAP.pdf (last accessed June 10, 2013).
33. **Fisher MC, Garner TW.** 2007. The relationship between the emergence of *Batrachochytrium dendrobatidis*, the international trade in amphibians and introduced amphibian species. *Fungal Biol Rev* **21**: 2–9.
34. **Smith FS, Sax FS, Lafferty KD.** 2006. Evidence for the role of infectious disease in species extinction and endangerment. *Conserv Biol* **20**:1349–1357.
35. **Daszak P, Cunningham AA.** 1999. Extinction by infection. *Trends Ecol Evol* **14**:279.
36. **Daszak P, Berger L, Cunningham AA, Hyatt AD, Green DE, Speare R.** 1999. Emerging infectious diseases and amphibian population declines. *Emerg Infect Dis* **5**:735–748.
37. **Schloegel LM, Hero JM, Berger L, Speare R, McDonald K, Daszak P.** 2006. The decline of the sharp-snouted day frog (*Taudactylus acutirostris*): the first documented case of extinction by infection in a free-ranging wildlife species? *Ecohealth* **3**:35–40.
38. **Duffy JE.** 2002. Biodiversity and ecosystem function: the consumer connection. *Oikos* **99**:201–219.
39. **McKinney ML, Lockwood JL.** 1999. Biotic homogenization: a few winners replacing many losers in the next mass extinction. *Trends Ecol Evol* **14**:450–453.
40. **Díaz S, Fargione J, Chapin FS III, Tilman D.** 2006. Biodiversity loss threatens human well-being. *PLoS Biol* **4**:e277. doi:10.1371/journal.pbio.0040277.
41. **Terborgh J, Lopez V, Nuñez P, Rao M, Shahabuddin G, Orihuela G, Riveros M, Ascanio R, Adler**

GH, Lambert TD, Balbas L. 2001. Ecological meltdown in predator-free forest fragments. *Science* **294**: 1923–1926.

42. **McMichael AJ.** 2004. Environmental and social influences on emerging infectious diseases: past, present and future. *Philos Trans R Soc Lond B Biol Sci* **359**:1049–1058.

43. **McCann KS.** 2000. The diversity-stability debate. *Nature* **405**:228–233.

44. **Begon M, Townsend CR, Harper JL.** 2006. *Ecology: from Individuals to Ecosystems*, 4th ed. Blackwell Publishing, Oxford, United Kingdom.

45. **Caut S, Casanovas JG, Virgos E, Lozano J, Witmer GW, Courchamp F.** 2007. Rats dying for mice: modelling the competitor release effect. *Austral Ecol* **32**:858–868.

46. **Heske EJ, Brown JH, Mistry S.** 1994. Long-term experimental study of a Chihuahuan Desert rodent community: 13 years of competition. *Ecology* **75**:438–445.

47. **Auffray JF, Renaud S, Claude J.** 2009. Rodent biodiversity in changing environments. *Kasetsart J (Nat Sci)* **43**:83–93.

48. **Pongsiri MJ, Roman J, Ezenwa VO, Goldberg TL, Koren HS, Newbold SC, Ostfeld RS, Pattanayak SK, Salkeld DJ.** 2009. Biodiversity loss affects global disease ecology. *BioScience* **59**:945–954.

49. **Chaisiri K, Chaeychomsri W, Siruntawineti J, Bordes F, Herbreteau V, Morand S.** 2010. Human-dominated habitats and helminth parasitism in Southeast Asian murids. *Parasitol Res* **107**:931–937.

50. **Mills JN.** 2006. Biodiversity loss and emerging infectious diseases: an example from the rodent-borne hemorrhagic fevers. *Biodiversity* **7**:9–17.

51. **Schmidt KA, Ostfeld RS.** 2001. Biodiversity and the dilution effect in disease ecology. *Ecology* **82**: 609–619.

52. **Clay CA, Lehmer EM, Jeor SS, Dearing MD.** 2009. Sin Nombre virus and rodent species diversity: a test of the dilution and amplification hypotheses. *PLoS One* **4**:e6467. doi:10.1371/journal.pone.0006467.

53. **Andrén H.** 1994. Effects of habitat fragmentation on birds and mammals in landscapes with different proportions of suitable habitat: a review. *Oikos* **71**:355–366.

54. **McCullough DR (ed).** 1996. *Metapopulations and Wildlife Conservation*. Island Press, Washington, DC.

55. **Wiens JA.** 1996. Wildlife in patchy environments: metapopulations, mosaics and management, p 53–84. *In* McCullough DR (ed), *Metapopulations and Wildlife Conservation*. Island Press, Washington, DC.

56. **Hastings A, Harrison S.** 1994. Metapopulation dynamics and genetics. *Annu Rev Ecol Syst* **25**:167–188.

57. **Medina-Vogel G, Merino LO, Monsalve Alarcón R, Vianna JA.** 2008. Coastal-marine discontinuities, critical patch size and isolation: implications for marine otter conservation. *Anim Conserv* **11**:57–64.

58. **Vianna JA, Ayerdi P, Medina-Vogel G, Mangel JC, Zeballos H, Apaza M, Faugeron S.** 2010. Phylogrography of the marine otter (*Lontra felina*): historical and contemporary factors determining its distribution. *J Hered* **101**:676–689.

59. **Medina-Vogel G, Boher F, Flores G, Santibañez A, Soto-Azat C.** 2007. Spacing behavior of marine otters (*Lontra felina*) in relation to land refuges and fishery wastes in central Chile. *J Mammal* **88**:487–494.

60. **Lafferty KD.** 2008. Effect of disease on community interactions and food web structure, p 205–222. *In* Ostfeld RS, Keesing F, Eviner VT (ed), *Infectious Disease Ecology: Effects of Ecosystems on Disease and of Disease on Ecosystems*. Princeton University Press, Princeton, NJ.

61. **Cully JF Jr, Williams ES.** 2001. Interspecific comparisons of sylvatic plague in prairie dogs. *J Mammal* **82**:894–905.

62. **Lomolino MV, Smith GA.** 2001. Dynamic biogeography of prairie dog (*Cynomys ludovicianus*) town near the edge of their range. *J Mammal* **82**:937–945.

63. **Collinge SK, Johnson WC, Ray C, Matchett R, Grensten J, Cully JF, Gage KL, Kosoy MY, Loye JE, Martin AP.** 2005. Landscape structure and plague occurrence in black-tailed prairie dogs on grasslands of the western USA. *Landsc Ecol* **20**:941–955.

64. **Gillespie TR, Chapman CA.** 2006. Prediction of parasite infection dynamics in primate metapopulations based on attributes of forest fragmentation. *Conserv Biol* **20**:441–448.

65. **Riley SP, Foley J, Chomel B.** 2004. Exposure to feline and canine pathogens in bobcat and gray foxes in urban and rural zones of a national park in California. *J Wildl Dis* **40**:11–22.

66. **Anderson JF, Andreadis TG, Vossbrinck CR, Tirrell S, Wakem EM, French RA, Garmendia AE, Van Kruiningen HJ.** 1999. Isolation of West Nile virus from mosquitoes, crows, and a Cooper's hawk in Connecticut. *Science* **286**:2331–2333.

67. **Sainsbury AW, Nettleton P, Gilray J, Gurnell J.** 2000. Grey squirrels have high seroprevalence to a parapoxvirus associated with deaths in red squirrels. *Anim Conserv* **3**:229–233.

68. **van Riper C, van Riper SG, Goff ML, Laird M.** 1986. The epizootiology and ecological significance of malaria in Hawaiian land birds. *Ecol Monogr* **56:**327–344.

69. **Cunningham AA, Daszak P, Rodriguez JP.** 2003. Pathogen pollution: defining a parasitological threat to biodiversity conservation. *J Parasitol* **89:**S78–S83.

70. **Cabello CC, Cabello CF.** 2008. [Zoonoses with wildlife reservoirs: a threat to public health and the economy]. *Rev Med Chil* **136:**385–393. (In Spanish.)

71. **Tabor GM.** 2002. Defining conservation medicine, p 8–16. *In* Aguirre AA, Ostfeld RS, Tabor GM, House C, Pearl MC (ed), *Conservation Medicine: Ecological Health in Practice.* Oxford University Press, New York, NY.

72. **Farr RW.** 1995. Leptospirosis. *Clin Infect Dis* **21:**1–6; quiz 7–8.

73. **Lagadec E, Gomard Y, Guernier V, Dietrich M, Pascalis H, Temmam S, Ramasindrazana B, Goodman SM, Tortosa P, Delagi K.** 2012. Pathgogenic *Leptospira* spp. in bats, Madagascar and Union of the Comoros. *Emerg Infect Dis* **18:**1696–1698.

74. **Levett P.** 2005. Leptospirosis, p 2789–2798. *In* Mandell GL, Bennett JE, Dolin R (ed), *Mandell, Douglas, and Bennett's Principles and Practice of Infectious Diseases,* 5th ed. Churchill Livingstone, Philadelphia, PA.

75. **Vinetz JM, Wilcox BA, Aguirre A, Gollin LX, Katz AR, Fujioka RS, Maly K, Horwitz P, Chang H.** 2005. Beyond disciplinary boundaries: leptospirosis as a model of incorporating transdisciplinary approaches to understand infectious disease emergence. *Ecohealth* **2:**291–306.

76. **Gaydos JK, Conrad PA, Gilardi KV, Blundell GM, Ben-David M.** 2007. Does human proximity affect antibody prevalence in marine-foraging river otters (*Lontra canadensis*)? *J Wildl Dis* **43:**116–123.

77. **Hanni KD, Mazet JA, Gulland FM, Estes J, Staedler M, Murray MJ, Miller M, Jessup DA.** 2003. Clinical pathology and assessment of pathogen exposure in southern and Alaskan sea otters. *J Wildl Dis* **39:** 837–850.

78. **Zunino E, Pizarro R.** 2007. [Leptospirosis: a literature review.] *Rev Chil Infectol* **24:**220–226 (In Spanish).

79. **Jaksic FM, Iriarte JA, Jiménez JE, Martínez DR.** 2002. Invaders without frontiers: cross-border invasions of exotic mammals. *Biol Invasions* **4:**157–173.

80. **Medina G.** 1997. A comparison of the diet and distribution of the southern river otter (*Lutra provocax*) and mink (*Mustela vison*) in Southern Chile. *J Zool* **242:**291–297.

81. **Fasola L, Chehébar C, Macdonald DW, Porro G, Cassini M.** 2009. Do alien North American mink compete for resources with native South American river otter in Argentinean Patagonia? *J Zool* **277:** 187–195.

82. **Ibarra JT, Fasola L, Macdonald DW, Rozzi R, Bonacic C.** 2009. Invasive American mink *Mustela vison* in wetlands of the Cape Horn Biosphere Reserve, southern Chile: what are they eating? *Oryx* **43:**87–90.

83. **Rozzi R, Sheriffs M.** 2003. El visón (*Mustela vison* Schreber: Carnivora: Mustelidae), un nuevo mamífero exótico para la isla Navarino. *An Inst Patagon* **31:**97–104.

84. **Medina-Vogel G.** 1996. Conservation status of *Lutra provocax* in Chile. *Pacific Conserv Biol* **2:**414–419.

85. **Medina-Vogel G, Kaufmann VS, Monsalve R, Gomez V.** 2003. The relationship between riparian vegetation, woody debris, stream morphology, human activity and the use of rivers by southern river otter in Chile. *Oryx* **37:**422–430.

86. **Medina-Vogel G, Gonzalez-Lagos C.** 2008. Habitat use and diet of endangered southern river otter *Lontra provocax* in a predominantly palustrine wetland in Chile. *Wildl Biol* **14:**211–220.

87. **Aued MB, Chehébar C, Porro G, Macdonald DW, Cassini MH.** 2003. Environmental correlates of the distribution of southern river otters *Lontra provocax*. *Oryx* **37:**413–421.

88. **Haydon DT, Laurenson MK, Sillero-Zubiri C.** 2002. Integrating epidemiology into population viability analysis: managing the risk posed by rabies and canine distemper to the Ethiopian wolf. *Conserv Biol* **16:** 1372–1385.

89. **Atlas R, Rubin C, Maloy S, Daszak P, Colwell R, Hyde B.** 2010. One Health—attaining optimal health for people, animals, and the environment. *Microbe* **5:**383–389.

90. **Dunn R.** 2010. Global mapping of ecosystem disservices: the unspoken reality that nature sometimes kills us. *Biotropica* **42:**555–557.

91. **Atlas RM, Maloy S (ed).** 2014. *One Health: People, Animals, and the Environment.* ASM Press, Washington, DC.

Zoonotic and Environmental Drivers of Emerging Infectious Diseases

One Health: People, Animals, and the Environment
Edited by Ronald M. Atlas and Stanley Maloy
© 2014 American Society for Microbiology, Washington, DC
doi:10.1128/microbiolspec.OH-0001-2012

Chapter 6

RNA Viruses: A Case Study of the Biology of Emerging Infectious Diseases

Mark E. J. Woolhouse,[1] Kyle Adair,[1] and Liam Brierley[1]

INTRODUCTION

Viruses account for only a small fraction of the 1400 or more different species of pathogen that plague humans—the great majority are bacteria, fungi, or helminths (1). However, as both the continuing toll of childhood infections such as measles and recent experience of AIDS and influenza pandemics illustrate, viruses are rightly high on the list of global public health concerns (2). Moreover, the great majority of newly recognized human pathogens over the past few decades have been viruses (3) and a large fraction of emerging infectious disease "events" have involved viruses (4).

There are two kinds of viruses: RNA viruses and DNA viruses. The latter largely consist, with the exception of a handful of pox- and herpesviruses, of viruses that have probably been present in and coevolved with humans for long periods of time. RNA viruses are very different. The majority of RNA viruses that infect humans are zoonotic, meaning that they can infect vertebrate hosts other than humans. Many of those that are not regarded as zoonotic are believed to have had recent (in evolutionary terms) zoonotic origins. So it is the RNA viruses that are of greatest interest in the context of One Health.

In this chapter, we review current knowledge of how RNA viruses in humans and other vertebrates are related, in terms of both of their evolution and their ecology, with the intention of trying to understand where human RNA viruses came from in the past and where new ones might emerge in the future. Until recently, research on these topics was essentially a series of case studies. Extraordinary work has been done detailing events such as the historical emergence of HIV-1 in Central Africa (5) and the more recent emergence of Nipah virus in Southeast Asia (6). But while every emergence event is a fascinating story in its own right, our aim here is to look beyond the specifics and to try to identify any underlying generalities that tell us something useful about the emergence of RNA viruses as a biological process.

We begin by comparing the RNA viruses reported to infect humans with RNA virus diversity as a whole and exploring the overlap between viruses in humans and viruses in other kinds of hosts. Next, we refine the analysis by distinguishing among viruses

---

[1]Centre for Immunity, Infection & Evolution, University of Edinburgh, Edinburgh EH9 3JT, United Kingdom.

according to their ability not just to infect humans but also to transmit from one human to another, which is a prerequisite for a virus being able to cause major epidemics and/or become an established, endemic human pathogen. We then consider in more detail the subset of human RNA viruses that can persist in human populations without the need for a nonhuman reservoir. Next, we attempt to identify characteristics of RNA viruses that allow them to cross the species barrier and those that predispose them to cause severe disease, as such viruses are of particular public health concern. We go on to discuss how new human RNA viruses arise (sometimes to subsequently disappear again). From the information assembled we construct a conceptual model of the relationship between RNA viruses in humans and other hosts. We consider how this model might be of practical value, concentrating on risk assessments for newly discovered viruses and also the much discussed topic of the design of surveillance programs for emerging infectious diseases.

DIVERSITY OF HUMAN RNA VIRUSES

The diversity of human RNA viruses was recently surveyed using a formal methodology (3), and we update that information here. All RNA viruses known to infect humans were included, with the exception of those only known to do so as the result of deliberate laboratory exposures.

In this chapter, we use virus species as designated by the Ninth Report of the International Committee for the Taxonomy of Viruses (ICTV) (7) (noting that this differs from earlier ICTV reports used in previous work and that it will doubtless change again in the not-too-distant future). ICTV designations may not always accurately reflect the biological meaning of a "species," i.e., reproductive isolation. The operational criteria used for RNA viruses may include any or all of (i) phylogenetic relatedness based on sequence data, (ii) serological cross-reactivity, (iii) host range, and (iv) transmission route. It is also important to note that any analysis at the level of a virus species implicitly ignores a great deal of biomedically relevant diversity. This point is best illustrated by the influenza A viruses: the epidemiology and public health importance of seasonal influenza A and the H5N1 or H7N9 "bird flu" variants are very different, but all are included within a single species. Less variable virus species than influenza A may still contain multiple serotypes and other functionally distinct subtypes. Despite these limitations, the species remains the most useful unit for studying virus diversity currently available.

Updating the earlier survey (3) with new taxonomic information (7) reveals 180 recognized species of RNA viruses that have been reported to infect humans. These viruses represent 50 genera and 17 families (with one genus, *Deltavirus*, currently unassigned to a family). It is not immediately obvious what we should make of this. Is 180 a large number or a small one? Should we be surprised that it is not much higher or that it is not much lower? We consider such questions further below. We can, at least, be sure that 180 is an underestimate. New human RNA virus species are still being discovered or recognized at a rate of approximately 2 per year, although recent work (8) has suggested that the pool of undiscovered species could be much smaller than previously proposed (3). Even if we still have very little idea of the number of species "out there," it is, as we will consider in detail later on, possible to say something about where "out there" is.

The possibility of large numbers of as yet unrecognized viruses also raises the specter of ascertainment bias. Certain kinds of RNA viruses may be underrepresented, perhaps dramatically so, among those currently recognized. These might be viruses from particular taxonomic groups, those associated with less severe disease or certain kinds of symptoms, or simply those that are rare and/or occur in less studied regions of the world. While this is clearly an issue, it is worth pointing out that both the rates and kinds of RNA viruses being discovered or recognized have been remarkably consistent for the past half century, despite massive changes in the technologies for virus detection and identification and considerable variability in the effort put into virus discovery in different places and at different times (3).

RNA VIRUSES OF HUMANS AND NONHUMANS

One striking observation is that 160 species of human-infective RNA virus species (89% of the total) are regarded as zoonotic; i.e., they can also infect other kinds of vertebrate hosts. (The definition of "zoonotic" ignores arthropod vectors; these are regarded as specialized transmission routes rather than alternative host species.) The nonhuman hosts usually (>90% of all zoonotic RNA virus species) include other mammals and less commonly (<40%) birds. Humans rarely, if ever, share their RNA viruses with anything else. Although the bias toward sharing viruses with other mammals is obvious, it is less clear whether we preferentially share viruses with particular kinds of mammals. Many human viruses (both RNA and DNA) are shared with ungulates, carnivores, rodents, primates, or bats (3), but our knowledge of the host range of most viruses is too incomplete for us to be confident about any underlying patterns. The remaining 20 RNA viruses are not known to naturally infect nonhuman hosts. However, most of these have close relatives that can infect other mammals. The only exceptions are hepatitis C, hepatitis delta, and rubella virus.

The overlap between the ability to infect humans and the ability to infect other mammals can be illustrated in other ways, too. Of the 62 recognized RNA virus genera containing species that can infect at least one kind of mammal, 50 (81%) contain species that can infect humans. And of the 19 recognized RNA virus families that contain species reported to infect mammals, all but 2 include species found in humans. The exceptions are the *Nodaviridae*, which are essentially insect viruses, and the *Arteriviridae*, which include species infecting a range of different mammals, notably including simian hemorrhagic fever virus.

The fact that human-infective species are distributed so widely among the RNA viruses of mammals strongly suggests that, in evolutionary terms, the ability to infect humans is very easily acquired by these viruses. It also implies that many, perhaps most, human RNA viruses need not have arisen by evolving from other human RNA viruses. This idea is supported by a recent analysis of the relationship between phylogeny and host range for three RNA virus families—*Paramyxoviridae*, *Caliciviridae*, and *Rhabdoviridae* —and two genera—*Alphavirus* and *Flavivirus*—which concluded that the majority of speciation events were associated with host species jumps (9). Note that this pattern contrasts markedly with the human DNA viruses, among which taxa such as the *Papillomaviridae* and the *Anelloviridae* appear to have undergone extensive diversification within humans.

THE PATHOGEN PYRAMID

The categorization of viruses based simply on their ability to infect humans fails to distinguish between a vast range of epidemiologies, from occasional very mild cases of Newcastle disease virus infection to pandemics of influenza A or HIV-1. A useful conceptual framework for thinking about this issue is the pathogen pyramid (10). The version of pyramid used here has four levels (Fig. 1).

Level 1 corresponds to human exposure, whether via ingestion, inhalation, the bite of an arthropod vector, or any other route. As discussed in the previous section, the most important sources of exposure are other mammals and, to a lesser degree, birds. There are no good estimates of the total diversity of mammal and bird viruses, but it seems likely that the human population is exposed to hundreds, perhaps thousands, of species on a regular basis. The major determinants of the rate of exposure to new viruses are the ecology and behavior of humans, the nonhuman virus reservoir(s), and (in some cases) arthropod vectors.

Level 2 corresponds to human infection, which we take to mean the ability to enter and replicate in human cells in vivo. For all (known) RNA viruses there are associated host responses, although not all infections necessarily lead to clinical symptoms of disease.

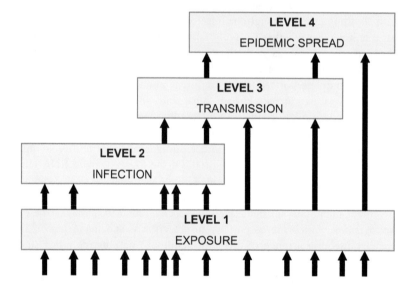

Figure 1. A representation of the pathogen pyramid. Each level of the pyramid represents a different degree of interaction between a virus and a human host. Level 1 corresponds to exposure of humans, level 2 to the ability to infect humans, level 3 to the ability to transmit from one human to another, and level 4 to the ability to cause epidemics or persist as an endemic infection. Arrows indicate pathways that viruses may take to reach each level. For example, a level 4 virus may arrive at that state directly, simply by exposure to the virus from a nonhuman reservoir. This is known as an "off-the-shelf" virus. Alternatively, it may initially enter the population as a level 2 or 3 virus—not capable of sustained transmission—but evolve the ability to transmit between humans at a sufficiently high rate to persist within a human population. This is known as a "tailor-made" virus. Adapted from reference 25. doi:10.1128/microbiolspec.OH-0001-2012.f1

Key determinants of the ability to infect humans include the route of entry (e.g., needle sharing has created a new entry route for blood-borne viruses) and the molecular biology of the human-virus interaction (discussed in more detail below). Of the 180 recognized species of RNA viruses that can infect humans, almost 60% (107 species) are restricted to level 2 (Fig. 2).

Level 3 corresponds to the ability both to infect humans *and* to transmit from one human to another. The ability to transmit refers to all kinds of transmission routes, including vectors. Less than half of human-infective RNA viruses (73 species in all) are able to transmit between humans. A minority of these (26 species) are restricted to level 3 (Fig. 2).

Level 4 corresponds to the ability to transmit sufficiently well that the virus can invade human populations, causing epidemics and/or establishing itself as an endemic human pathogen. In epidemiological parlance, this corresponds to the condition that R_0 is >1 within the human population, where R_0 is the basic reproduction number, defined as the number of secondary cases generated by a single primary case introduced into a large population of naïve hosts. In contrast, level 3 viruses have an R_0 of <1 in humans, which implies that although self-limiting outbreaks are possible, the infection cannot "take off" and cause a major epidemic. Although R_0 is partly determined by the transmissibility of the virus, it is also a function of the behavior and demography of the human host population; for example, changes in living conditions, travel patterns, and sexual behavior (for sexually transmitted viruses) can all greatly influence R_0. More generally, the term "crowd diseases" implies that certain human viruses (and other pathogens) can only become established once critical host population densities have been reached (10). Our best estimate is that there are 47 level 4 RNA virus species in humans (Fig. 2).

A useful exercise is to consider what kinds of viruses are found at levels 2, 3, and 4 in the pyramid. There appear to be three major determinants of this: (i) taxonomy (at the level of both family and genus), (ii) transmission route (especially the distinction between vector-borne transmission and other routes), and (iii) host range (expressed here as the ability to infect different mammalian orders). These three factors are not independent (1); in particular, there are very few vector-borne viruses with narrow host ranges (11).

Nonetheless, several patterns can be identified. First, only two vector-borne viruses are found at the top of the pyramid (level 4): yellow fever and dengue (Fig. 2). It is not immediately apparent why this should be so; we will consider this point further later on. Second, viruses with a host range that is, as far as we know, restricted to primates are rarely found lower down on the pyramid (levels 2 and 3), with a few exceptions such as the simian foamy viruses. The obvious implication is that if a virus is capable of infecting and transmitting from our closest relatives, then it is very likely to have the same capabilities in us. Patterns are also apparent in the taxonomy of human-infective viruses: for example, the *Bunyaviridae*, *Rhabdoviridae*, *Arenaviridae*, and *Togaviridae* (with the exception of rubella, which is atypical of that group) are not represented at level 4 at all. This reflects the fact that these four families are made up of viruses that are vector borne and/or are not primate specialists.

Finally, it is worth noting that the "shape" of the pathogen pyramid for RNA viruses differs from that for nonviral human pathogens. Most strikingly, much smaller fractions of recognized species of bacteria, fungi, protozoa, or helminths are capable of extensive spread in human populations (i.e., are found at level 4). On the other hand, human DNA

LEVEL 4

Aichi   Betacoronavirus 1   Dengue   Hepatitis A   Hepatitis C   Hepatitis E   Hepatitis delta   Human astrovirus
Human coronavirus 229E, HKU1, NL63   Human enterovirus A-D   HIV-1 and -2   Human metapneumovirus
Human parainfluenza 1-4   Human parechovirus   Human picobirnavirus   Human respiratory syncytial virus
Human rhinovirus A-C   Human torovirus   Influenza A-C   Mammalian orthoreovirus   Measles   Mumps
Norwalk   PTLV 1-3   Rotavirus A-C   Rubella   Sapporo   SARS-related coronavirus   Theilovirus   Yellow fever

LEVEL 3

Andes   Barmah Forest   Bwamba   Chikungunya   Colorado tick fever   Crimean-Congo hemorrhagic fever
Guanarito   Junin   Lake Victoria Marburg   Lassa   Lymphocytic choriomeningitis   Machupo
Nelson Bay orthoreovirus   Nipah   O'nyong-nyong   Oropouche   Rabies   Reston Ebola   Ross River
Sabia   Semliki forest   Sudan Ebola   Venezuelan equine encephalitis   West Nile   Zaire Ebola   Zika

LEVEL 2

African green monkey simian foamy   Aroa   Australian bat lyssavirus   Avian metapneumovirus   Bagaza
Banna   Bayou   Black Creek Canal   Borna disease   Bovine enterovirus   Bovine viral diarrhea 1
Bunyamwera   Californian encephalitis   Candiru   Caraparu   Catu   Chandipura   Changuinola
Chapare   Dhori   Dobrava-Belgrade   Dugbe   Duvenhage   Eastern equine encephalitis   Edge Hill
Encephalomyocarditis   Equine rhinitis A-B   European bat lyssavirus 1-2   Everglades   Foot-and-mouth disease
Gadgets Gully   Getah   Great Island   Guama   Guaroa   Hantaan   Hendra   Highlands J   Ilheus
Irkut   Isfahan   Japanese encephalitis   Kairi   Kokobera   Kyasanur Forest disease   Laguna Negra
Langat   Lebombo   Ljungan   Louping ill   Macaque simian foamy   Maraba   Marituba   Madrid   Nyando
Mayaro   Mokola   Mucambo   Murray Valley encephalitis   New York   Newcastle disease   Ntaya   Powassan
Omsk hemorrhagic fever   Oriboca   Orungo   Parainfluenza 5   Pichinde   Piry   Pixuna   Seoul
Punta Toro   Puumala   Rift Valley fever   Rio Bravo   Rio Negro   Saaremaa   Sandfly fever Naples   St. Louis encephalitis   Tacaiuma
Shuni   Simian foamy   Simian virus 41   Sin Nombre   Sindbis   Tonate   Tula   Uganda S
Tai Forest Ebola   Tembusu   Thailand   Thogoto   Tick-borne encephalitis   Vesicular stomatitis Indiana   Vesicular stomatitis New Jersey
Una   Usutu   Uukuniemi   Vesicular stomatitis Alagoas   Whataroa   Whitewater Arroyo   Wyeomyia
Wesselsbron   Western equine encephalitis

viruses are even more concentrated at the top of the pyramid, with almost 90% of species at level 4. These patterns could simply be an artifact of our incomplete knowledge of virus diversity at lower levels of the pyramid, but they could also reflect real biological differences between viruses and other kinds of pathogens: viruses (especially DNA viruses) may be more likely to speciate within humans, or viruses (especially RNA viruses) that jump the species barrier into humans may be more capable of spreading in human populations or of rapidly evolving that capability (see below).

HUMAN-ADAPTED RNA VIRUSES

There is a semantic argument that only those viruses that are capable of persisting in human populations in the absence of a nonhuman reservoir should be described as "human" viruses. In our terminology these are, by definition, the level 4 viruses, comprising 47 species, 20 of which are not known to have any natural hosts other than humans. These 47 viruses—referred to here as "human adapted"—represent 12 families and 29 genera. Their most striking common characteristic is that almost all of them are transmitted by ingestion, inhalation, or direct contact; just 2 are transmitted by vectors.

There are several possible routes for a virus to reach level 4 on the pathogen pyramid (indicated by the arrows in Fig. 1). One possibility is that humans are exposed to a virus that is already capable of effective transmission between humans; i.e., the virus is pre-adapted to humans (noting that this does not preclude further adaptation once the virus has entered the human population). These have been termed "off-the-shelf" viruses. Such viruses may be rare, perhaps extremely rare, variants of the population in the nonhuman reservoir, in which case the main determinants of the rate at which such viruses enter the human population is the amount of genetic variability within the reservoir and the rate at which humans are exposed to the preadapted variants.

Another possibility is that the virus first enters the human population with limited ability to transmit between humans (i.e., level 3) but that it is able to evolve that ability before the otherwise self-limiting chain of infections dies out (12). These have been termed "tailor-made" viruses. Key determinants of the rate at which such viruses invade the human population are the frequency of primary infections and the virus mutation rate. We note that for a level 2 virus to evolve human transmissibility, this would have to happen during the course of a primary infection. Such infections presumably give evolution relatively little material to work with, and it may be that level 2 viruses are "dead ends" in an evolutionary sense as well as an epidemiological sense. For example, rabies infections are relatively common in humans and are likely to have been so for thousands of years, but human-transmissible variants have failed to materialize (with the proviso that rabies is technically a level 3 pathogen because of rare instances of human-to-human transmission via organ transplants).

Figure 2. All currently recognized human-infective RNA viruses categorized with respect to their ability to infect and transmit from humans (levels 2, 3, and 4 of the virus pyramid—see Fig. 1) and distinguished in terms of transmission route (green for vector-borne transmission, blue for other routes) and nature of diagnostic evidence (the viruses not in boldface type have only been reported in humans using serology-based methods). doi:10.1128/microbiolspec.OH-0001-2012.f2

The origins of the human-adapted RNA viruses are of considerable interest, not least as a possible pointer to the likely sources of future viral threats to human health. It has previously been noted (10) that we have information on the origins of only a small minority of human pathogens, including RNA viruses. However, as stated above, it seems likely that many of them arose by species jumps from other mammals or (less often) birds, perhaps followed by some diversification within humans (e.g., human enteroviruses or parainfluenza viruses). The direct transmission routes used by most of these viruses are consistent with their being crowd diseases; that is, in contrast to vector-borne viruses, the basic reproduction number increases with human population density.

MECHANISMS

As explained above, whether a virus is found at level 2, 3, or 4 of the pyramid reflects its ability to transmit from one human to another. Human demography and behavior play a key role in this, but of course, intrinsic properties of the virus are also crucial.

The first consideration is the ability of the virus to infect humans at all. Given the importance of this topic, we know surprisingly little about it. In effect, the question comes down to factors that restrict host range. Empirically, it does seem that the species barriers between different mammals, including humans, are very leaky: the majority of known mammal RNA viruses are capable of infecting multiple species. Only two studies (3, 13), however, have looked systematically at mechanisms, showing that use of a phylogenetically conserved receptor to gain entry to host cells is a necessary but not sufficient condition for a virus to be able to infect both humans and nonprimates. This result appears robust, but the data are incomplete because the cell receptor has yet to be identified for the majority of human viruses.

Gaining entry to host cells is only the first step in initiating an infection. The virus must also be capable of replicating in host cells, being released from host cells, evading the innate immune response, and perhaps becoming systemic. All of these processes depend on the specifics of the molecular interplay between virus and host, and all can contribute to the species barrier and host range restriction (14). The species barrier may be quantitative rather than qualitative, perhaps expressed by the need for a higher infective dose. In one of very few experimental studies of the species barrier (15), it was found that the 50% lethal dose for rabies virus obtained from foxes was up to a million times lower for foxes than it was for cats and dogs. Similarly, there is evidence that human influenza A viruses can replicate in chimpanzees but do so at a much lower rate (14).

The ability to get into (i.e., infect) a host does not equate with the ability to get out of (i.e., transmit from) that host. A key determinant of the ability to transmit is the virus's capacity to invade and replicate in cells of particular tissues, notably the lower gastrointestinal tract, the upper respiratory tract, the urogenital tract, or possibly the blood or skin. In a few cases, the determinants of tissue tropisms are well understood. For example, H5N1 influenza A transmits well from ducks and poultry but not from humans. This is because it utilizes a variant of the sialic acid receptor in the host cell membrane that occurs in the upper respiratory tract of ducks and poultry but is confined to the lower respiratory tract of humans (14).

Tissue tropisms inevitably play a key role in determining the route of virus transmission (e.g., respiratory, fecal-oral, or arthropod vector). It has been suggested that altering tissue tropism is harder for a virus to achieve than switching host species (9). This idea is borne out by the observation that transmission route tends to be a relatively deep-rooted trait in virus phylogenies, often to the level of family, in marked contrast to host range, which tends to be far more labile.

These few mechanistic and ecological insights fall well short of a proper understanding of why some kinds of viruses tend to occur at higher or lower levels of the pathogen pyramid. Host relatedness seems to play a role; hence, viruses from other primates do seem more likely to be transmissible in humans than those acquired from nonprimates, an idea supported by other studies of host relatedness and pathogen transmissibility (16). But not all highly transmissible human viruses have been acquired from other primates. Transmission route is also important; vector-borne viruses in particular seem to be relatively good at infecting humans but relatively poor at being transmitted by humans (17). It is possible that although humans are frequently exposed to vector-borne viruses, some of which are capable of setting up an infection, these viruses are not easily able to adapt to a new host (perhaps because any adaptation to a new vertebrate host must not compromise their interaction with the invertebrate vector [14]). Those that have adapted to humans—dengue and yellow fever—are ones that probably originated in other primates.

VIRULENCE

In public health terms the ability of a virus to spread through human populations is, of course, only part of the story; human RNA viruses also vary enormously in the degree of harm they cause, a characteristic referred to as virulence. In the context of human infections we generally regard a pathogen as virulent if it has a high case-fatality ratio or if infection routinely results in severe clinical disease. On this basis, HIV-1, severe acute respiratory syndrome coronavirus (SARS-CoV), and rabies would be regarded as virulent, whereas parainfluenza and rhinoviruses would not.

Pathogen virulence is a very complex phenomenon, reflecting properties of the pathogen, the host, and the interaction between them. It has been variously proposed that virulence is influenced by transmission route, host range, level of the pathogen pyramid, and the time that the pathogen and the host have had to coevolve (see reference 18 for an introduction to a large body of literature). These characteristics are not independent, so hypothesis testing is not straightforward, although some theories do look promising. For example, the only two recent instances of newly emerging level 4 pathogens—HIV-1 and SARS-CoV—are/were both spectacularly virulent, in line with ideas that the virulence of novel host-pathogen combinations need not be near any evolutionary optimum. The only two level 4 RNA viruses that are vector borne—dengue and yellow fever—are also relatively virulent, in line with ideas that vector-borne diseases can be more virulent because an ambulant host is not needed for transmission. There are also good examples of very virulent RNA viruses, such as rabies, for which humans are effectively dead-end hosts, in line with ideas that such infections are not subject to any evolutionary constraints because they do not contribute to the next generation of infections. On the other hand, many level 2 viruses, such as Newcastle disease virus, Sindbis virus, and others, result in only mild infections, so rabies may just lie at one end of a broad spectrum.

Another idea is that viruses acquired from particular kinds of reservoirs, primates versus nonprimates or mammals versus birds, might be especially virulent. The evidence, however, is inconsistent in this regard. It is true that some highly virulent human viruses, such as HIV-1 and dengue, were acquired from or are shared with other primates, our closest relatives. On the other hand, some highly virulent viruses are ultimately acquired from hosts much more distantly related to humans, such as H5N1 influenza A from birds or SARS and Nipah viruses from bats.

This important topic would clearly benefit from a systematic survey of the virulence of human RNA viruses (none has been published to date), which could be used to construct formal tests of the various hypotheses about pathogen virulence to be found in the evolutionary biology literature.

EMERGENCE AND THE CHANGING CAST OF RNA VIRUSES

New RNA virus species continue to be discovered, identified, or recognized in humans. Recent examples include Nelson Bay orthoreovirus, Irkut virus, primate T-lymphotropic virus 3, human coronavirus HKU1, and human rhinovirus C. Moreover, there is usually a backlog of reports of new human viruses that have yet to be formally recognized as species. Not all of these viruses will have recently invaded human populations; many will turn out to be long-standing human pathogens that have only recently been recognized or accepted as "species."

It is therefore important to understand that the continued accumulation of recognized human RNA virus species may reflect less the possibility that genuinely new viruses are continually emerging, most likely acquired from nonhuman reservoirs, than the fact that we are still getting to grips with the taxonomic diversity of viruses that have been with us for some time. This distinction between viruses that we have only just discovered and viruses that have only just discovered us is, of course, crucial in the context of emerging infectious diseases. If most of the so-called new viruses are not new at all, then this implies that events such as the advent of HIV/AIDS in the early 1980s or the curtailed SARS epidemic in 2003 may be just unusual, one-off occurrences with their own specific causes. If, on the other hand, genuinely new viruses are appearing all the time, then the HIVs and SARS-CoVs are more accurately regarded as just the highly visible tip of a much larger iceberg. Without a much more detailed and thorough understanding of the phylogenies and origins of all human viruses, not just those with high public health profiles, we cannot resolve this question.

Perhaps the most striking feature of recently discovered RNA viruses is that they tend to be much like the RNA viruses that we already knew about. They are members of the same virus families, have the same transmission routes, and share the same kinds of nonhuman hosts. If these newly recognized viruses are indeed emerging, then it seems as though there is nothing special about emergence, at least from a biologist's perspective. Even if this is correct, it is still often suggested that the *rate*, if not the biology, of pathogen emergence is higher in the early 21st century than it has been in the past. This reflects the notion that a variety of so-called drivers of emergence, ranging from human population growth to changes in farming methods, are combining to create a "perfect storm." This idea is difficult to evaluate critically. Arguably there have been only a handful of global emergence events in the past century, notably those involving HIV-1, variants of influenza A, and SARS-CoV. This is not a strikingly large number given that many of the other 40 or so human-adapted RNA viruses may have emerged only in the past few millennia. Of course, it could be argued that less dramatic events such as the geographical spread of West Nile virus or outbreaks of Ebola are more frequent now than they have been in the past, but that claim is even harder to test with any rigor.

Another side to this issue is rarely discussed. One recent study (8) reports that while the number of virus species accumulates, at the same time many of those recognized in past years or decades seem to have disappeared, these making up about one-third of the total. There is, of course, one well-known example of the eradication of a human RNA virus through human intervention, SARS-CoV, accompanying the even more impressive story of the eradication of smallpox, a DNA virus. However, there are many more examples of viruses that seem to have disappeared of their own accord, an unexpected observation worthy of careful consideration. There are several possibilities. First of all, rare infections, especially those with mild or common clinical presentations, may simply have been missed or no one has bothered to report them. Another possibility is that reports from earlier times are unreliable; for example, it is striking that no human cases of foot-and-mouth disease have been noticed since a handful of reports in the mid-1960s. But it seems likely that many of the missing viruses have indeed disappeared, at least temporarily, from humans, even if they are still present in nonhuman reservoirs. Some, of course, could reappear in humans at some point in the future: this has happened for the bat lyssaviruses, for example, and is a worrying possibility for SARS-CoV.

The implication of these missing viruses is that the extant diversity of human RNA viruses is perhaps closer to 100 species than the figure of 180 given earlier. The number of missing species corresponds, very roughly, to an average loss rate of 1 per year (8). Another way of expressing this is that there would have to be one new or rediscovered species of human RNA virus reported every year just to maintain the level of diversity that we are aware of at present.

A CONCEPTUAL MODEL

All of the above is consistent with the following conceptualization of the relationship between RNA viruses that can infect humans and those found in other kinds of hosts, particularly other mammals. Rather than being distinct groups, viruses of humans and viruses of other mammals are readily interchanged over evolutionary time. Some of the viruses that cross the species barrier into humans persist and may become human-adapted viruses, though this seems to be a relatively rare occurrence. Many of the others remain as zoonoses, and yet others disappear again. The repertoire of human viruses is therefore not fixed but is dynamic, over time scales measured in decades (8). However, this process is far from random. Although humans share their RNA viruses with many different mammalian taxa, those from other primates appear most likely to be capable of spreading through human populations. Similarly, although almost every family of viruses found in mammals contains species found in humans, some virus families seem to be capable of, at best, limited spread in human populations. This conceptual model is illustrated diagrammatically in Fig. 3.

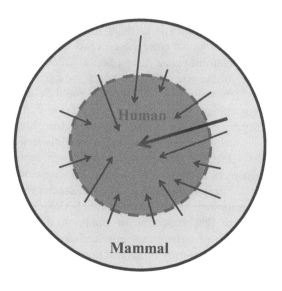

Figure 3. A schematic representation of the relationship between human viruses and viruses from other mammals. Human viruses are depicted as a subset of mammal viruses, only partially protected by a species barrier. There are frequent minor incursions of zoonotic viruses (small arrows), and many of these may not persist in human populations. Occasionally there may be a much more significant event (large arrow) whereby a mammal virus proves capable of establishing itself as a new human virus, perhaps involving adaptation to infect and transmit from humans.
doi:10.1128/microbiolspec.OH-0001-2012.f3

SURVEILLANCE AND RISK ASSESSMENT

Our conceptual model has practical implications for both disease surveillance and risk assessment, especially in the context of newly emerging infectious diseases.

The importance of early detection of potential epidemics or pandemics cannot be overstressed, a point made by several major studies (2). The early detection through clinical surveillance of SARS, coupled with effective intervention based on case isolation and quarantine, prevented a potentially catastrophic pandemic (19). A matter of some debate is whether or not surveillance should be extended into the nonhuman reservoirs of infection from which novel human pathogens are most likely to emerge—a concept sometimes referred to as "getting ahead of the curve."

It helps, of course, if we know what we are looking for and where best to look for it (20). We currently have only the beginnings of answers to these questions. Viruses, especially respiratory viruses, are often picked out as the most obvious threat to global public health (2). New viruses are very likely to have a zoonotic origin, almost certainly acquired from mammals or birds. Emergence events are most likely to occur in regions—so-called hot spots—that combine high human population densities with high densities of domestic animals and/or a high diversity of wildlife (4). All of this information is useful but falls well short of a recipe for designing a feasible global surveillance system (20).

One strategy to increase the likelihood of early detection is to implement sentinel surveillance in people in close, high-risk contact with animal populations, such as bush meat hunters or slaughterhouse workers. In tandem with recent advances in the technologies available for virus detection—especially those based on high-throughput nucleic acid sequencing—such programs should at least improve our knowledge of the diversity of viruses "out there" that humans are exposed to, a process sometimes referred to as "chatter" (10). Pathogen discovery programs, particularly in understudied taxa such as wild rodents and bats (21), should also add greatly to our knowledge of potential threats to human health.

Once a novel or previously unknown virus is identified, it is obviously important to assess any potential risk to public health. Initial assessments are generally based on the kind of comparative biology approach discussed here. A recent example of this is Schmallenberg virus, a novel virus first detected in sheep and cattle in northern Europe in 2011. Schmallenberg is a member of *Orthobunyavirus*, a diverse genus of vector-borne bunyaviruses that are found in a variety of hosts but especially in ungulates. Given these characteristics, and despite the fact that some distantly related orthobunyaviruses—notably Oropouche virus—do cause disease in and may even be transmitted by humans, Schmallenberg was provisionally designated low risk to humans and no human cases have yet been found (22). The even more recently reported Middle East respiratory syndrome (MERS) coronavirus (23) has rightly caused much more concern.

CONCLUDING REMARKS

Emerging diseases caused by RNA viruses are a One Health issue. There is a continuous interchange, over both epidemiological and evolutionary time scales, between viruses in humans and viruses in other animals that we cannot ignore. RNA viruses that pose serious threats to global public health have arisen repeatedly by jumping into humans from other animals. This has been going on for millennia and it continues today, as fast as ever and perhaps even faster. We have to anticipate that new viral threats will emerge in coming years or decades and we need to be prepared to rise to these new challenges as they appear.

It is worth pointing out that the first virus was discovered in nonhuman animals (foot-and-mouth disease virus at the very end of the 19th century) before they were identified in humans. The same is true (24) for several important kinds of viruses, such as retroviruses (and lentiviruses specifically), rotaviruses, papillomaviruses, and coronaviruses. A corollary of this is that veterinary rather than medical expertise may, at least initially, be our best source of knowledge about newly discovered viruses.

We have discussed the need for more effective surveillance for novel viruses but concluded that although attempts to characterize the kinds of viruses most likely to emerge are useful, precise prediction is not a realistic objective, for now at least. On the other hand, there could be considerable benefit from a better understanding of RNA virus diversity in the most important host species. At present we do not even have a complete inventory of the viruses in humans, and while we have some knowledge of the viruses in major livestock species, we know very little about the viruses present in wild mammals or birds. These gaps can and should be filled: we need to know what is out there now, and what might be waiting around the corner.

Acknowledgments. We thank Conor O'Halloran for assistance with data collation. We are grateful to past and present members of Epigroup and numerous collaborators for many fruitful discussions. This work is part of the VIZIONS project funded by a Wellcome Trust Strategic Award.

Citation. Woolhouse MEJ, Adair K, Brierley L. 2013. RNA viruses: a case study of the biology of emerging infectious diseases. Microbiol Spectrum 1(1):OH-0001-2012. doi:10.1128/microbiolspec.OH-0001-2012.

REFERENCES

1. **Taylor LH, Latham SM, Woolhouse MEJ.** 2001. Risk factors for human disease emergence. *Philos Trans R Soc Lond B Biol Sci* **356:**983–989.

2. **King DA, Peckham C, Waage JK, Brownlie J, Woolhouse MEJ.** 2006. Epidemiology. Infectious diseases: preparing for the future. *Science* **313:**1392–1393.

3. **Woolhouse MEJ, Scott FA, Hudson Z, Howey R, Chase-Topping M.** 2012. Human viruses: discovery and emergence. *Philos Trans R Soc Lond B Biol Sci* **367:**2864–2871.

4. **Jones KE, Patel NG, Levy MA, Storeygard A, Balk D, Gittleman JL, Daszak P.** 2008. Global trends in emerging infectious diseases. *Nature* **451:**990–993.

5. **Sharp PM, Hahn BH.** 2010. The evolution of HIV-1 and the origin of AIDS. *Philos Trans R Soc Lond B Biol Sci* **365:**2487–2494.

6. **Epstein JH, Field HE, Luby S, Pulliam JR, Daszak P.** 2006. Nipah virus: impact, origins, and causes of emergence. *Curr Infect Dis Rep* **8:**59–63.

7. **King AM, Adams MJ, Carstens EB, Lefkowitz EJ (ed).** 2012. *Virus Taxonomy: Ninth Report of the International Committee for the Taxonomy of Viruses.* Elsevier, Amsterdam, The Netherlands.

8. **Woolhouse MEJ, Adair K.** 2013. The diversity of human RNA viruses. *Future Virol* **8:**159–171.

9. **Kitchen A, Shackelton LA, Holmes EC.** 2011. Family level phylogenies reveal modes of macroevolution in RNA viruses. *Proc Natl Acad Sci USA* **108:**238–243.

10. **Wolfe ND, Dunavan CP, Diamond J.** 2007. Origins of major human infectious diseases. *Nature* **447:** 279–283.

11. **Woolhouse MEJ, Taylor LH, Haydon DT.** 2001. Population biology of multihost pathogens. *Science* **292:** 1109–1112.

12. **Antia R, Regoes RR, Koella JC, Bergstrom CT.** 2003. The role of evolution in the emergence of infectious diseases. *Nature* **426:**658–661.

13. **Bae SE, Son HS.** 2011. Classification of viral zoonosis through receptor pattern analysis. *BMC Bioinformatics* **12:**96. doi:10.1186/1471-2105-12-96.

14. **Kuiken T, Holmes EC, McCauley J, Rimmelzwaan GF, Williams CS, Grenfell BT.** 2006. Host species barriers to influenza virus infections. *Science* **312:**394–397.

15. **Blancou J, Aubert MF.** 1997. [Transmission of rabies virus: importance of the species barrier]. *Bull Acad Natl Med* **181:**301–312 (In French.)

16. **Streicker DG, Turmelle AS, Vonhof MJ, Kuzmin IV, McCracken GF, Rupprecht CE.** 2010. Host phylogeny constrains cross-species emergence and establishment of rabies virus in bats. *Science* **329:** 676–679.

17. **Woolhouse MEJ, Adair K.** 2013. Ecological and taxonomic variation among human RNA viruses. *J Clin Virol* [Epub ahead of print.] doi:10.1016/j.jcv.2013.02.019.

18. **Ebert D, Bull J.** 2008. The evolution and expression of virulence, p 153–167. *In* Stearns SC, Koella JC (ed), *Evolution in Health and Disease,* 2nd ed. Oxford University Press, Oxford, United Kingdom.

19. **World Health Organization Multicentre Collaborative Network for Severe Acute Respiratory Syndrome Diagnosis.** 2003. A multicentre collaboration to investigate the cause of severe acute respiratory syndrome. *Lancet* **361:**1730–1733.

20. **Morse SS, Mazet JA, Woolhouse M, Parrish CR, Carroll D, Karesh WB, Zambrana-Torrelio C, Lipkin WI, Daszak P.** 2012. Prediction and prevention of the next pandemic zoonosis. *Lancet* **380:** 1956–1965.

21. **Drexler JF, Corman VM, Müller MA, Maganga GD, Vallo P, Binger T, Gloza-Rausch F, Rasche A, Yordanov S, Seebens A, Oppong S, Adu Sarkodie Y, Pongombo C, Lukashev AN, Schmidt-Chanasit J, Stöcker A, Carneiro AJ, Erbar S, Maisner A, Fronhoffs F, Buettner R, Kalko EK, Kruppa T, Franke CR, Kallies R, Yandoko ER, Herrler G, Reusken C, Hassanin A, Krüger DH, Matthee S, Ulrich RG, Leroy EM, Drosten C.** 2012. Bats host major mammalian paramyxoviruses. *Nat Commun* **3:** 796. doi:10.1038/ncomms1796.

22. **Ducomble T, Wilking H, Stark K, Takla A, Askar M, Schaade L, Nitsche A, Kurth A.** 2012. Lack of evidence for Schmallenberg virus infection in highly exposed persons, Germany, 2012. *Emerg Infect Dis* **18:**1333–1335.

23. **Cotten M, Lam TT, Watson SJ, Palser AL, Petrova V, Grant P, Pybus OG, Rambaut A, Guan Y,**

Pillay D, Kellam P, Nastouli E. 2013. Full-genome deep sequencing and phylogenetic analysis of novel human betacoronavirus. *Emerg Infect Dis* **19:**736–742.

24. **Palmarini M.** 2007. A veterinary twist on pathogen biology. *PLoS Pathog* **3:**e12. doi:10.1371/journal.ppat.0030012.

25. **Woolhouse M, Antia R.** 2008. Emergence of new infectious diseases, p 215–228. *In* Stearns SC, Koella JC (ed), *Evolution in Health and Disease*, 2nd ed. Oxford University Press, Oxford, United Kingdom.

One Health: People, Animals, and the Environment
Edited by Ronald M. Atlas and Stanley Maloy
© 2014 American Society for Microbiology, Washington, DC
doi:10.1128/microbiolspec.OH-0006-2012

Chapter 7

Factors Impacting the Control of Rabies

Louis H. Nel[1]

INTRODUCTION

Rabies is a classical zoonosis that has been known to man for ages. The disease can be caused by several viral species in the *Lyssavirus* genus, but the original lyssavirus, the rabies virus (RABV) itself, is by far the most important from a zoonosis perspective. The extreme neurotropism of RABV and the evolutionarily conserved elements and structures of the mammalian brain suggest that this virus evolved an ultimate niche for replication, simultaneously exploiting classical social behavior of a wide diversity of hosts among the chiropters and carnivores. Substantial evidence indicates that RABV originated in bats and later switched hosts to yield globally disseminated canine rabies. Following the revolutionary work of Louis Pasteur, control and elimination of dog rabies was achieved in Europe, but widespread colonial introduction of European strains of dog RABV to other parts of the world occurred. Thus, dog rabies spread rapidly in the 1900s, and today the vast majority of the tens of thousands of annual human rabies cases stem from dog rabies, which has become endemic in the entire developing world. The fact that human rabies is preventable, through control in the dog reservoir on one hand and through effective prophylaxis in cases of exposure on the other hand, is an indictment of public health strategies and practices. This article discusses some of the many drivers that have contributed to the recurrent neglect of rabies in the modern world, as well as evolving One Health-based rabies control partnerships and initiatives that have been progressive, productive, and promising of true global benefits.

RHABDOVIRUSES

The majority of all viruses, in particular those that are zoonotic and hence relevant within the One Health context, are RNA viruses. Among RNA virus families, most animal viruses possess membranes (envelopes) (Fig. 1) acquired during their exit from infected cells, which then also facilitate entry into new host cells. In contrast, the vast majority of plant viruses do not have lipid membranes, given the architecture of plant cells, but there are two important exceptions. One is the *Bunyaviridae* (Rift Valley fever virus, Crimean Congo hemorrhagic fever virus, etc.), while the other is the

---

[1]Department of Microbiology and Plant Pathology, Faculty of Natural and Agricultural Sciences, University of Pretoria, Pretoria 0001, South Africa.

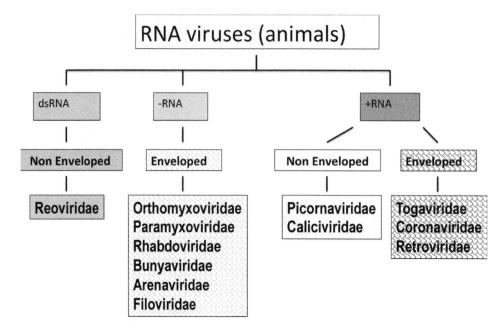

Figure 1. Genome type and membrane presence of the major families of animal RNA viruses. dsDNA, double-stranded DNA. doi:10.1128/microbiolspec.OH-0006-2012.f1

Rhabdoviridae. There are a vast number of different rhabdoviruses that infect an astonishing array of hosts within the insect, plant, fish, and mammalian orders (1). However, not only are the rhabdoviruses of insects the most numerous within the family, but those rhabdoviruses of hosts other than insects are mostly transmitted by insects. A peculiar exception to insect transmissibility is the topic of this article, the lyssaviruses, of which RABV is the type species. Rabies, together with its unique transmission mechanism, is a classical zoonosis that has horrified humans for ages (2).

LYSSAVIRUS DIVERSITY

The *Lyssavirus* genus comprises 12 species, many of which have been discovered in recent years (Table 1). With the discovery of new viruses came the realization of the extensive diversity within the genus and the likelihood that more species remain to be discovered. However, it is the original lyssavirus, RABV, that is by far the most important from a zoonosis perspective (3–5).

THE EMERGENCE AND EVOLUTION OF RABV

Canine rabies has in all likelihood existed since antiquity, with ancient documents describing a disease transmissible from dogs to man with epidemiological and clinical features that closely resemble rabies (6). More recently, with the advancement of sequence analysis and modeling, the principle of RABV host switching from chiropters to carnivores was demonstrated with the use of molecular clocks (7). The interpretation of

Table 1. Known lyssaviruses and their associated hosts and geographic distribution[a]

Viral species	Main reservoir hosts	Other hosts documented	Known distribution
Rabies virus	Carnivores and chiropters (insectivorous and hematophagous)	Variety of mammals including man	Universal; only a few countries are rabies free
Lagos bat virus	Chiropters (frugivorous)	Carnivores, insectivorous bat	Africa, widespread
Mokola virus	Shrews	Variety of mammals including man	Africa, widespread
Duvenhage virus	Chiropters (insectivorous)	Man	Africa, southeastern countries
European bat lyssavirus-1	Chiropters (insectivorous)	Variety of mammals including man	Western and Eastern Europe, Russia
European bat lyssavirus-2	Chiropters (insectivorous)	Man	Western Europe
Australian bat lyssavirus	Chiropters (frugivorous and insectivorous)	Man	Australia
Aravan virus	Chiropters (insectivorous)	NA[b]	Kyrgyzstan
Khujand virus	Chiropters (insectivorous)	NA	Tajikistan
Irkut virus	Chiropters (insectivorous)	NA	Siberia
West Caucasian bat virus	Chiropters (insectivorous)	NA	Caucasus Mountains
Shimoni bat lyssavirus	Chiropters (insectivorous)	NA	Kenya
Bokeloh bat lyssavirus	Chiropters (insectivorous)	NA	Germany
Ikoma lyssavirus	African civet	NA	Tanzania

[a]Bokeloh bat and Ikoma lyssaviruses are tentatively included as new species.
[b]NA, not applicable.

molecular clocks in RNA virus evolution requires much care, considering the propensity of RNA viruses to mutate rapidly, the formation of quasispecies, and the subsequent positive or adaptive selection (8). Nevertheless, the approach is useful in determining ancestral links and pathways of divergence, although attempts to precisely date such events may be less dependable.

With the exception of the African Mokola virus (9, 10), all lyssavirus species are exclusively viruses of bats or, in the case of RABV, occur in bats and terrestrial mammals. For one recently discovered lyssavirus, Ikoma, only one case is known to date (civet cat, Tanzania), and it is not possible to conclude on the likely reservoir species (11). As far as the bat lyssaviruses are concerned, most recent insights suggest a propensity for specific RABV variants to most efficiently spill over to bat species that are phylogenetically close to the parental host species, regardless of spatial and other ecological factors (12). Furthermore, those lyssaviruses of bats occurring in tropical and subtropical climates (as opposed to temperate regions of the world) evolve at a significantly faster rate, probably due to more sustained yearlong bat activity (13). This factor is likely to have been a key contributor to the diversity of lyssaviruses found in the tropical and subtropical regions of Africa (14, 15). Considering the above and given the genetic diversity of the bat lyssaviruses, as opposed to the relative closely related assemblage of terrestrial RABV, the evidence for the spillover from bats to yield globally disseminated canine rabies is substantial. In the modern day, such events are well documented. A decade-long record of the spillovers of a bat variant of RABV into skunks and foxes, with subsequent propagation within the spillover host species, provides one of the best showcases of the natural frequency of such events (16).

RABIES VIRUS: AN OPPORTUNIST PAR EXCELLENCE

The extreme neurotropism of RABV and the evolutionarily conserved elements and structures of the mammalian brain suggest that this virus evolved an ultimate niche for replication. To reach this niche, furtive evasion of immune responses is achieved while transport within immune-privileged neuronal systems is rapid and uninterrupted (17). After utilizing the neuronal tissues of the brain for extensive replication, the virus transports to the salivary glands (primarily, but also to other locations). Here efficient replication is followed by viral passage into the oral cavity, with high numbers of infectious virions accumulating in saliva. Thus, efficient transmission is guaranteed should saliva and virus be exposed to mucosal tissues or breach the dermal protection of a new host in another way. In dogs and other carnivores, this is in fact often achieved through the ability of the virus, during neurovirulent infection of the brain, to render the infected animal aggressive, warranting biting events that allow virus entry into new hosts. Given the transmission mechanism, it is evident that RABV very efficiently exploits the classical social behavior of mammals. Such reservoir species belong in particular, but not exclusively, to the *Carnivora* and the *Chiroptera* orders (3, 18, 19). The entire process, inclusive of neurotropism, neurovirulence, evasion/exploitation of host immunity, glandular passage, and direct-contact transmission, is highly efficient (Fig. 2).

PATHOGENICITY AND IMMUNE EVASION OR AMBIVALENCE AND THE BLOOD-BRAIN BARRIER

Following a transmission event, i.e., passage of virus through the dermis or otherwise into cellular tissues of a susceptible host, it is possible, but still undetermined, that virus may replicate in nonneuronal cells after receptor-mediated entry. One likely receptor for such purpose is nicotinic acetylcholine (20). Nicotinic acetylcholine, given its postsynaptic location, is unlikely to serve for entry into motor neurons, but enriches RABV at the neuromuscular junction and could be used to infect muscle cells. Another good receptor candidate is p75 neurotrophin (p75NTR), which is widespread on neuronal as well as nonneuronal cells, including muscles (21). p75NTR expression renders resistant cells permissive, but on the other hand, there is no difference in disease progression in p75NTR-deficient and wild-type mice (22). One study has shown that RABV and European bat lyssavirus-1 bind to p75NTR, while other bat lyssaviruses do not (23). It is also understood that dog RABV strains are highly specific for neurons while bat strains can also infect astrocytes, but much remains to be clarified with regard to the disease progression of bat lyssaviruses in their respective reservoirs. For RABV, perhaps the most likely receptor for neuronal entry is neuronal cell adhesion molecule (NCAM) (24). This molecule is widespread on all peptide hormone-producing cells and neurons, where its presynaptic location renders it an ideal receptor candidate for RABV. The expression of NCAM renders virus-resistant cells permissive, providing some experimental evidence. In NCAM-deleted transgenic mice, animals remain susceptible to RABV infection, but the disease is markedly delayed, indicating a role for NCAM, albeit not essential (24). It thus appears that RABV receptors may be ubiquitous and that different receptors and coreceptors are involved, depending on RABV strain and lyssavirus species. These aspects are not well understood and are likely to play a major role in the puzzling

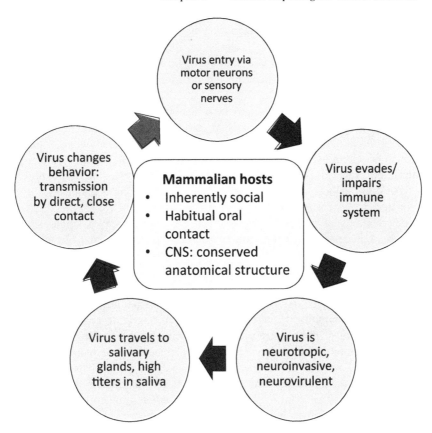

Figure 2. The rabies cycle. Lyssaviruses are uniquely adapted to effectively exploit the ecological and anatomical characteristics of their primary mammalian hosts and vectors. CNS, central nervous system. doi:10.1128/microbiolspec.OH-0006-2012.f2

differences in tropism, pathogenicity, and infection outcomes of different lyssavirus species and RABV variants.

Once the synaptic cleft has been bridged, RABV moves from the axon terminal toward the neuron cell body (site of virus replication and subsequent crossing of the synaptic cleft to reach the next-in-line neuron). The mode of transport, in this retrograde direction, was thought to be enabled by interaction of viral proteins with the dynein light chain 8 (25, 26), but later findings disputed this concept, suggesting that the light chain 8 instead impacts on a transcriptional level (27). Nevertheless, axonal travel directed toward the brain is fast (50 to 100 mm/day), and the strict unidirectional traverse has also made RABV an ideal tool as a tracer in studies of neuronal networks and anatomy (28).

Replication of lyssaviruses involves the synthesis of five subgenomic mRNAs, one for each of the viral proteins (3′-N-P-M-G-L-5′). The order of genes on the RNA genome determines the corresponding number of transcripts, with the rate of transcription gradually declining from the 3′ to the 5′ end of the genome (14). The relative copy numbers of individual proteins are thus well regulated and important in maintaining viral phenotype. For example, changing the position or copy numbers of the *G* gene on the viral RNA with corresponding higher rates of *G* transcription has been shown to have an attenuating effect on the virus phenotype (28, 29). However, although it has been shown that pathogenicity could correlate inversely with the rate of *G* expression in some studies (29, 30), other recent findings discredited this concept, illustrating the fact that the factors that influence lyssavirus virulence are multiple and complex (31). While the influence of G copy numbers on virus pathogenicity may be in doubt, various studies have demonstrated that G is likely to be a major determinant of pathogenicity. For example, Ito et al. (32) demonstrated that a nonpathogenic RABV is converted into a pathogenic virus through three mutations within the *G* gene and that these mutations affect pathogenicity through their impact on virus cell-cell spread in the CNS. Classically, a single mutation at Arg-333 in RABV G has been associated with attenuation, playing a major role in vaccine development (33, 34). It has become clear that various proteins, inclusive of G, P, and M, can be determinants of pathogenicity and that the importance of single amino acid changes should be considered within a larger and cooperative context of the entire viral genotype.

Apart from the role of individual proteins and domains on these proteins, there is substantial evidence that RABV pathogenicity correlates inversely with the rate of replication and the capacity to induce neuronal apoptosis. Among others, RABV uniquely evades host innate immunity by selective targeting of interferon-activated signal transduction and activator of transcription (STAT) proteins by the viral phosphoprotein (P). STAT signaling is inhibited in various ways (17). It appears that such unique mechanisms of immune evasion are conserved among all lyssaviruses (35). There seems to be an ambivalent role for the innate immune response to RABV pathogenesis (36). Transgenic mice that overexpress LGP2 (a regulator of RIG1-mediated innate immunity) and thus have an impairment of innate immunity have improved survival from rabies. Such intervention actually favors RABV elimination from the brain. Thus, RABV appears to exploit innate immunity to develop an immunoevasive strategy. The mouse blood-brain barrier (BBB) remains firmly closed in the case of infection with a virulent RABV strain, while the BBB opens when infection is with an attenuated RABV strain (37). This loss of BBB integrity is more extensive in the cerebellum than the cerebral cortex, and with the possible exception of CD8, immune effectors for virus clearance more commonly target the cerebellum. The observation that attenuated RABV infection promotes RABV-specific antibody entry into CNS tissues, and that passively administered RABV-specific antibodies can cross the BBB under certain conditions, has specific relevance for future rabies therapy (38).

CONTROL OF DOG RABIES AND EMERGENCE OF WILDLIFE RABIES IN THE DEVELOPED WORLD

The establishment of rabies cycles in dogs became an important public health concern in the New World starting in the 1800s. Following the revolutionary work of Louis Pasteur, subsequent developments in rabies vaccinology allowed for the eradication of New World dog rabies—first in the United Kingdom and Western Europe and later in North America (39, 40). However, an important caveat was to follow: the emergence of wildlife rabies. In Europe, it was the red fox that became the principal rabies vector and reservoir, while raccoons, skunks, various fox species and coyotes, and other species became important reservoirs in North America (39, 41, 42). Extensive vaccination and breakthroughs in oral vaccination allowed for the eradication of fox rabies in Western Europe, but wildlife rabies persists in North America, where its control through oral vaccination campaigns remains exceedingly costly (43, 44).

EMERGENCE OF DOG RABIES IN THE DEVELOPING WORLD AND THE BURDEN OF HUMAN RABIES

At the time when control and elimination of dog rabies was achieved in the New World, widespread colonial introduction of European strains of dog RABV to other parts of the world occurred (45). Thus, dog rabies spread rapidly in the 1900s, and today the vast majority of the tens of thousands of annual human rabies cases stem from dog rabies, which has become endemic in the entire developing world. In Africa, several hundred million people are estimated to be at risk of endemic dog rabies, with more than 30,000 human deaths annually. In Asia, current estimates indicate as many as 40,000 human deaths annually (46). The fact that human rabies is entirely preventable, through control in the dog reservoir on the one hand and through effective prophylaxis in cases of exposure on the other hand, is a major indictment of public health strategies and practices in the developing world.

FACTORS IMPACTING THE CONTROL OF RABIES

Why then has a highly fatal but preventable zoonosis progressively established itself as a neglected disease throughout Africa and Asia? Many factors contribute, but the lack of priority is perhaps most strongly driven by institutional juggling of the responsibility for rabies control and poor awareness or appreciation of the public health impact of rabies. Considering classical priorities in the developing world, it is worth reflecting that rabies is not associated with any agricultural importance. The impetus for effective control would likely be greater if rabies had a major economic impact. To an extent this is the case in some countries where the laboratory-confirmed rabies cases in cattle (incidental, spillover hosts) regularly outnumber those cases confirmed in dogs and other carnivores (rabies reservoirs) (14, 47). The veterinary neglect of dogs is exacerbated by the fact that dogs are typically unrestricted and free roaming in areas of Asia, Africa, and Latin America where dog rabies is endemic. These animals are excluded from classical health care systems, as only a small minority of owned and restricted dogs are of interest to private veterinarians and veterinary services (48). The resources needed for primary health care of large, free-roaming dog populations are significant and may not seem warranted for a disease that is seen as an issue of public health. On the public health side, misdiagnosis is common (49, 50), as rabies frequently presents with a variety of non-specific clinical symptoms, including paralysis, which occurs in as many as one-third of cases (51, 52, 72). Apart from overlapping symptoms, the degree of professional ignorance of rabies in some areas where dog rabies is endemic is often puzzling (49, 53). It is also true that rabies primarily affects rural community types, characterized by poverty, remote location, poor infrastructure, and negligible health care. Collectively, poor surveillance and diagnosis in the animal reservoir and misdiagnosis, ignorance, and insufficient services on the medical side combine to fuel the circle of neglect (Fig. 3), allowing

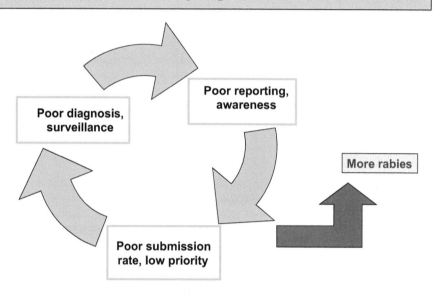

Figure 3. The perpetuation of a neglected zoonosis. Rabies is a classically under-estimated disease in the developing world, where dog rabies is endemic, given nonspecific clinical symptoms, poor surveillance, and lack of laboratory diagnosis. doi:10.1128/microbiolspec.OH-0006-2012.f3

for the progression of rabies. Estimates published as long ago as 2005 indicated that the disease threatened more than 3 billion people in Asia and Africa and in more than 150 countries and territories (54).

On the global health agenda, a loss of newsworthiness and geopolitical issues may well have influenced advocacy and disease priority. Dog rabies, although spectacularly persistent and opportunistic, is prevalent only in the developing world and does not necessarily demand the same attention as some new diseases with pandemic potential, such as those associated with novel strains of influenza or coronaviruses. In reality, mortality due to rabies, which occurs mostly in children and without any other health risk factors, outstrips many other infectious diseases that are perceived to be more important (54, 55), and rabies also has the highest case-fatality ratio of all infectious diseases of humans (52). Thus the World Health Organization (WHO) recognizes rabies as notifiable. Unfortunately, a few countries where rabies is particularly prevalent—such as India—do not (56), and structures for publication of rabies statistics by the WHO were not well supported by many member countries. The World Organisation for Animal Health (Office International des Epizooties, or OIE) also regards rabies as notifiable, with publication of statistics on the World Animal Health Information Database (WAHID) (57), but statistics from countries where dog rabies is endemic generally do not correlate with even the most conservative estimates (46, 58).

The inevitable neglect of a disease associated with poverty and for which the primary reservoir is not livestock is perhaps predictable, and thus rabies is a classic example of a disease for which any hope of future control is dependent on the unconditional execution and instruction of the "One Health" paradigm on global, regional, and national levels.

ASPIRATIONS FOR A RABIES-FREE WORLD AND EVOLUTION OF NEW PARTNERSHIPS

A number of diverse groups and organizations that are independent from broader United Nations bodies or reference organizations such as the WHO or the OIE focus on rabies activities in different parts of the world. For example, the Latin-America National Rabies Directors Network (REDIPRA, established in 1983) is an important coalition for the region. The Rabies in the Americas Association was formed in 1990 and among others hosts an annual Rabies in the Americas (RITA) meeting, the largest annual rabies conference that consistently attracts a global audience. In Europe, Rabies in Eurasia meetings took place under the auspices of the OIE in Kiev (2003) and Paris (2007), but more recently the Middle East and Central Eastern Europe Rabies Expert Bureau (MEEREB, 2010) was also formed. Focusing on the problem of rabies in Asia, the Rabies in Asia Foundation (RIA, 2006) and the Asia Rabies Expert Bureau (AREB, 2004) are also new initiatives. The Southern and Eastern African Rabies Group (SEARG) was formed in 1992 as a coalition of anglophone countries of the continent. In francophone Africa, the Africa Rabies Expert Bureau (AFROREB, 2008), driven by Sanofi Pasteur, was more recently established. While these organizations epitomize the effort of rabies champions, experts, and interest groups, more is needed to curb dog rabies and thus prevent human rabies. For the parts of the world where dog rabies is endemic, only REDIPRA and the Pan American Health Organization in Latin America can claim tangible successes in rabies control through a One Health approach. There is no pan-Asian or pan-African approach to rabies control, underlining these parts of the world as the problem areas where almost all cases of human rabies occur. Since rabies is so effectively controlled in the developed world, but a serious problem across the entire continents of Africa and Asia, it is clear that a global approach is needed to promote and address the realities of the persistent progression of dog rabies among the world's poor.

The Alliance for Rabies Control was formed in Scotland in 2006 and became the Global Alliance for Rabies Control (GARC) in 2007, in that year also launching as one of its first major initiatives the inaugural World Rabies Day (WRD). WRD, sanctioned by the United Nations, falls on September 28 (the anniversary of Louis Pasteur's death) and has been remarkably successful in promoting rabies initiatives across the world. Since the inaugural event, participatory activities and the numbers of countries involved in subsequent WRD initiatives have consistently increased in leaps and bounds from year to year, clearly illustrating the need for such messages in communities across the world (59). The principal objective and achievement of WRD remains advocacy and the generation of widespread awareness of rabies and its true burden—the key first step toward the quest for and implementation of any (or better) disease control measures. Indeed, 2007 also saw the launching of a GARC rabies control program in Bohol, Philippines, that in due course proved to be quite successful and led the way for other similar initiatives. GARC also established the Partners for Rabies Prevention (PRP) in 2008, as a widely representative group of rabies stakeholders and experts who endeavor to support leading public-private rabies control activities across the world. In essence, PRP provides a uniquely uniting enterprise that allows for collective strategic thinking and generation of ideas and plans through the utility of diverse skills, experiences, and capabilities of the global spectrum of partners. As one of the first undertakings, PRP developed and launched a blueprint for rabies elimination and control, in a quest to meaningfully assist in potential or existing national and international rabies interventions. This blueprint is essentially a novel and dynamic operational toolkit for rabies elimination that is entirely built on the principles of the One Health concept (60).

New vigor and global partnering to address the neglect of dog rabies in the developing world gradually resulted in several projects that have the core objective of demonstrating human rabies prevention through dog rabies control and eventual elimination. Three such large-scale demonstration projects are supported and partially funded by the Bill & Melinda Gates Foundation and administered by the WHO and represent a significant step in raising the profile of rabies in the developing world (61, 62). The project sites are located in Asia (Philippines, Visayas Islands) and Africa (southeastern Tanzania and KwaZulu-Natal Province, South Africa). These programs will serve as a platform for generating information on the unique challenges and solutions facing each site, with a view to extending these projects to neighboring regions. It is estimated that eliminating rabies in these three areas will save in excess of 50 million people from the constant fear of rabies (62).

The selection and establishment of these programs was based on detailed plans that promised success in demonstrating effective control and elimination of dog rabies. Apart from dog rabies endemicity, other criteria included (i) a good record of rabies surveillance; (ii) disease burden in dogs and humans well supported by laboratory diagnosis; (iii) a general understanding of the epidemiology of rabies in the region; (iv) potential to benefit other countries in the region, based on demographic and geographic similarities; and (5) proven, government-driven efforts or commitment to control the disease in dogs (see, for example, references 63–65).

Rabies is a complex disease, and the components of programs to control the disease are therefore equally multifaceted. Thus, one of the intentions of these demonstration projects has been the development or implementation of research into new technologies and biologics to improve strategies for dog rabies control. For these programs, typical research activities include, among others aspects of vaccinology, epidemiology, diagnostics, animal primary health, human health, dog ecology, dog population management, and knowledge, attitudes, and practices of the affected communities. Generally, the benefits gained from international interest, participation, and contributions to these control programs were evident from early on (63), and success in one of the fundamental goals of the Gates Foundation/WHO programs, i.e., human rabies prevention, has already been reported (58, 73). The aim of these projects is to demonstrate and enable a paradigm shift toward an ideal One Health approach in dealing with rabies. Clearly, maintaining isolated rabies-free regions in Africa or Asia will be nearly impossible and pan-continental strategies, grown from successful regions/programs, will be necessary for sustained control. Such a lofty ideal will be incredibly challenging to fulfill. However, the largest hurdle to the elimination of dog and human rabies remains the lack of political priority or will and not the lack of methodology, biologics, or funding.

As catalysts for national and global approaches to dog rabies control and human rabies prevention, demonstration or pilot programs are essential. Thus, apart from the Gates Foundation/WHO programs, several other valuable endeavors have followed the One Health-based dog rabies control successes of the developed world and more recently of Latin America. Quite a few of these have been focused on parts of Asia, one of which, in Bohol, was mentioned previously as an early initiative after the formation of GARC. This is a program that explicitly sought to elicit community-based advocacy, planning, and execution of rabies control actions. Since its inception, many partners—other than GARC and the provincial government—have contributed with treasure and/or talent (66). The successes within this program illustrate modern-day successes in rabies control in keeping with the One Health paradigm and should be inspirational to others concerned with the devastation of rabies in the entirety of Southeast Asia.

In Sri Lanka, the World Society for the Protection of Animals (WSPA), the Blue Paw Trust, and the Colombo Municipal Council formed a partnership to address management of the Colombo dog population, including vaccination of the entire dog population and creating rabies awareness (67). In Indonesia, rabies was recently introduced in Bali. Toward the end of 2009, a coordinated and effective rabies control program developed and supported mass vaccination projects (59, 68).

THE FUTURE

A key concept from the programs described above, and those that will follow in the aspiration for a world free of dog rabies, is a clear comprehension of the complexity of a classical zoonosis that can only be addressed with a One Health approach that embraces both human and animal public health doctrines inclusive of scientific method and research, community and governmental function, communication and education, and secured priority funding.

Many drivers contribute to the recurrent neglect of rabies in the modern world (Fig. 3). Important key words reflect classical features of neglect: (i) "a lack of" priority, supplies (vaccines or affordable biologics), capacity (local and beyond), data (to understand burden), models (to demonstrate feasibility), persistence (toward sustainability), and awareness (about the disease or options for control); and (ii) "poor or insufficient" notifiability of rabies, availability of educational materials and initiatives, communication among stakeholders, technology transfer from research to practice, and ability to interest major funding bodies.

Rabies remains endemic throughout the developing world and, for all the reasons discussed, loses visibility as it falls between authorities concerned with human health and with animal health. Poor epidemiological surveillance and inconsistent reporting—including to the responsible global authoritative bodies—have created a lack of rabies awareness and lack of appreciation of the burden that it conveys to the peoples of the world. The absence of reliable and sustained rabies data compromises the priority that the control of rabies should be given, to the extent that the ultimate objective of eradication will always be difficult to justify on national levels or to global funding agencies.

The above issues need to be effectively addressed if the cycle of neglect is to be overcome. To a large extent the new global partnerships and road maps, with resultant pilot and demonstration programs, are exactly focused on these considerations that have been identified as the major drivers of the current-day dog rabies crisis. For example, the value and importance of dog ecology and welfare, inclusive of new inventions such as effective and appropriate immune contraception and the quest for efficacious and cost-effective vaccines for oral vaccination of dogs, are key paradigms in the global rabies expert community. The demand for better surveillance is supported by the offering of new diagnostic tests that are as reliable as the classical gold standard but faster and simpler to perform (69). The value of molecular epidemiology with added possibilities to determine and predict transmission pathways is and should be promoted, as this will have a major impact on the fine-tuning of operational steps during rabies control campaigns.

It is true that recent rabies control partnerships and initiatives have been progressive, productive, and promising of true global benefits. However, as with any disease control program, big or small, collective persistence will be required to ensure consistent progress and sustainability of early successes. Herein lies a significant challenge. For stakeholders and experts concerned with rabies, it will be important to qualify and advocate the burden that this disease inflicts on humanity. As an opportunistic virus, rabies continues to spread into an expanding global dog reservoir, and the dynamics of the impacts of the disease need to be reassessed in line with its past and continued neglect. Such assessment is the cornerstone of responsible global advocacy toward achieving and maintaining appropriate priority on the national and international agendas for meaningful disease control. Although an earlier estimate of the burden of rabies was a useful exercise (54), it was primarily based on evidence from fragmented areas/countries in Africa and Asia and is in danger of becoming outdated as rabies rapidly progresses in the modern era. Therefore, a priority of the PRP and GARC had been to reevaluate the universal burden of rabies, inclusive of prophylaxis costs, disability-adjusted life year (DALY) scores, and economic burden models that would allow for meaningful evaluation within the entire spectrum of public health interests and priorities. But while rabies is a serious public health issue, it remains, in the developing world, primarily a disease of dogs. Its agricultural impact is fairly minimal—so the economic burden, while not zero, is perhaps easily dismissed when compared with those presented by a plethora of livestock diseases. Thus the necessity for the veterinary sector to buy into the One Health paradigm remains a primary mission. It is in this regard that international, national, and/or local organizations promoting animal welfare (WSPA, Humane Society International, International Fund for Animal Welfare, etc.) have become important players, by advocating and implementing appropriate practices for the care, treatment, and management of dog populations in areas where dog rabies is endemic. In addition, the OIE has recently released its Fifth Strategic Plan, which includes the One Health approach, committing to improved cooperation with human-animal-environment interfaces (70). This uniformity will require true collaboration between medical, veterinary, and wildlife sectors—the One Health approach. Because of the need for consistent and transparent data (74), appropriate actions and changes will be necessary and feasible. In addition, pathways for rabies control will have to be pan-continental and rely on promising declarations of global cooperation between the OIE, WHO, and the Food and Agricultural Organization of the United Nations (71), as they hone respective disease-fighting coordination mechanisms.

CONCLUDING REMARKS

Rabies control is a long-term goal that cannot be driven by economics alone. Those countries and regions willing to attempt elimination of rabies will have to realize that the substantial investment required will yield slow, albeit inevitable returns. The One Health model perfectly applies to rabies and reminds us that, even in the modern world, collective thinking is capable of producing simple but novel concepts that will allow for the solving of age-old and new public health problems, given appropriate and sustained institutional and sociopolitical support.

Citation. Nel LH. 2013. Factors impacting the control of rabies. Microbiol Spectrum 1(2):OH-0006-2012. doi:10.1128/microbiolspec.OH-0006-2012.

REFERENCES

1. **Hogenhout SA, Redinbaugh MG, Ammar el-D.** 2003. Plant and animal rhabdovirus host range: a bug's view. *Trends Microbiol* **11:**264–271.
2. **Baer GM.** 2007. The history of rabies, p 1–22. *In* Jackson AC, Wunner WH (ed), *Rabies*, 2nd ed. Elsevier/Academic Press, Amsterdam, The Netherlands.
3. **King AA, Turner GS.** 1993. Rabies: a review. *J Comp Pathol* **108:**1–39.
4. **Nel L.** 2005. Vaccines for lyssaviruses other than rabies. *Expert Rev Vaccines* **4:**533–540.
5. **Malerczyk C, Nel LH, Gniel D, Blumberg L.** 2010. Rabies in South Africa and the FIFA Soccer World Cup: travelers' awareness for an endemic but neglected disease. *Hum Vaccin* **6:**385–389.
6. **Fales FM.** 2010. Chapter 2: Mesopotamia. *Handb Clin Neurol* **95:**15–27.
7. **Badrane H, Tordo N.** 2003. Host switching in *Lyssavirus* history from the Chiroptera to the Carnivora orders. *J Virol* **75:**8096–8104.
8. **Domingo E, Sheldon J, Perales C.** 2012. Viral quasispecies evolution. *Microbiol Mol Biol Rev* **76:**159–216.
9. **Nel L, Jacobs J, Jaftha J, von Teichman B, Bingham J, Olivier M.** 2000. New cases of Mokola virus infection in South Africa: a genotypic comparison of southern African virus isolates. *Virus Genes* **20:**103–106.
10. **Sabeta CT, Markotter W, Mohale DK, Shumba W, Wandeler AI, Nel LH.** 2007. Mokola virus in domestic mammals, South Africa. *Emerg Infect Dis* **13:**1371–1373.
11. **Marston DA, Horton DL, Ngeleja C, Hampson K, McElhinney LM, Banyard AC, Haydon D, Cleaveland S, Rupprecht CE, Bigambo M, Fooks AR, Lembo T.** 2012. Ikoma lyssavirus, highly divergent novel lyssavirus in an African civet. *Emerg Infect Dis* **18:**664–667.
12. **Streicker DG, Turmelle AS, Vonhof MJ, Kuzmin IV, McCracken GF, Rupprecht CE.** 2010. Host phylogeny constrains cross-species emergence and establishment of rabies virus in bats. *Science* **329:**676–679.
13. **Streicker DG, Lemey P, Velasco-Villa A, Rupprecht CE.** 2012. Rates of viral evolution are linked to host geography in bat rabies. *PLoS Pathog* **8:**e1002720.
14. **Nel LH, Rupprecht CE.** 2007. Emergence of lyssaviruses in the Old World: the case of Africa. *Curr Top Microbiol Immunol* **315:**161–193.
15. **Markotter W, Kuzmin I, Rupprecht CE, Nel LH.** 2008. Phylogeny of Lagos bat virus: challenges for lyssavirus taxonomy. *Virus Res* **135:**10–21.
16. **Kuzmin IV, Shi M, Orciari LA, Yager PA, Velasco-Villa A, Kuzmina NA, Streicker DG, Bergman DL, Rupprecht CE.** 2012. Molecular inferences suggest multiple host shifts of rabies viruses from bats to mesocarnivores in Arizona during 2001–2009. *PLoS Pathog* **8:**e1002786.
17. **Schnell MJ, McGettigan JP, Wirblich C, Papaneri A.** 2010. The cell biology of rabies virus: using stealth to reach the brain. *Nat Rev Microbiol* **8:**51–61.
18. **Rupprecht CE, Hanlon CA, Hemachudha T.** 2002. Rabies re-examined. *Lancet Infect Dis* **2:**327–343.
19. **Scott T, Hasse R, Nel L.** 2012. Rabies in kudu (*Tragelaphus strepsiceros*). *Berl Munch Tierarztl Wochenschr* **125:**236–241.

20. **Lentz TL, Burrage TG, Smith AL, Crick J, Tignor GH.** 1982. Is the acetylcholine receptor a rabies virus receptor? *Science* **215:**182–184.

21. **Tuffereau C, Bénéjean J, Blondel D, Kieffer B, Flamand A.** 1998. Low-affinity nerve-growth factor receptor (P75NTR) can serve as a receptor for rabies virus. *EMBO J* **17:**7250–7259.

22. **Tuffereau C, Schmidt K, Langevin C, Lafay F, Dechant G, Koltzenburg M.** 2007. The rabies virus glycoprotein receptor p75NTR is not essential for rabies virus infection. *J Virol* **81:**13622–13630.

23. **Tuffereau C, Desmézières E, Bénèjean J, Jallet C, Flamand A, Tordo N, Perrin P.** 2001. Interaction of lyssaviruses with the low-affinity nerve-growth factor receptor p75NTR. *J Gen Virol* **82**(Pt 12)**:**2861–2867.

24. **Thoulouze MI, Lafage M, Schachner M, Hartmann U, Cremer H, Lafon M.** 1998. The neural cell adhesion molecule is a receptor for rabies virus. *J Virol* **72:**7181–7190.

25. **Jacob Y, Badrane H, Ceccaldi PE, Tordo N.** 2000. Cytoplasmic dynein LC8 interacts with lyssavirus phosphoprotein. *J Virol* **74:**10217–10222.

26. **Raux H, Flamand A, Blondel D.** 2000. Interaction of the rabies virus P protein with the LC8 dynein light chain. *J Virol* **74:**10212–10216.

27. **Tan GS, Preuss MA, Williams JC, Schnell MJ.** 2007. The dynein light chain 8 binding motif of rabies virus phosphoprotein promotes efficient viral transcription. *Proc Natl Acad Sci USA* **104:**7229–7234.

28. **Bentivoglio M, Mariotti R, Bertini G.** 2010. Neuroinflammation and brain infections: historical context and current perspectives. *Brain Res Rev* **66:**152–173.

29. **Faber M, Pulmanausahakul R, Hodawadekar SS, Spitsin S, McGettigan JP, Schnell MJ, Dietzschold B.** 2002. Overexpression of the rabies virus glycoprotein results in enhancement of apoptosis and antiviral immune response. *J Virol* **76:**3374–3381.

30. **Faber M, Li J, Kean RB, Hooper DC, Alugupalli KR, Dietzschold B.** 2009. Effective preexposure and postexposure prophylaxis of rabies with a highly attenuated recombinant rabies virus. *Proc Natl Acad Sci USA* **106:**11300–11305.

31. **Wirblich C, Schnell MJ.** 2011. Rabies virus (RV) glycoprotein expression levels are not critical for pathogenicity of RV. *J Virol* **85:**697–704.

32. **Ito Y, Ito N, Saito S, Masatani T, Nakagawa K, Atoji Y, Sugiayma M.** 2010. Amino acid substitutions at positions 242, 255 and 268 in rabies virus glycoprotein affect spread of viral infection. *Microbiol Immunol* **54:**89–97.

33. **Mebatsion T.** 2001. Extensive attenuation of rabies virus by simultaneously modifying the dynein light chain binding site in the P protein and replacing Arg333 in the G protein. *J Virol* **75:**11496–11502.

34. **Dietzschold B, Schnell M, Koprowski H.** 2005. Pathogenesis of rabies. *Curr Top Microbiol Immunol* **292:** 45–56.

35. **Wiltzer L, Larrous F, Oksayan S, Ito N, Marsh GA, Wang LF, Blondel D, Bourhy H, Jans DA, Moseley GW.** 2012. Conservation of a unique mechanism of immune evasion across the *Lyssavirus* genus. *J Virol* **86:**10194–10199.

36. **Chopy D, Pothlichet J, Lafage M, Mégret F, Fiette L, Si-Tahar M, Lafon M.** 2011. Ambivalent role of the innate immune response in rabies virus pathogenesis. *J Virol* **85:**6657–6668.

37. **Phares TW, Kean RB, Mikheeva T, Hooper DC.** 2006. Regional differences in blood-brain barrier permeability changes and inflammation in the apathogenic clearance of virus from the central nervous system. *J Immunol* **176:**7666–7675.

38. **Hooper DG, Roy A, Kean RB, Phares TW, Barkhouse DA.** 2011. Therapeutic immune clearance of rabies virus from the CNS. *Future Virol* **6:**387–397.

39. **Wandeler AI.** 2008. The rabies situation in Western Europe. *Dev Biol (Basel)* **131:**19–25.

40. **Centers for Disease Control and Prevention.** 2007. *US declared canine-rabies free. September 7, 2007.* Centers for Disease Control and Prevention, Atlanta, GA. http://www.cdc.gov/news/2007/09/canine_rabies .html (last accessed April 28, 2013).

41. **Velasco-Villa A, Reeder SA, Orciari LA, Yager PA, Franka R, Blanton JD, Zuckero L, Hunt P, Oertli EH, Robinson LE, Rupprecht CE.** 2008. Enzootic rabies elimination from dogs and reemergence in wild terrestrial carnivores, United States. *Emerg Infect Dis* **14:**1849–1854.

42. **Blanton JD, Palmer D, Rupprecht CE.** 2010. Rabies surveillance in the United States during 2009. *J Am Vet Med Assoc* **237:**646–657.

43. **Rupprecht CE, Barrett J, Briggs D, Cliquet F, Fooks AR, Lumlertdacha B, Meslin FX, Müler T, Nel LH, Schneider C, Tordo N, Wandeler AI.** 2008. Can rabies be eradicated? *Dev Biol (Basel)* **131:** 95–121.

44. **Blanton JD, Palmer D, Dyer J, Rupprecht CE.** 2011. Rabies surveillance in the United States during 2010. *J Am Vet Med Assoc* **239:**773–783.

45. **Nel LH, Markotter W.** 2007. Lyssaviruses. *Crit Rev Microbiol* **33:**301–324.

46. **Global Alliance for Rabies Control.** 2011. *Annual number of deaths from rabies hits 70,000 worldwide. September 28, 2011.* Global Alliance for Rabies Control, Manhattan, KS. http://www.rabiescontrol.net /news/news-archive/annual-number-of-deaths-from-rabies-hits-70000-worldwide.html (last accessed April 28, 2013).

47. **SEARG—Southern and Eastern African Rabies Group.** 2013. http://www.searg.info/doku.php? id=meetings (last accessed April 28, 2013).

48. **Lembo T, Attlan M, Bourhy H, Cleaveland S, Costa P, de Balogh K, Dodet B, Fooks AR, Hiby E, Leanes F, Meslin FX, Miranda ME, Müller T, Nel LH, Rupprecht CE, Tordo N, Tumpey A, Wandeler A, Briggs DJ.** 2011. Renewed global partnerships and redesigned roadmaps for rabies prevention and control. *Vet Med Int* **2011:**923149.

49. **Cohen C, Sartorius B, Sabeta C, Zulu G, Paweska J, Mogoswane M, Sutton C, Nel LH, Swanepoel R, Leman PA, Grobbelaar AA, Dyason E, Blumberg L.** 2007. Epidemiology and molecular virus characterization of reemerging rabies, South Africa. *Emerg Infect Dis* **13:**1879–1886.

50. **Mallewa M, Fooks AR, Banda D, Chikungwa P, Mankhambo L, Molyneux E, Molyneux ME, Solomon T.** 2007. Rabies encephalitis in a malaria-endemic area of Malawi, Africa. *Emerg Infect Dis* **13:** 136–139.

51. **Weyer J, Szmyd-Potapczuk AV, Blumberg LH, Leman PA, Markotter W, Swanepoel R, Paweska JT, Nel LH.** 2011. Epidemiology of human rabies in South Africa, 1983–2007. *Virus Res* **155:**283–290.

52. **World Health Organization.** 2005. *WHO Expert Consultation on Rabies: First Report.* WHO technical report series, **931.** World Health Organization, Geneva, Switzerland.

53. **Dodet B, Africa Rabies Bureau (AfroREB).** 2009. The fight against rabies in Africa: from recognition to action. *Vaccine* **27:**5027–5032.

54. **Knobel DL, Cleaveland S, Coleman PG, Fèvre EM, Meltzer MI, Miranda ME, Shaw A, Zinsstag J, Meslin FX.** 2005. Re-evaluating the burden of rabies in Africa and Asia. *Bull World Health Organ* **83:** 360–368.

55. **Zeng H, Pappas C, Katz JM, Tumpey TM.** 2011. The 2009 pandemic H1N1 and triple-reassortant swine H1N1 influenza viruses replicate efficiently but elicit an attenuated inflammatory response in polarized human bronchial epithelial cells. *J Virol* **85:**686–696.

56. **Menezes R.** 2008. Rabies in India. *CMAJ* **178:**564–566.

57. **World Organisation for Animal Health (OIE).** 2011. *World Animal Health Information Database (WAHID) Interface.* OIE, Paris, France. http://www.oie.int/wahis_2/public/wahid.php/Wahidhome/Home (last accessed April 28, 2013).

58. **Nel LH, Scott TP, Wright N, Mollentze N, Markotter W, Sabeta CT, le Roux K.** 2011. Rabies and rabies control in African regions, p 51–58. *In Rabies Control — Towards Sustainable Prevention at the Source.* Compendium of the OIE Global Conference on Rabies Control, Incheon-Seoul, Korea, 7 to 9 September 2011. OIE, Paris, France.

59. **Global Alliance for Rabies Control.** 2013. *World Rabies Day September 28, 2013.* Global Alliance for Rabies Control, Manhattan, KS. http://www.worldrabiesday.org/ (last accessed April 28, 2013).

60. **Lembo T, Partners for Rabies Prevention.** 2012. The blueprint for rabies prevention and control: a novel operational toolkit for rabies elimination. *PloS Negl Trop Dis* **6:**e1388.

61. **Bill & Melinda Gates Foundation.** 2008. *Grant OPP49679—World Health Organization.* Bill & Melinda Gates Foundation, Seattle, WA. http://www.gatesfoundation.org/How-We-Work/Quick-Links /Grants-Database/Grants/2008/11/OPP49679 (last accessed June 26, 2013).

62. **World Health Organization.** 2010. *Bill & Melinda Gates Foundation fund WHO-coordinated project to control and eventually eliminate rabies in low-income countries.* World Health Organization, Geneva, Switzerland. www.who.int/rabies/bmgf_who_project/en/index.html (last accessed April 28, 2013).

63. **Nel L, Le Roux K, Atlas R.** 2009. Rabies control program in South Africa. *Microbe* **4:**61–65.

64. **Coetzee P, Nel LH.** 2007. Emerging epidemic dog rabies in coastal South Africa: a molecular epidemiological analysis. *Virus Res* **126:**186–195.

65. **Coetzee P, Weyer J, Paweska JT, Burt FJ, Markotter W, Nel LH.** 2008. Use of a molecular epidemiological database to track human rabies case histories in South Africa. *Epidemiol Infect* **136:** 1270–1276.

66. **Global Alliance for Rabies Control.** 2010. *Alliance for Rabies Control—Projects overview—Philippines.* Global Alliance for Rabies Control, Manhattan, KS. http://www.rabiescontrol.net/assets/files/resources /newsletters/GARCnewsletter20.pdf (last accessed 26 June 2013).

67. **World Society for the Protection of Animals.** 2010. *Humane and sustainable dog population management in Colombo; mid-project review June 2007–June 2010.* World Society for the Protection of Animals, London, United Kingdom. http://www.fao.org/fileadmin/user_upload/animalwelfare/Case% 20Study_Colombo.pdf (last accessed 26 June 2013).

68. **World Society for the Protection of Animals.** 2010. *Case study: Gianyar's mass vaccination project.* World Society for the Protection of Animals, London, United Kingdom. http://www.wspa-international.org /images/CaseStudy-GianyarRabies_ENG.pdf (last accessed April 28, 2013).

69. **Niezgoda M, Rupprecht CE.** 2006. Standard operating procedure for the direct rapid immunohisto-chemistry test for the detection of rabies virus antigen, p 1–16. National Laboratory Training Network Course. U.S. Department of Health and Human Services, Centers for Disease Control and Prevention, Atlanta, GA.

70. **World Organisation for Animal Health (OIE).** 2011. *The Fifth Strategic Plan.* OIE, Paris, France. http://www.oie.int/about-us/director-general-office/strategic-plan/ (last accessed April 28, 2013).

71. **Food and Agriculture Organization of the United Nations,Animal Production and Health Division.** 2012. *FAO, OIE and WHO recommit to defend against diseases at the animal-human-ecosystems interfaces.* Food and Agriculture Organization of the United Nations, Rome, Italy. http://www.fao.org/ag/againfo /home/en/news_archive/2011_Tripartite_against_Diseases.html (last accessed April 28, 2013).

72. **Gadre G, Satishchandra P, Mahadevan A, Suja MS, Madhusudana SN, Sundaram C, Shankar SK.** 2010. Rabies viral encephalitis: clinical determinants in diagnosis with special reference to paralytic form. *J Neurol Neurosurg Psychiatry* **81:**812–820.

73. **le Roux K, Nel LH.** 2011. Local governments, municipalities and dog rabies control, p 145–149. *In Rabies Control — Towards Sustainable Prevention at the Source.* Compendium of the OIE Global Conference on Rabies Control, Incheon-Seoul, Korea, 7 to 9 September 2011. OIE, Paris, France.

74. **Nel LH.** 2013. Discrepancies in data reporting for rabies, Africa. *Emerg Infect Dis* **19:**529–533.

One Health: People, Animals, and the Environment
Edited by Ronald M. Atlas and Stanley Maloy
© 2014 American Society for Microbiology, Washington, DC
doi:10.1128/microbiolspec.OH-0010-2012

Chapter 8

Emergence of Influenza Viruses and Crossing the Species Barrier

Zeynep A. Koçer,[1] Jeremy C. Jones,[1] and Robert G. Webster[1]

INTRODUCTION

Influenza is a respiratory disease affecting humans, a limited number of other mammals, and birds. Of the three genera of orthomyxoviruses affecting humans, influenza viruses B and C established permanent lineages in ancient times, whereas influenza A viruses continue to emerge from zoonotic reservoirs and cause annual epidemics and, at irregular intervals, pandemics. Aquatic birds of the world are natural reservoirs for 16 of the 17 known influenza subtypes, and 1 subtype has been characterized from bats. Only three hemagglutinin subtypes (H1, H2, and H3) have caused pandemics in humans; the H1 and H3 subtypes are currently circulating in swine; and the H3 subtype is currently the only remaining epidemic subtype in horses and appears to be establishing a permanent lineage in dogs. All 16 subtypes of influenza viruses in the aquatic bird reservoir occur as low-pathogenicity strains that replicate predominantly in the intestinal tract and cause limited symptoms of overt disease. Subtypes H5 and H7 have the unique ability to evolve into highly pathogenic strains that are lethal in gallinaceous poultry and have the propensity for transitory interspecies transmission to mammals.

The available evidence indicates that all of the influenza pandemics in humans and other mammals have originated from the aquatic bird reservoir. Such events are relatively rare in humans; the occurrence of four pandemics in the past century indicates that there is a barrier to the free exchange of influenza viruses between aquatic bird reservoirs and humans. In this article, we discuss the nature of the proposed species barrier, the intermediate hosts, and the properties of influenza viruses that make them a threat to both veterinary and human public health. The applicability of the concept of "One World—One Health" to influenza is incontrovertible. Characterization of the 2009 H1N1 unequivocally shows that each of the eight gene segments comprising the pandemic viruses in humans can be traced back to the wild bird reservoir and that these viruses were transmitted to humans via swine and subsequently transmitted back to swine. Thus, the early detection and control of influenza requires the collaborative effort of an integrated team comprising virologists, ecologists, veterinarians, and human public health officials.

---

[1]Department of Infectious Diseases, Division of Virology, St. Jude Children's Research Hospital, Memphis, TN 38105.

The present challenge in pandemic preparedness is to identify the influenza viruses in natural reservoirs that have the potential to cause the next lethal disease in domestic poultry or cause a pandemic in humans or other mammals.

GENOMIC FEATURES OF INFLUENZA A VIRUSES

Influenza A viruses are enveloped, single-stranded, negative-sense RNA viruses belonging to the family *Orthomyxoviridae*. The 13.5-kb genome consists of 8 segments coding for 12 proteins (1), 2 of which are surface glycoproteins hemagglutinin (HA) and neuraminidase (NA), required for host cell recognition via receptor binding and the release of virus from the host cell, respectively. Influenza A viruses are further divided into 17 HA and 10 NA subtypes based on the antigenicity of the 2 surface glycoproteins. The remaining proteins, known as internal proteins, are required for the synthesis and packaging of new virions. Viral RNA is replicated via an RNA-dependent RNA polymerase encoded by a viral polymerase complex (PB1, PB2, and PA). PB1-F2 is a small protein that is transported to the mitochondria and nucleus and induces apoptosis in the host cell (2). PA-X protein is expressed from a second open reading frame on the same segment and is obtained by ribosomal frameshifting. PA-X modulates the host response by decreasing viral pathogenicity (3). The other major proteins are nucleoprotein (NP), matrix (M), and nonstructural (NS) proteins, which are involved in the transport of viral RNA from the nucleus to the cytoplasm and in encapsidation before the virus progeny leaves the infected cell (Fig. 1). The virus acquires its envelope from the host cell membrane via a budding process (4).

Of the three types (A, B, and C) of influenza viruses found in nature, influenza A viruses are the most prevalent and are the principal type that infects both avian and mammalian species, including humans. Thus, they represent a unique risk in terms of zoonotic transmission among a variety of hosts. Influenza A viruses are believed to have been in evolutionary stasis with their natural host reservoir for many centuries (5). Nevertheless, rapid genetic changes in the virus genome are inevitable due to virus-driven and host-driven forces. The changes caused by virus-driven forces are due to the segmented nature of the genome and error-prone nature of RNA polymerase. Host-driven forces include neutralizing antibodies produced by the host immune system and receptor specificity. Genetic variants resistant to antiviral drugs also contribute to the evolution of influenza A viruses.

Although some gene sequences retain a higher degree of conservation, mutations can occur in any gene segment of influenza A viruses. Mutant variants of influenza A viruses arise in each replication cycle, as the RNA-dependent RNA polymerase cannot proofread the newly synthesized gene segments. The majority of mutations are not tolerated in the viral population, but a few may confer a fitness advantage by facilitating the establishment of a virus in a new host (adaptation, transmission, modulation of host response, etc.). Genetic variants with mutations at the antigenic sites on HA and NA genes are usually well tolerated, as they provide a selective advantage for the newly produced mutants to escape recognition by the host immune system. The mutation rates at the antigenic sites are significantly higher (6.7×10^{-3} substitutions per nucleotide per year for HA and 3.2×10^{-3} substitutions per nucleotide per year for NA) than at other genes (6). These point mutations (nucleotide substitutions, insertions, or deletions) result in amino

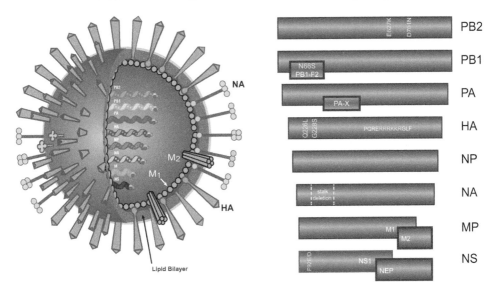

Figure 1. Influenza A virus structure and molecular determinants conferring pathogenesis and host range. Influenza A is an enveloped, negative-sense RNA virus with an eight-segment genome. The virion is studded with surface glycoproteins HA and NA and the M2 ion channel. Pathogenesis and transmission are mediated by multiple genes. Predominant molecular characteristics conferring these traits are diagrammed on each gene product above and as follows. HA: Sialic acid binding restrictions are partially mediated by residues 226 and 228 at the receptor binding site. The presence or absence of a multibasic cleavage site influences the cleavability of the virus by a broader range of enzymes, which leads to high pathogenicity of the virus in host species by causing a systemic infection (13). NA: Sialidase activity is specific to the binding restrictions of the HA protein and cleaves sialic acid residues, permitting release (14); deletions in the stalk region may confer adaptation to domestic poultry (13). PB2: Positions 627 (76) and 701 (22) are associated with enhanced replication in mammals. The immunomodulatory potential of changes or expression of the following proteins may contribute to early and productive replication in a new host. NS1: Position F92E/D confers cytokine resistance in mammalian hosts (77). PB1-F2: Position N66S is associated with increased virulence and cytokine dysregulation in mice (78). PA-X: Expression of this protein may lessen immunopathology during viral infection (3). doi:10.1128/microbiolspec.OH-0010-2012.f1

acid substitutions that affect the antigenicity of the virus, a process known as antigenic drift. Only a few point mutations can be sufficient to make the surface glycoproteins unrecognizable by the host immune system, resulting in the circulation of new antigenic variants in host populations.

Genetic variants also arise by antigenic shift, which occurs when a host cell is coinfected with more than one strain of influenza A viruses. In this case, it is likely that a virion packaged in the host cell contains segments from viruses of different origins. Antigenic shift occurs mainly in influenza A viruses, with which coinfection is more likely due to the broad range of hosts affected. Antigenic shift results in the emergence of new HA-NA combinations and antigenic variants by reassortment of antigenic sites from different virus strains. Reassortment of other gene segments is also likely during coinfection, which results in viruses consisting of mixed gene constellations from different origins. True recombination is much rarer than antigenic drift or antigenic shift; to date, it has been reported in only a few cases, as it can occur only within and between gene segments of certain strains of influenza A viruses (4).

Viruses produced by point mutations, reassortment, antigenic drift, and antigenic shift may have greater selective advantage than parental viral strains because newly produced genetic variants can escape recognition by the host immune system or can develop resistance to antiviral drugs. Furthermore, mutant variants might confer a selective advantage in zoonotic transmission of viral strains among different host systems. Therefore, the viral evolutionary process can have dramatic consequences for public and veterinary health due to lack of existing population immunity, especially in the absence of available vaccines or antivirals. The continuous but independent evolution of influenza A viruses due to biological, ecological, and geographic barriers is a major concern from the One Health perspective, considering the zoonotic potential of the disease. Thus, understanding the genomic nature of influenza A viruses will contribute to the efforts made for public and veterinary health.

RESERVOIRS FOR INFLUENZA A VIRUSES

Influenza A viruses are known for their ability to infect a variety of host species, including humans, swine, mink, horses, marine mammals, cats, dogs, and wide range of wild and domestic birds. However, the *Anseriformes* (ducks, geese, and swans) and *Charadriiformes* (gulls, terns, sandpipers, and waders) are considered the major reservoirs for influenza A viruses in nature. All 16 HA and 9 NA antigenic subtypes of influenza A viruses and their numerous HA-NA combinations have been detected in aquatic bird reservoirs (5, 7). The recent identification of a new antigenic subtype (H17) of influenza A virus from bats (8) indicates that there could be yet-undiscovered reservoirs for influenza A viruses (Fig. 2).

Ducks are the major host species in terms of sustainability, evolution, and spread of influenza A viruses. According to surveillance studies conducted in the Northern Hemisphere, low-pathogenicity avian influenza viruses (LPAIVs) are highly prevalent in juvenile birds, with the prevalence peaking before the birds migrate from north to south in early fall and then gradually dropping to low levels in spring (5, 7). This year-round presence of influenza A viruses in duck populations confirms that ducks are the major reservoir for influenza A viruses. Although most HA subtypes have been isolated from ducks, the predominant subtypes are H3, H4, and H6.

Shorebirds, including gulls, sandpipers, and terns, are susceptible to infections by LPAIVs. The majority of the HA subtypes, including H13 and H16, but not H14 and H15, have been isolated from shorebirds during active surveillance studies at Delaware Bay on the northeast seaboard of the United States. H1, H3, H7, H9, H10, and H11 are the predominant subtypes isolated from shorebird species (9). Influenza A viruses appear to be more diverse in shorebirds than ducks.

The isolation frequency of influenza A viruses from passerine birds is not as high as that for waterfowl and shorebirds. Although passerine birds can be infected and spread the virus to other birds (especially as seen in high-pathogenicity avian influenza virus [HPAIV] outbreak areas), the evolutionary role of passerine birds in influenza

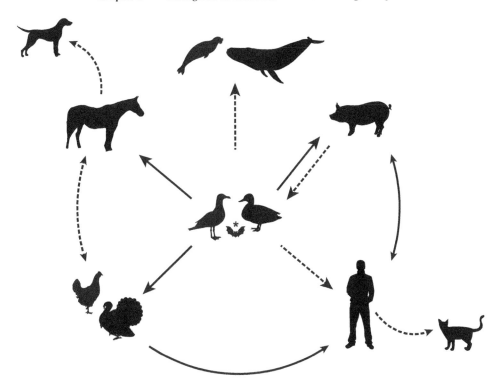

Figure 2. Transmission and host range of influenza A viruses. Wild aquatic birds, and possibly bats, serve as the reservoir for influenza A viruses. Well-established transmission events from the reservoir to other host species are represented by solid lines with directionality indicated by arrowheads. Less frequent transmission or events for which data are anecdotal are represented by dotted lines. *bats. Molecular characterization only. doi:10.1128/microbiolspec.OH-0010-2012.f2

sustainability remains unresolved. The presence of influenza A viruses in passerine birds is a controversial topic, as it has been almost impossible to isolate the viruses from field samples by known culture techniques. However, the number of positive samples determined by molecular detection methods has been significantly high in the *Passeriformes* (particularly starlings and sparrows) in the United States (10). The infectivity of an influenza virus isolated from starlings and the viral shedding via feces after experimental infection (11) raised the concern that passerine birds might transmit the disease to domestic poultry. In addition to wild waterfowl, shorebirds, and passerines, both LPAIVs and HPAIVs have also been isolated from captive birds, zoo animals, and domestic and commercially raised poultry species.

On the basis of geographic and ecological separation of host species and major migratory flyways around the world, two main lineages of avian influenza A viruses have been identified: North American and Eurasian lineages. Although these two lineages are separated by geographic barriers, limited mixing of the lineages occurs via the migratory birds moving through overlapping flyways between Alaska and Far East Russia (7); however, mixing of the viruses from two lineages on a complete-genome level is a very rare event (9). The isolation of H13N9 from gulls in Argentina suggests that a separate lineage of influenza A viruses evolved in South America independently of the other two known lineages (12).

Many waterfowl and shorebirds migrate because of seasonal changes. The migration distance can be short (e.g., around the same region) or long (e.g., intercontinental). Migratory birds contribute significantly to the spread and transmission of LPAIVs, which generally do not cause symptoms in birds and are excreted in large amounts in the feces. Therefore, the virus is carried along the flyway and can be spread to other wild and domestic birds on the way. The breeding and nonbreeding areas, wintering sites, and all other stopover locations along the flyway are convenient places for epizootics to launch, as bird populations reach a high density at some time points.

With the changing environmental and geographic conditions of the planet, the emergence of new strains and new reservoirs is inevitable. Influenza A viruses will also take action to stay in the game and ensure the survival of the fittest, like all other organisms in the evolutionary process. From the perspective of the One Health initiative, extensive global surveillance studies are essential to comprehend the ecology and evolution of influenza A viruses in wild and domestic birds as well as other host species, including possible new reservoirs. Thus, monitoring the distribution of current subtypes around the world, identifying new antigenic variants and/or reassortants, and studying changes in geographic and ecological barriers between the host species will facilitate the urgent actions that need to be taken to ensure public and veterinary health.

INFLUENZA VIRUSES: CROSSING THE SPECIES BARRIER

Although all HA and NA subtypes have been isolated from migratory waterfowl, the number of viruses that move from this reservoir into other animals is relatively small. The idea of a species barrier that prevents the movement of viruses from the reservoir into other hosts is an important concept in influenza biology. Viruses that replicate in avian species often display reduced or inefficient replication in mammals, and the barriers that inhibit transmission between these groups are spatial, physiological, and molecular in origin (13). Spatially, the physical separation of host species from the wild bird reservoir may prevent initial contact and infection, but the continual growth and spread of human populations and their domesticated animals has narrowed this division. This is particularly evident in developing countries where local markets house domesticated and wild birds with other species in a constrained area (14).

Physiological differences between birds and mammals serve as a second barrier. In birds, influenza viruses replicate primarily in the enteric tract at temperatures of 40 to 41°C. In contrast, mammalian viruses replicate most commonly in the upper respiratory tract (32°C) and the bronchioles (37°C). Thus, avian viruses may be impaired in the ability to establish productive infection in mammalian airways due to the lower temperatures in these tissues (15).

Molecular characteristics, such as receptor specificity of the virus, present a final barrier to successful interspecies transmission. Influenza HA binds the terminal sialic acid residues on host cell carbohydrates. Avian influenza viruses preferentially bind sialic acids with α(2-3) linkages to the underlying galactose, whereas human viruses bind sialic acids with α(2-6) linkages. Other viruses, such as those that infect or are isolated from pigs, may bind both receptors (13). In humans, epithelial cells of the upper airway predominantly express α(2-6) linkages and may restrict replication of avian viruses, whereas swine airways possess both receptor types and allow infection of both mammalian and avian viruses (16). Virus NA activity also has specificity to cleave sialic acid linkages that corresponds with the HA receptor specificity (14). The combination of these factors represents a major obstacle the virus must overcome to recognize and enter the cells of a new host. Specific residues and glycosylations in the receptor-binding domain of the HA protein may further complicate this interaction (17, 18). Even if the virus gains the ability to bind to the host cell of a different species, changes in internal proteins such as the PB2 polymerase and immunomodulatory activities of NS1, PB1-F2, or PA-X may further influence its ability to replicate and cause disease in a new host (17) (Fig. 2). Despite the hurdles that exist for viruses attempting to emerge from a wild bird reservoir, the high mutation rate inherent in the replication process facilitates the genesis of novel variants with potential to transmit to a wide variety of poultry and mammals.

From Wild Birds to Poultry

Influenza A viruses infect a wide variety of domesticated gallinaceous birds including chickens, turkeys, quail, and pheasant. They can be divided in two categories: LPAIVs and HPAIVs. The vast majority of viruses exhibit an LPAIV phenotype, and the most prevalent HA subtypes are H3, H6, H9, and H10 (19). To date, only two subtypes (H5 and H7) have evolved to become highly pathogenic. LPAIV forms of these subtypes are currently circulating in poultry populations, while HPAIV forms cause severe outbreaks at certain locales.

The introduction of LPAIVs into poultry likely comes from aquatic and/or migratory birds, which are naturally attracted to dams or watercourses on or near farms. Shedding of the virus into the water and sharing of this contaminated water source with flocks facilitate the initial infection. Lack of proper biosecurity measures (particularly in developing countries) and the movement of people, equipment, and feed in and out of the farms contribute to spread and persistence. Further spread of the disease occurs when an infected bird is taken to a live bird market or housed with uninfected birds on the farm. Transmission of LPAIVs from bird to bird leads to genetic changes that alter its fitness and potential to cause an outbreak or increase its pathogenicity.

In H5 and H7 influenza viruses, several mechanisms and genetic changes have been identified that are important for a shift from LPAIV to HPAIV in poultry. The major genetic change takes place at the cleavage site of the HA protein by insertion or substitution of multiple amino acids. LPAIVs possess a single arginine at the cleavage site, whereas HPAIVs contain multiple basic amino acids (arginine/lysine). This small change in the amino acid motif at the cleavage site can dramatically change the virulence of the virus by allowing the HA protein to be cleaved by a wider variety of proteases found in different cell types. This increases virus tropism and leads to systemic infection. The ability of the virus to replicate in various organs significantly increases the mortality. The change from LPAIV to HPAIV might also occur through recombination between the HA protein and an internal gene (20, 21). Additional genetic changes, such as deletion in the stalk region of the NA protein, might play a role in the adaptation of these viruses to chickens. It has also been shown that a mutation from aspartic acid to asparagine at position 701 of the PB2 protein contributes to the change from LPAIV to HPAIV (Fig. 1) (22).

The conversion from LPAIV to HPAIV in poultry might take several days to several years before causing an outbreak. Although disease signs vary for birds infected with HPAIVs, the major signs are ruffled feathers, edema of the head and face, sinusitis, respiratory signs, excessive lacrimation, decreased egg production, huddling, paralysis, incoordination, torticollis, cyanosis of unfeathered skin (especially of the combs and wattles), diarrhea, and nervous disorders (5, 23). HPAIV infections often progress rapidly and result in high mortality. Once the virus becomes highly pathogenic, it might reenter migratory waterfowl and wild birds around the outbreak area and even transmit to humans in case of direct contact with the infected or dead birds.

Although not HPAIVs, the H9N2 influenza A viruses have become a major concern for outbreaks in chickens, turkeys, ostriches, pheasant, and quail in Asia, Europe, North America, and the Middle East since the 1990s (24). The virus has become endemic in many countries, and vaccination efforts on poultry farms are not sufficient to control or eradicate the disease.

The outbreaks caused by LPAIVs and HPAIVs in domestic and commercial poultry result in the slaughter of millions of birds and a considerable economic loss. The degree of loss varies depending on the number of domestic and commercial poultry farms in close vicinity to an outbreak and the precautionary biosecurity measures taken. Proper biosecurity measures to avoid spread of the outbreak include monitoring the health of birds on a regular basis for disease symptoms, keeping the shared food and water sources clean, and taking extra precautions while transferring equipment and supplies between farms so as to avoid mechanical transfer of the disease. In addition, active surveillance studies should be conducted at both poultry farms and live bird markets, especially in areas at high risk of influenza A outbreaks.

Swine

Influenza infection in pigs manifests clinically as fever, lethargy, anorexia, and weight loss, and virus is shed by coughing and sneezing. The nasal discharge and aerosol droplets are highly communicable, and intraherd spread is often exacerbated by housing livestock in small, confined areas (25). Although mortality is rare, infected animals may exhibit reproductive disorders and stunting of growth, which increases time to market and contributes to an agricultural economic burden (26).

Pigs play a crucial role in influenza evolution and transmission by serving as a platform to breach spatial, physiological, and molecular aspects of the species barrier. Because pigs are a popular livestock worldwide, their interaction with other influenza hosts such as birds (wild and domestic) and humans is common. Physiological features such as warmer temperatures in the upper respiratory tract (36 to 37°C) than that in humans may facilitate replication of avian viruses (25). Respiratory epithelia of pigs also contain both the human-type [α(2-6)] and avian-type [α(2-3)] influenza receptors. Thus, pigs are susceptible to infection with both human and avian influenza viruses. In the event of a coinfection with both types of viruses, reassortment may occur and resulting variants can be transmitted back to an immunologically naïve human host (27). The concept of pigs as a "mixing vessel" has emerged as a partial explanation for the ability of viruses to breach the influenza species barrier and may contribute to the generation of new epidemic and pandemic viruses. Numerous cases of antigenic mixing and cross-species infections (both human and avian) from pigs have been reported, lending credence to the mixing vessel hypothesis (25–28). A recent example is the 2009 H1N1 pandemic, in which a swine virus introduced into the human population was shown to be a triple reassortant with gene segments from human, avian, and swine influenza viruses (29).

Experimentally, pigs are susceptible to most HA subtypes (H1 to H13). However, only viruses of H1, H3, N1, and N2 subtypes have a sustained presence in pig populations. Much of our understanding of the epizootic nature of swine influenza viruses comes from surveillance data from the North American and European herds during the past century. Clinical signs of influenza in pigs were first observed in North America during the 1918 pandemic. In 1930, Shope and colleagues identified the causative agent as an H1N1 influenza virus that is commonly referred to as "classical swine H1N1" (25, 26). Most reports identify this virus as being genetically similar to the progenitor pandemic 1918 H1N1 virus, and it may have passed from birds into pigs (30). The classical swine H1N1 virus maintained epizootic and relatively genetically stable circulation in North American swine populations for nearly 70 years (26). During this time period, sporadic cases of human infection or seropositivity were reported, but they were usually a result of close contact with swine. An exception was an outbreak of H1N1 at Fort Dix, NJ, in 1976, in which the virus was of swine origin and infected more than 200 trainees, causing 12 hospitalizations and 1 death. A national immunization campaign was initiated, but proved unnecessary as the virus did not spread beyond the facility. Immediate contact with pigs was not reported among the infected trainees, though the possibility of introduction of the virus from an incoming trainee could not be ruled out (28).

In Europe, the first reported swine influenza isolates in 1938 and again in the late 1970s were viruses closely related to H1N1s currently circulating in humans. In both cases, isolated viruses contained only human influenza-like genes, providing further evidence that wholly human influenza viruses could be transferred into pigs. The latter half of the 20th century witnessed the introduction of classical swine H1N1 (possibly from import of North American pigs) into European herds. However, an important divergence from classical swine H1N1 dominance occurred in 1976 when an entirely avian H1N1 was transferred, likely from wild ducks, into Belgian and German herds. This "avian-like swine H1N1" continued to circulate and quickly became the dominant lineage in Europe (25).

The predominance of H1N1 viruses in North American and European swine was overshadowed in the late 20th century when reassortment events gave rise to the novel subtype H3N2. In both North America (1997) and Europe (1973), genetic profiles of early H3N2 viruses suggested transmission from humans into pigs. Later triple-reassortant isolates contained mixtures of influenza genes from swine, human, and avian hosts, and there have been instances of reassortment between the H3N2 viruses and cocirculating swine H1N1 (25–27). In the latter case, such cocirculation gave rise to "second-generation" reassortant viruses of the novel subtype H1N2. Although H1N2 has rarely been isolated outside of pigs, infections in mink (31), humans (32), and turkeys (triple-reassortant H1N2) (33) have occurred in the past decade.

In recent years, viruses outside the commonly circulating swine subtypes (H1N1, H3N2, and H1N2) have caused disease in pigs. In Canada (1999), H4N6 viruses with genes exclusively of avian origin were likely passed to pigs from local ducks, and the resulting virus proved efficient at spreading among pigs (26). In the United States (2006), two H2N3 viruses were isolated from sick pigs on two separate farms. Although the H4N6 and H2N3 isolates did not spread outside the respective isolation zones, each virus displayed genetic signatures (receptor binding and structure) of adaptation to mammals and represented the possible introduction of a new HA subtype into swine populations (26, 34).

Endemic and epizootic infections of pigs with influenza viruses represent a significant risk to global health given the role of this species in generating novel influenza reassortants. Continual surveillance is key to both limiting spread and identifying new virus threats.

Horses

As in other mammalian hosts, equine influenza is a localized upper respiratory tract infection causing fever, coughing, and lethargy. It is a significant burden to the equestrian community and thoroughbred industry because outbreaks can delay competitive events and activities (35, 36). Respiratory epithelia of horses are dominated by $\alpha(2\text{-}3)$ receptors, suggesting a preferential susceptibility to avian viruses (37). Viruses readily spread to closely housed horses via nasal discharge and respiratory droplets expelled by persistent coughing (35). Equestrian events and competitions often serve as outbreak sites when animals from various geographic locations are brought together. To combat this spread, vaccination strategies are widely used in North America and Europe (36).

Equine influenza was first reported in 1956 with an outbreak of H7N7 virus in Prague, but it has not been isolated in more than 30 years and has likely disappeared from horse populations (38, 39). Susceptibility of horses to the H7 subtype and isolation of H7 LPAIVs and HPAIVs from domestic poultry and birds over the past decade suggest that reemergence of the H7 subtype in horses is a valid risk that needs to be explored.

The H3N8 subtype, initially isolated from horses in Miami, FL, in 1963, is the sole subtype that continually circulates and causes sporadic epizootic outbreaks worldwide. In most cases, a breach in biosecurity involving unvaccinated animals has been implicated in the outbreaks rather than introduction of a virus from another host (36). However, introduction of influenza to horses from a possible avian source was documented in 1989 in northeastern China. More than 13,000 animals were infected, resulting in a mortality rate of 20%. Genetic analysis of these viruses suggested a common avian progenitor, likely a result of transmission from Central Asian ducks into herds (40), yet this virus did not persist or spread outside the region.

In the past decade, outbreaks of equine-like H3N8 in dogs have been documented in several countries, including the United Kingdom, United States, and Australia. There is evidence of cross-species transmission from horses to dogs in at least three instances, which may have occurred due to housing or transport of dogs in close contact with infected horses or by feeding dogs meat from infected horses (37).

The presence of avian-like receptors in the respiratory epithelia and past evidence of cross-species infection by avian viruses demonstrate that horses are potential recipients of other influenza subtypes. Experimental evidence of the ability of equine isolates to infect humans (41) and the recent spread into dogs highlight the role of horses in the transmissibility and evolution of influenza.

Other Species

Although it occurs less commonly, aquatic mammals can serve as hosts for multiple subtypes of influenza virus. In 1979 to 1980, a severe outbreak of H7N7 virus was reported in harbor seals in New England. Shortly thereafter, an H4N5 (1982) virus was isolated from a sick seal in the same region. Both viruses were composed of genes entirely from avian influenza sources (42, 43). Over the next decade, H4N6 (1991) and H3N3 (1992) viruses were isolated from seals in Massachusetts and were closely related to circulating North American avian influenza viruses. These isolates caused varying degree of illness, from neurological replication and mortality (H7N7) to acute lung replication and increased incidence of stranding noted within the time periods of isolation (43). Serological analyses of Arctic ringed seals (1984 to 1998) and South American fur seals demonstrated varying degrees of seropositivity (2 to 27%) to influenza viruses of different subtypes (44, 45). In addition to seals, viruses have also been isolated from striped whales in the South Pacific (H1N2; 1978) and pilot whales in New England (H13N2/9; 1984), and seropositivity of Canadian beluga whales has been reported (1991) (45–47). In each instance, genotypic analyses suggest possible virus introduction from wild birds, likely as a result of the shared habitats of seals and various species of shorebirds. To date, infections in water mammals remain transient, with limited evidence to suggest seal-to-seal spread of these viruses. However, a recent harbor seal H3N8 isolate (New England, 2011) had molecular features and receptor-binding properties that indicated adaptation to mammals, increasing the potential for intraspecies transmission (48).

Natural infections in mink have been reported for H10N4 (Sweden, 1984), H5N1 (Sweden, 2006), H3N2 (Canada, 2006), and H1N2 (United States, 2010) (31, 49). The H10N4 virus was likely introduced into mink on a farm setting from wild mallard ducks. The H3N2 virus was a triple reassortant and may have come from uncooked feed containing infected pig tissues (including lung). Additionally, mink have been experimentally infected with influenza viruses of avian, human, swine, and equine origin. Their evolutionary ancestor, the ferret, shares this property and is the gold standard for modeling influenza infections and transmission.

Seroprevalence and natural influenza infection of wild and domestic felids has been reported for subtypes H1N1, H3N2, and H5N1, whereas experimental infection studies show that domestic cats are susceptible to a wide range of influenza viruses of avian and human origin. Infection with highly pathogenic avian H5N1 was thought to have occurred by ingestion of bird meat of previously infected animals and has since been experimentally recapitulated (50). The presence of influenza viruses from various subtypes in aquatic mammals, mink, and felids demonstrates the potential for broad host adaptation and warrants further study into the potential of these hosts to mediate antigenic mixing and interspecies transmission.

Humans

Humans are a highly mobile species with an expanding population and living environment. Interaction with wild animals is an increasingly common occurrence that escalates the threat of emerging infectious diseases, particularly novel influenza viruses from the wild bird reservoir. Common agricultural livestock, including chickens and pigs, serves as the intermediate host of influenza viruses and further elevates the risk of transmission of viruses into the human population. Thus, influenza infection in humans is an excellent example of the interplay between human and animal health and its importance to the spread and interspecies transmission of pathogens.

Despite vaccination programs and antiviral therapies, influenza viruses remain endemic in humans. Infecting approximately 5 to 15% of the world population annually, and causing 36,000 deaths every year in the United States alone, influenza remains a significant public health and economic burden (51). Infections are most commonly acute and limited to the upper respiratory tract. The virus receptor predominant in the human upper respiratory tract is the α(2-6) linkage. Thus, humans are less susceptible to avian viruses than are other mammalian hosts such as pigs and horses. However, α(2-3) linkages become more abundant in the lower lung, possibly allowing replication of highly virulent avian viruses such as H5N1 (52). In healthy adults, the virus incubation period is 2 to 5 days, followed by 5 to 8 days of replication with associated clinical signs such as fever, fatigue, general body aches, and nasal congestion. In rare cases, infection may be associated with conjunctivitis, pneumonia, and secondary bacterial infections, or with gastrointestinal symptoms in children. The virus is shed in high titers via respiratory discharge from sneezing and coughing and is highly communicable (51, 53). Influenza viruses circulate in yearly epidemics, often during winter months, in the Northern and Southern Hemispheres. Currently, two subtypes of influenza A are endemic in humans (H1N1 and H3N2), and one subtype (H2N2) has disappeared from the human population (51).

All three subtypes that previously circulated or are currently circulating in humans have caused one or more pandemics. Before the 20th century, evidence of influenza pandemics was recorded largely on the basis of clinical symptoms or outbreaks of respiratory illness (30). Advances in microbiology, medicine, and record keeping allowed a more thorough study of the first pandemic of the 20th century. The 1918 Spanish influenza, caused by the H1N1 virus, was the most severe pandemic in terms of morbidity and mortality in recent history. An estimated 20 million to 40 million people were killed worldwide, but the high mortality rate may have been due to the medical care of the time and the high incidence of bacterial coinfections (30, 54). The exact origin of the virus remains unclear. The surface proteins from human isolates are most similar to those from classical swine isolates, leading to the hypothesis that virus entry into humans occurred via an intermediate pig host. However, this hypothesis is complicated by the facts that surface proteins from the human isolate retained avian-like characteristics and that the disease in pigs was not clinically documented until after the virus had circulated in humans for several months. The latter observation suggests that humans may have transmitted the virus to pigs (30, 55, 56). Regardless of its origin, the pandemic progenitor likely emerged from the avian reservoir and entered pigs and humans, and two lineages (human H1N1 and classical swine H1N1) persisted in their respective populations for several decades subsequently (55, 56).

The human H1N1 virus was supplanted 4 decades later by a new pandemic virus (H2N2) that had acquired avian surface proteins H2 and N2 on the backbone of the previous pandemic virus. The 1957 Asian influenza was replaced a decade later by a new pandemic. The 1968 H3N2 Hong Kong influenza virus had again acquired an avian surface protein (H3) on the backbone of the previous pandemic strain. Both the 1957 and

1968 pandemics were less severe than the 1918 pandemic. This drop in morbidity and mortality was likely because of advances in medicine and antimicrobial agents rather than drastic changes in the virulence and communicability of the viruses themselves (57). In 1977, a pseudopandemic (Russian influenza) and reemergence of the H1N1 subtype in humans may have been the result of accidental release of the virus from freezer storage (56). The H3N2 and H1N1 subtypes have continued to circulate endemically in humans on a yearly basis.

The first influenza pandemic of the 21st century was marked by intensive study of viral genetics and epidemiology, concluding that the pandemic swine influenza (H1N1) was a reassortant virus that was transmitted from pigs into humans. The virus was a so-called triple reassortant and contained genes of classical swine (H1, NP, and NS), Eurasian avian-like swine H1N1 (N1 and M), human H3N2 (PB1), and avian (PB2 and PA) origin. The virus is believed to have circulated in North American swine for nearly 2 decades before emerging in humans (29). Initial cases of respiratory disease were reported in late March 2009 in Mexico, with confirmed cases in the United States first reported in April 2009. By May the virus had spread worldwide, and on July 11, 2009, the World Health Organization (WHO) officially declared a pandemic. Infection rates with the pandemic H1N1 (pH1N1) virus were elevated in traditional high-risk groups such as the very young and elderly and also in pregnant women, the obese, and those younger than 18 years of age. The latter group comprised more than 60% of pH1N1 infections reported in the United States, recalling the infectivity patterns seen with the 1918 pandemic virus. However, the pH1N1 was clinically milder than previous pandemics. The pandemic was declared to have ended in August 2010, after infection rates of 11 to 21% in 218 countries and more than 18,000 laboratory-confirmed deaths. However, mortality in developing countries may have been significantly underreported and the global deaths from pH1N1 may have been significantly higher (29, 58). The relatively "mild" morbidity and low mortality of the pH1N1 virus may be due to several factors such as rapid vaccine production and implementation, use and efficacy of current antivirals, and advances in public health and modern medical care.

The pH1N1 virus serves as an excellent example of the threat of zoonotic transmission and reassortment capabilities of influenza viruses. The virus itself harbored influenza virus genes from three major hosts: birds, pigs, and humans. The genes donated from the swine viruses were themselves a result of reassortment from classical swine and European avian-like swine viruses (29). Together, and possibly through careful mixing within the pig, these elements created a virus that was robust and fit as well as highly infectious and communicable in humans. That the pH1N1 virus may have circulated for years in swine without detection further highlights the need for constant surveillance of influenza viruses and their potential to emerge in various hosts. The past 15 years has seen the emergence of HPAIVs of subtypes H5 and H7 as well as H9 LPAIVs in human hosts without prior adaptation. The endemic nature of these viruses in poultry in many parts of the world is a troubling prospect for the generation of potential pandemic culprits.

HIGHLY PATHOGENIC H5N1 INFLUENZA—AN UNPRECEDENTED EVENT

The emergence of highly pathogenic H5N1 influenza virus in the 1990s in Southeast Asia, its subsequent spread to domestic poultry and mammals in more than 60 Eurasian countries, and its reintroduction into migratory waterfowl is a testament to the need for the One Health concept, which integrates ecology with veterinary and human medicine (59). It is noteworthy that this avian influenza virus was first detected in a child in Hong Kong in 1997 (60), most probably acquired from exposure to poultry in a live bird market. Retrospective studies indicate that the eight gene segments in the H5N1 influenza virus were of Eurasian avian origin. The wild bird precursor H5N1 LPAIV was presumably transmitted to domestic waterfowl in southern China and then spread to chickens through the live bird market system. Subsequent epidemiological studies have implicated exposure to live poultry markets as a major risk factor for acquiring H5N1 influenza virus (61). Transition of the H5N1 LPAIV to its HPAIV phenotype likely occurred during circulation in commercial chicken farms. After the H5N1 HPAIV emerged in commercial poultry, it was probably transmitted back to waterfowl through live poultry markets in the coastal region of southern China and has served as the continuing source of H5N1 HPAIV for the region (62). The absence of overt disease signs in chickens and other gallinaceous poultry in live bird markets in Hong Kong during the initial outbreak was a puzzling feature. One possible explanation is that the lethality of H5N1 was being masked by cocirculating H9N2 influenza viruses, as the initial H5N1 virus contained "internal" gene segments closely homologous with the G1 lineage of H9N2 influenza viruses.

Culling of all poultry in Hong Kong resulted in an immediate cessation of poultry and human infections. Six of 18 human infections were fatal. The original H5N1 was eradicated, but multiple genotypes of H5N1 reemerged from aquatic birds in southern China with the following chronology of events.

- 2002: Infection of exotic waterfowl in Hong Kong parks
- 2003: Infection of a family of three in Fujian, China
- 2003 to 2004: Spread to poultry and humans in Japan, South Korea, Vietnam, Thailand, Lao PDR, and Cambodia
- 2005: Infection of bar-headed geese and waterfowl at Qinghai Lake, China, with subsequent spread to the Indian subcontinent, Africa, and Europe

To date, 63 countries have been affected by the H5N1 virus. The H5N1 HPAIV was eradicated in most countries in Europe as well as Japan, Thailand, and South Korea by quarantine, culling of poultry, and compensation. In contrast, in countries that opted for control by vaccination (China, Vietnam, Indonesia, and Egypt), the virus has become endemic, with sporadic outbreaks occurring in poultry in neighboring countries. Although vaccines are not being used in the Indian subcontinent, widespread outbreaks seen in Bangladesh and sporadic outbreaks in bordering countries suggest that the H5N1 virus is endemic in poultry in this region. The H5N1 HPAIV has continued to evolve and has multiple distinguishable clades based on the sequence of the hemagglutinin. The following are continuing concerns about the future evolution of high-pathogenicity H5N1 viruses.

- Acquisition of mutations that will make the virus transmissible in mammals, as recently demonstrated in ferrets (63, 64), with the possibility of a pandemic in humans
- Perpetuation in the aquatic bird reservoir with minimal disease signs

- Establishment of a stable lineage in swine, the intermediate host
- Transmission to the Americas by either migratory waterfowl or smuggled birds

These concerns embrace the fields of ecology, veterinary sciences, and human public health, emphasizing the importance of using an integrated approach for the pandemic preparedness efforts to control H5N1 influenza.

CONTROL STRATEGIES

The effort to understand and control interspecies transmission of influenza needs to begin with surveillance within the virus reservoir as well as in each susceptible host. Understanding the patterns and identities of viruses circulating in each host (wild birds, domestic poultry, swine, and humans) is the first step to developing methods to adequately control the viruses. Risk assessment of viruses identified in surveillance efforts can further define virus characteristics and the threats posed to birds and mammals. These steps are essential to develop the most common control strategy for influenza, vaccination. Influenza vaccines for both humans and animals are most commonly egg-propagated, inactivated viruses that produce a protective neutralizing antibody to the HA protein (65). A successful vaccine depends on several key factors: (i) antigenic similarity of vaccine seeds to circulating strains, (ii) immunogenicity of the selected virus, and (iii) strain suitability to high-titer growth in eggs (66). Failure of any of these factors can delay lead production or fail to stop spread within populations.

Influenza viruses remain endemic in humans despite readily available vaccines and antivirals. However, annual vaccination with a trivalent (H3N2, H1N1, and influenza B) influenza vaccine is an important public health effort to limit influenza morbidity, mortality, and associated economic and productivity losses (65–67).

The degree to which livestock vaccination confers protection varies, depending on the species and geographic location of animals. Poultry vaccination, especially against H5 LPAIVs and HPAIVs, is most common in areas where these viruses are endemic, including South and Central Asia and parts of the Middle East. Development of avian H5 vaccines is particularly challenging because of continual virus evolution, maternal antibody interference, and the fact that vaccination may limit morbidity and mortality but not prevent animals from shedding virus. Thus, vaccination may not be the most effective method of control in domestic poultry. Alternate or secondary measures may be necessary to control an outbreak or address endemicity. Quarantine and/or culling of affected animals may quickly and successfully eradicate infection but cause a significant economic burden to farms. Monetary compensation for culled flocks is one option to address this problem and potentially increase compliance with an eradication campaign (68).

Current swine influenza vaccines provide at least partial protection against H3N2, H1N1, and H1N2 viruses and may limit intraherd spread. However, the susceptibility of swine to many types of influenza viruses, as well as their potential to pass new variants to other hosts, indicates that vaccination does not eliminate all risk. Thus, the surveillance of circulating swine viruses in tandem with traditional vaccine control measures is essential to identify novel viruses emerging from this host (69).

The horse population is highly mobile because of the competitive nature of the equine industry. Routine vaccination in countries where equine influenza is endemic (e.g., United States and United Kingdom) and immediate vaccination of horses imported into countries where the disease is not endemic is an important step in limiting outbreaks and virus dissemination (35, 36). In recent years, transmission of equine influenza viruses into dogs has led to the development and licensing of canine H3N8 vaccines (70).

Two classes of antiviral drugs are currently used to control existing influenza infections: entry blockers (amantadine and rimantadine) and neuraminidase inhibitors (oseltamivir and zanamivir) (71). Joint statements from the WHO, Food and Agricultural Organization, and World Organisation for Animal Health recommend these antivirals for human use only. The emergence of amantadine-resistant H5N1 HPAIVs, possibly through treatment of poultry with this drug, further justifies the exclusion of livestock from treatment with current antivirals (72). Human H1N1 and H3N2 viruses are highly resistant to entry blockers, and resistance to neuraminidase inhibitors in both human seasonal and pH1N1 viruses is on the rise (71, 73). Thus, continued pursuit of novel influenza antivirals should be given high priority.

The combined approach of surveillance, risk assessment, vaccination, and additional biocontainment measures such as culling and isolation of affected animals is a thorough and effective means to limit interspecies transmission and creation of new influenza viruses.

RISK ASSESSMENT AND RISK MANAGEMENT FOR INFLUENZA A: MORE THAN MEETS THE EYE

The reservoir for influenza A viruses in nature is enormous, considering all aquatic ecosystems and the bird populations residing in those habitats. In addition, rapid genetic changes in the viral genome due to replication errors and the segmented nature of the virus make prediction of future epidemics and pandemics of influenza A viruses difficult. The zoonotic potential of influenza A viruses significantly increases their importance in terms of public and veterinary health. With the emergence of each pandemic wave, influenza experts from multidisciplinary fields have been working to develop a risk assessment and management program to evaluate the potential risk of influenza A viruses in nature.

Risk assessment and risk management efforts should be conducted as part of both pandemic preparedness and postpandemic evaluation (74). Continuous active surveillance is an indispensable part of prepandemic action. In addition, it is essential to comprehend the biological and genetic aspects of influenza A viruses, such as the molecular changes required for adapting to a new host and/or for transmission among different host systems, the efficiency of sustainability of the virus in a new host population, and the new set of selective pressures imposed on viruses as a result of inevitable changes in environmental conditions (e.g., temperature and humidity).

Risk assessment is conducted by the WHO, the Centers for Disease Control and Prevention (CDC), and external influenza experts. The current risk assessment strategy is based solely on the antigenicity of the virus, and the main result of these endeavors is the development of annual influenza vaccines. The CDC is currently developing the Influenza Risk Assessment Tool (IRAT) with the help of external influenza experts, which evaluates "the potential pandemic risk posed by influenza A viruses that currently circulate in animals but not in humans." According to the evaluation criteria of IRAT, each virus can be categorized as low risk, moderate risk, or high risk. Viruses are assessed on the basis of their properties (e.g., genomic variation, receptor binding, transmission in experimental animals, and antiviral treatment susceptibility/resistance), the attributes of the population (e.g., existing population immunity, disease severity and pathogenesis, and antigenic relationship to vaccine candidates), and ecology and epidemiology (e.g., global distribution of the virus in animals, infection in animal species, and human infections) (75).

Overall, establishment of an efficient risk assessment and management program for contemporary and prospective influenza A viruses will accelerate the understanding of the ecology and evolution of these viruses as well as the infection and transmission dynamics among different host species. Information gleaned from these efforts has direct implications for planning and responses to epidemics and pandemics. Thus, the bridge between scientific agencies and governments should remain strong to facilitate interactive communication and mediate implementation of risk management programs for the sake of national and global health interests.

CONCLUDING REMARKS

In the 21st century, the populations of humans and their domesticated livestock are increasing at an unprecedented rate. Such expansion consumes resources from local environments and encroaches upon natural ecosystems. Concomitantly, the effects of global climate change, including rising temperatures and sea levels, are gradually altering these ecosystems and the wild species that inhabit them. Where these two phenomena collide, the potential for emergence of novel influenza viruses is high. The core components of the One Health concept—human and animal health and environmental awareness—are directly applicable to influenza evolution and zoonotic transmission. From the human perspective, clinicians, epidemiologists, and virologists must examine viruses that have circulated in the past to predict what may emerge in epidemic or pandemic form in the future. The identification of emerging viruses has direct implications for vaccine development and antiviral susceptibility, both of which are key control strategies in the public health arena. A similar endeavor, with the inclusion of veterinarians and agricultural workers, is necessary to address the animal health component. Because of the zoonotic nature of influenza viruses, the data collected by experts in each field are important for understanding the pathogenesis of new viruses and their ability to transmit between various human and animal hosts. The acquisition of these data begins with active influenza surveillance from the environments from which these viruses may emerge. While human surveillance of annual circulating viruses is a recognized process for vaccine generation in many countries, animal surveillance outside of endemic and outbreak zones should be increased in practice and scope. This includes sampling of wild birds within natural flyways and aquatic environments as well as agricultural animals on both small and large farms. While we most commonly recognize and focus on the ability of influenza viruses to become highly pathogenic and virulent, the reverse trend is equally possible. A likely evolutionary trait of an influenza virus is to decrease virulence in a host, thus maintaining and facilitating spread. For these reasons, surveillance of not only diseased but also healthy humans and animals should not be overlooked. For humans, this includes incorporation of seroanalysis in current diagnostic protocols. In agricultural settings, surveillance of healthy poultry and swine is absolutely necessary to identify low-pathogenicity viruses that are circulating and simmering asymptomatically in livestock.

The genetic instability of influenza viruses, combined with their wide host range and potential to transmit between individual hosts, facilitates the genesis of novel viruses with varying degrees of pathogenicity and virulence. It has become increasingly evident that focus in any one area or on any single host, be it human or animal, is not sufficient to accurately understand the role that influenza plays in the health of each of these groups. This is highlighted by the emergence and transmission of virulent H5 and H7 viruses from birds directly to humans in the past decade, as well as the recent H1N1 pandemic, which contained influenza genes donated from wild birds, swine, and humans.

Thus, the future for controlling influenza viruses and other emerging infectious diseases depends on collaboration between ecologists, virologists, veterinarians, and physicians with the aim of predicting the pathogenicity of benign disease agents in their reservoir and host species.

Acknowledgments. The authors wish to acknowledge support from the National Institute of Allergy and Infectious Diseases, National Institutes of Health (contract number HHSN 26600700005C), and ALSAC. We thank Vani Shanker for critical review of this manuscript.

Citation. Koçer ZA, Jones JC, Webster RG. 2013. Emergence of influenza viruses and crossing the species barrier. Microbiol Spectrum 1(2):OH-0010-2012. doi:10.1128/microbiolspec.OH-0010-2012.

REFERENCES

1. **Strauss JH, Strauss EG.** 2002. *Viruses and Human Disease*, p 147–156. Academic Press, San Diego, CA.
2. **Chen W, Calvo PA, Malide D, Gibbs J, Schubert U, Bacik I, Basta S, O'Neill R, Schickli J, Palese P, Henklein P, Bennink JR, Yewdell JW.** 2001. A novel influenza A virus mitochondrial protein that induces cell death. *Nat Med* **7:**1306–1312.
3. **Jagger BW, Wise HM, Kash JC, Walters KA, Wills NM, Xiao YL, Dunfee RL, Schwartzman LM, Ozinsky A, Bell GL, Dalton RM, Lo A, Efstathiou S, Atkins JF, Firth AE, Taubenberger JK, Digard P.** 2012. An overlapping protein-coding region in influenza A virus segment 3 modulates the host response. *Science* **337:**199–204.
4. **Steinhauer DA, Skehel JJ.** 2002. Genetics of influenza viruses. *Annu Rev Genet* **36:**305–332.
5. **Webster RG, Bean WJ, Gorman OT, Chambers TM, Kawaoka Y.** 1992. Evolution and ecology of influenza A viruses. *Microbiol Rev* **56:**152–179.
6. **Smith FL, Palese P.** 1989. Variation in influenza virus genes: epidemiological, pathogenic, and evolutionary consequences, p 319–359. *In* Krug RM (ed), *The Influenza Viruses*. Plenum, New York, NY.
7. **Olsen B, Munster VJ, Wallensten A, Waldenström J, Osterhaus AD, Fouchier RA.** 2006. Global patterns of influenza A virus in wild birds. *Science* **312:**384–388.
8. **Tong S, Li Y, Rivailler P, Conrardy C, Castillo DA, Chen LM, Recuenco S, Ellison JA, Davis CT, York IA, Turmelle AS, Moran D, Rogers S, Shi M, Tao Y, Weil MR, Tang K, Rowe LA, Sammons S, Xu X, Frace M, Lindblade KA, Cox NJ, Anderson LJ, Rupprecht CE, Donis RO.** 2012. A distinct lineage of influenza A virus from bats. *Proc Natl Acad Sci USA* **109:**4269–4274.
9. **Krauss S, Obert CA, Franks J, Walker D, Jones K, Seiler P, Niles L, Pryor SP, Obenauer JC, Naeve CW, Widjaja L, Webby RJ, Webster RG.** 2007. Influenza in migratory birds and evidence of limited intercontinental virus exchange. *PLoS Pathog* **3:**e167.
10. **Fuller TL, Saatchi SS, Curd EE, Toffelmier E, Thomassen HA, Buermann W, DeSante DF, Nott MP, Saracco JF, Ralph C, Alexander JD, Pollinger JP, Smith TB.** 2010. Mapping the risk of avian influenza in wild birds in the US. *BMC Infect Dis* **10:**187.
11. **Nestorowicz A, Kawaoka Y, Bean WJ, Webster RG.** 1987. Molecular analysis of the hemagglutinin

genes of Australian H7N7 influenza viruses: role of passerine birds in maintenance or transmission? *Virology* **160**:411–418.

12. **Pereda AJ, Uhart M, Perez AA, Zaccagnini ME, La Sala L, Decarre J, Goijman A, Solari L, Suarez R, Craig MI, Vagnozzi A, Rimondi A, König G, Terrera MV, Kaloghlian A, Song H, Sorrell EM, Perez DR.** 2008. Avian influenza virus isolated in wild waterfowl in Argentina: evidence of a potentially unique phylogenetic lineage in South America. *Virology* **378**:363–370.

13. **Neumann G, Kawaoka Y.** 2006. Host range restriction and pathogenicity in the context of influenza pandemic. *Emerg Infect Dis* **12**:881–886.

14. **Kuiken T, Holmes EC, McCauley J, Rimmelzwaan GF, Williams CS, Grenfell BT.** 2006. Host species barriers to influenza virus infections. *Science* **312**:394–397.

15. **Scull MA, Gillim-Ross L, Santos C, Roberts KL, Bordonali E, Subbarao K, Barclay WS, Pickles RJ.** 2009. Avian influenza virus glycoproteins restrict virus replication and spread through human airway epithelium at temperatures of the proximal airways. *PLoS Pathog* **5**:e1000424.

16. **Ito T, Kawaoka Y.** 2000. Host-range barrier of influenza A viruses. *Vet Microbiol* **74**:71–75.

17. **Fukuyama S, Kawaoka Y.** 2011. The pathogenesis of influenza virus infections: the contributions of virus and host factors. *Curr Opin Immunol* **23**:481–486.

18. **Baigent SJ, McCauley JW.** 2003. Influenza type A in humans, mammals and birds: determinants of virus virulence, host-range and interspecies transmission. *Bioessays* **25**:657–671.

19. **Alexander DJ.** 2000. A review of avian influenza in different bird species. *Vet Microbiol* **74**:3–13.

20. **Suarez DL, Senne DA, Banks J, Brown IH, Essen SC, Lee CW, Manvell RJ, Mathieu-Benson C, Moreno V, Pedersen JC, Panigrahy B, Rojas H, Spackman E, Alexander DJ.** 2004. Recombination resulting in virulence shift in avian influenza outbreak, Chile. *Emerg Infect Dis* **10**:693–699.

21. **Pasick J, Handel K, Robinson J, Copps J, Ridd D, Hills K, Kehler H, Cottam-Birt C, Neufeld J, Berhane Y, Czub S.** 2005. Intersegmental recombination between the haemagglutinin and matrix genes was responsible for the emergence of a highly pathogenic H7N3 avian influenza virus in British Columbia. *J Gen Virol* **86**:727–731.

22. **Li Z, Chen H, Jiao P, Deng G, Tian G, Li Y, Hoffmann E, Webster RG, Matsuoka Y, Yu K.** 2005. Molecular basis of replication of duck H5N1 influenza viruses in a mammalian mouse model. *J Virol* **79**: 12058–12064.

23. **Spickler AR, Trampel DW, Roth JA.** 2008. The onset of virus shedding and clinical signs in chickens infected with high-pathogenicity and low-pathogenicity avian influenza viruses. *Avian Pathol* **37**: 555–577.

24. **Food and Agriculture Organization of the United Nations (FAO).** 2012. *Understanding avian influenza.* Agriculture Department, Animal Production and Health Division, FAO, Rome, Italy. http://www.fao.org/avianflu/documents/key_ai/key_book_preface.htm (last accessed July 23, 2012).

25. **Kuntz-Simon G, Madec F.** 2009. Genetic and antigenic evolution of swine influenza viruses in Europe and evaluation of their zoonotic potential. *Zoonoses Public Health* **56**:310–325.

26. **Olsen CW.** 2002. The emergence of novel swine influenza viruses in North America. *Virus Res* **85**: 199–210.

27. **Ma W, Lager KM, Vincent AL, Janke BH, Gramer MR, Richt JA.** 2009. The role of swine in the generation of novel influenza viruses. *Zoonoses Public Health* **56**:326–337.

28. **Myers KP, Olsen CW, Gray GC.** 2007. Cases of swine influenza in humans: a review of the literature. *Clin Infect Dis* **44**:1084–1088.

29. **Christman MC, Kedwaii A, Xu J, Donis RO, Lu G.** 2011. Pandemic (H1N1) 2009 virus revisited: an evolutionary retrospective. *Infect Genet Evol* **11**:803–811.

30. **Taubenberger JK, Reid AH, Janczewski TA, Fanning TG.** 2001. Integrating historical, clinical and molecular genetic data in order to explain the origin and virulence of the 1918 Spanish influenza virus. *Philos Trans R Soc Lond B Biol Sci* **356**:1829–1839.

31. **Yoon KJ, Schwartz K, Sun D, Zhang J, Hildebrandt H.** 2012. Naturally occurring *Influenza A virus* subtype H1N2 infection in a Midwest United States mink (*Mustela vison*) ranch. *J Vet Diagn Invest* **24**: 388–391.

32. **Komadina N, Roque V, Thawatsupha P, Rimando-Magalong J, Waicharoen S, Bomasang E, Sawanpanyalert P, Rivera M, Iannello P, Hurt AC, Barr IG.** 2007. Genetic analysis of two influenza A (H1) swine viruses isolated from humans in Thailand and the Philippines. *Virus Genes* **35**: 161–165.

33. **Suarez DL, Woolcock PR, Bermudez AJ, Senne DA.** 2002. Isolation from turkey breeder hens of a reassortant H1N2 influenza virus with swine, human, and avian lineage genes. *Avian Dis* **46:** 111–121.

34. **Ma W, Vincent AL, Gramer MR, Brockwell CB, Lager KM, Janke BH, Gauger PC, Patnayak DP, Webby RJ, Richt JA.** 2007. Identification of H2N3 influenza A viruses from swine in the United States. *Proc Natl Acad Sci USA* **104:**20949–20954.

35. **Cullinane A, Elton D, Mumford J.** 2010. Equine influenza—surveillance and control. *Influenza Other Respi Viruses* **4:**339–344.

36. **Elton D, Bryant N.** 2011. Facing the threat of equine influenza. *Equine Vet J* **43:**250–258.

37. **Daly JM, MacRae S, Newton JR, Wattrang E, Elton DM.** 2011. Equine influenza: a review of an unpredictable virus. *Vet J* **189:**7–14.

38. **Sovinova O, Tumova B, Pouska F, Nemec J.** 1958. Isolation of a virus causing respiratory disease in horses. *Acta Virol* **2:**52–61.

39. **Webster RG.** 1993. Are equine 1 influenza viruses still present in horses? *Equine Vet J* **25:**537–538.

40. **Guo Y, Wang M, Kawaoka Y, Gorman O, Ito T, Saito T, Webster RG.** 1992. Characterization of a new avian-like influenza A virus from horses in China. *Virology* **188:**245–255.

41. **Kasel JA, Couch RB.** 1969. Experimental infection in man and horses with influenza A viruses. *Bull W H O* **41:**447–452.

42. **Hinshaw VS, Bean WJ, Webster RG, Rehg JE, Fiorelli P, Early G, Geraci JR, St Aubin DJ.** 1984. Are seals frequently infected with avian influenza viruses? *J Virol* **51:**863–865.

43. **Callan RJ, Early G, Kida H, Hinshaw VS.** 1995. The appearance of H3 influenza viruses in seals. *J Gen Virol* **76**(Pt 1):199–203.

44. **Blanc A, Ruchansky D, Clara M, Achaval F, Le Bas A, Arbiza J.** 2009. Serologic evidence of influenza A and B viruses in South American fur seals (*Arctocephalus australis*). *J Wildl Dis* **45:**519–521.

45. **Nielsen O, Clavijo A, Boughen JA.** 2001. Serologic evidence of influenza A infection in marine mammals of Arctic Canada. *J Wildl Dis* **37:**820–825.

46. **Hinshaw VS, Bean WJ, Geraci J, Fiorelli P, Early G, Webster RG.** 1986. Characterization of two influenza A viruses from a pilot whale. *J Virol* **58:**655–656.

47. **Lvov DK, Zdanov VM, Sazonov AA, Braude NA, Vladimirtceva EA, Agafonova LV, Skljanskaja EI, Kaverin NV, Reznik VI, Pysina TV, Oserovic AM, Berzin AA, Mjasnikova IA, Podcernjaeva RY, Klimenko SM, Andrejev VP, Yakhno MA.** 1978. Comparison of influenza viruses isolated from man and from whales. *Bull W H O* **56:**923–930.

48. **Anthony SJ, St Leger JA, Pugliares K, Ip HS, Chan JM, Carpenter ZW, Navarrete-Macias I, Sanchez-Leon M, Saliki JT, Pedersen J, Karesh W, Daszak P, Rabadan R, Rowles T, Lipkin WI.** 2012. Emergence of fatal avian influenza in New England harbor seals. *MBio* **3:**e00166-12.

49. **Gagnon CA, Spearman G, Hamel A, Godson DL, Fortin A, Fontaine G, Tremblay D.** 2009. Characterization of a Canadian mink H3N2 influenza A virus isolate genetically related to triple reassortant swine influenza virus. *J Clin Microbiol* **47:**796–799.

50. **Harder TC, Vahlenkamp TW.** 2010. Influenza virus infections in dogs and cats. *Vet Immunol Immunopathol* **134:**54–60.

51. **Clark NM, Lynch JP III.** 2011. Influenza: epidemiology, clinical features, therapy, and prevention. *Semin Respir Crit Care Med* **32:**373–392.

52. **Peiris JS, Cheung CY, Leung CY, Nicholls JM.** 2009. Innate immune responses to influenza A H5N1: friend or foe? *Trends Immunol* **30:**574–584.

53. **Nicholson KG, Wood JM, Zambon M.** 2003. Influenza. *Lancet* **362:**1733–1745.

54. **Shanks GD, Brundage JF.** 2012. Pathogenic responses among young adults during the 1918 influenza pandemic. *Emerg Infect Dis* **18:**201–207.

55. **Reid AH, Fanning TG, Hultin JV, Taubenberger JK.** 1999. Origin and evolution of the 1918 "Spanish" influenza virus hemagglutinin gene. *Proc Natl Acad Sci USA* **96:**1651–1656.

56. **Taubenberger JK, Hultin JV, Morens DM.** 2007. Discovery and characterization of the 1918 pandemic influenza virus in historical context. *Antivir Ther* **12**(4 Pt B):581–591.

57. **Horimoto T, Kawaoka Y.** 2005. Influenza: lessons from past pandemics, warnings from current incidents. *Nat Rev Microbiol* **3:**591–600.

58. **Pada S, Tambyah PA.** 2011. Overview/reflections on the 2009 H1N1 pandemic. *Microbes Infect* **13:** 470–478.

59. **Capua I, Alexander DJ.** 2007. Animal and human health implications of avian influenza infections. *Biosci Rep* **27**:359–372.

60. **de Jong JC, Claas EC, Osterhaus AD, Webster RG, Lim WL.** 1997. A pandemic warning? *Nature* **389**:554.

61. **Kung NY, Morris RS, Perkins NR, Sims LD, Ellis TM, Bissett L, Chow M, Shortridge KF, Guan Y, Peiris MJ.** 2007. Risk for infection with highly pathogenic influenza A virus (H5N1) in chickens, Hong Kong, 2002. *Emerg Infect Dis* **13**:412–418.

62. **Chen H, Deng G, Li Z, Tian G, Li Y, Jiao P, Zhang L, Liu Z, Webster RG, Yu K.** 2004. The evolution of H5N1 influenza viruses in ducks in southern China. *Proc Natl Acad Sci USA* **101**:10452–10457.

63. **Imai M, Watanabe T, Hatta M, Das SC, Ozawa M, Shinya K, Zhong G, Hanson A, Katsura H, Watanabe S, Li C, Kawakami E, Yamada S, Kiso M, Suzuki Y, Maher EA, Neumann G, Kawaoka Y.** 2012. Experimental adaptation of an influenza H5 HA confers respiratory droplet transmission to a reassortant H5 HA/H1N1 virus in ferrets. *Nature* **486**:420–428.

64. **Herfst S, Schrauwen EJ, Linster M, Chutinimitkul S, de Wit E, Munster VJ, Sorrell EM, Bestebroer TM, Burke DF, Smith DJ, Rimmelzwaan GF, Osterhaus AD, Fouchier RA.** 2012. Airborne transmission of influenza A/H5N1 virus between ferrets. *Science* **336**:1534–1541.

65. **Ellebedy AH, Webby RJ.** 2009. Influenza vaccines. *Vaccine* **27**(Suppl 4):D65–D68.

66. **Schultz-Cherry S, Jones JC.** 2010. Influenza vaccines: the good, the bad, and the eggs. *Adv Virus Res* **77**: 63–84.

67. **Szucs TD.** 1999. Influenza. The role of burden-of-illness research. *Pharmacoeconomics* **16**(Suppl 1):27–32.

68. **Kapczynski DR, Swayne DE.** 2009. Influenza vaccines for avian species. *Curr Top Microbiol Immunol* **333**:133–152.

69. **Vincent AL, Ma W, Lager KM, Janke BH, Richt JA.** 2008. Swine influenza viruses: a North American perspective. *Adv Virus Res* **72**:127–154.

70. **US Department of Agriculture Animal and Plant Health Inspection Service (APHIS).** APHIS issues conditional license for canine influenza virus vaccine. June 23, 2009. APHIS, Washington, DC. http://www. aphis.usda.gov/newsroom/content/2009/06/caninevacc.shtml (last accessed July 31, 2012).

71. **Saladino R, Barontini M, Crucianelli M, Nencioni L, Sgarbanti R, Palamara AT.** 2010. Current advances in anti-influenza therapy. *Curr Med Chem* **17**:2101–2140.

72. **World Health Organization (WHO).** 2005. Use of antiviral drugs in poultry, a threat to their effectiveness for the treatment of human avian influenza. November 11, 2005. WHO, Geneva, Switzerland. http://www. who.int/foodsafety/micro/avian_antiviral/en/ (last accessed July 31, 2012).

73. **Das K.** 2012. Antivirals targeting influenza A virus. *J Med Chem* **55**:6263–6277.

74. **Dowdle WR.** 2006. Influenza pandemic periodicity, virus recycling, and the art of risk assessment. *Emerg Infect Dis* **12**:34–39.

75. **Centers for Disease Control and Prevention (CDC).** 2012. Influenza Risk Assessment Tool (IRAT). June 21, 2012. CDC, Atlanta, GA. http://www.cdc.gov/flu/pandemic-resources/tools/risk-assessment.htm (last accessed July 25, 2012).

76. **Shinya K, Hamm S, Hatta M, Ito H, Ito T, Kawaoka Y.** 2004. PB2 amino acid at position 627 affects replicative efficiency, but not cell tropism, of Hong Kong H5N1 influenza A viruses in mice. *Virology* **320**: 258–266.

77. **Seo SH, Hoffmann E, Webster RG.** 2002. Lethal H5N1 influenza viruses escape host anti-viral cytokine responses. *Nat Med* **8**:950–954.

78. **Conenello GM, Zamarin D, Perrone LA, Tumpey T, Palese P.** 2007. A single mutation in the PB1-F2 of H5N1 (HK/97) and 1918 influenza A viruses contributes to increased virulence. *PLoS Pathog* **3**:1414–1421.

One Health: People, Animals, and the Environment
Edited by Ronald M. Atlas and Stanley Maloy
© 2014 American Society for Microbiology, Washington, DC
doi:10.1128/microbiolspec.OH-0020-2013

Chapter 9

One Health and Food-Borne Disease: *Salmonella* Transmission between Humans, Animals, and Plants

Claudia Silva,[1] Edmundo Calva,[1] and Stanley Maloy[2]

INTRODUCTION

There are >2,600 recognized serovars of *Salmonella enterica*. Many of these *Salmonella* serovars have a broad host range and can infect a wide variety of animals, including mammals, birds, reptiles, amphibians, and insects. In addition, *Salmonella* can grow in plants and can survive in protozoa, soil, and water. Hence, reducing human infections will require the reduction of *Salmonella* in animals and limitation of transmission from the environment.

SALMONELLA IN ANIMALS AND HUMANS

The species *S. enterica* is subdivided into seven subspecies, designated by roman numerals. The majority of *Salmonella* human pathogens belong to subspecies I isolates, whereas the other subspecies are mainly associated with cold-blooded vertebrates (1, 2). There are >2,600 serovars of *S. enterica*. The serovars differ widely in their ability to infect different mammals and birds, and can be divided into three groups based upon their host range: broad-host-range or generalist, host-adapted, and host-restricted serovars (3–5). Host-restricted serovars are associated exclusively with one particular host species. For example, *S. enterica* serovars Typhi, Paratyphi A, Paratyphi C, and Sendai cause disease only in humans; Abortusovis is restricted to goats and sheep; Gallinarum and Pullorum are restricted to poultry; Typhisus is restricted to swine; and Abortusequi is restricted to horses. Other serovars are adapted to a particular host but retain the ability to cause disease in alternative hosts. For example, *S.* Choleraesuis and *S.* Dublin are host-adapted serovars associated with severe systemic disease in cattle and pigs, respectively, but they infrequently cause disease in other mammalian hosts, including humans. The host-restricted and host-adapted serovars produce systemic infection in their natural hosts, but there is limited or no evidence of gastroenteritis. These serovars migrate rapidly from the intestine to the reticuloendothelial system, where they reside in intracellular niches (e.g., macrophages) and often persist in the host to produce a carrier state. The establishment of a

[1]Departamento de Microbiología Molecular, Instituto de Biotecnología, Universidad Nacional Autónoma de México, Cuernavaca, Morelos 62210, Mexico; [2]Center for Microbial Sciences, San Diego State University, San Diego, CA 92182-1010.

chronic infection in the carrier permits shedding of a relatively low bacterial load for an extended period of time. In contrast, broad-host-range serovars, such as *S.* Typhimurium and *S.* Enteritidis, can infect a wide range of animals, from insects to reptiles, birds, and mammals. Although capable of causing systemic disease in certain animals, broad-host-range serovars usually induce a self-limiting gastroenteritis in infected hosts (6).

Only about 50 of the subspecies I serovars are isolated as animal and human pathogens (6). Most human salmonellosis cases are food borne, often derived indirectly from animal or human fecal contamination. However, infections are also acquired through direct or indirect animal contact in homes, veterinary clinics, zoological gardens, farm environments, or other public and private settings. Clinically sick animals may pose the greatest risk to humans because they are more likely to shed *Salmonella* organisms at higher concentrations than are apparently healthy animals. However, asymptomatic carriers can shed *Salmonella* organisms for long periods of time. A recent review (6) describes the variety of sources of *Salmonella* transmission from mammals, birds, reptiles, amphibians, fish, and invertebrates to humans; the distribution of the most common human *Salmonella* serovars among animals; and the distribution of these infections in different geographic regions.

Salmonella organisms occur naturally in the gastrointestinal tract of many reptiles as a part of their normal intestinal microbiota and are commonly shed in their feces (6). Although reptiles often carry *Salmonella* subspecies II, III, and IV, other serovars of subspecies I commonly associated with human salmonellosis, notably *S.* Typhimurium and *S.* Enteritidis, also occur in reptiles. The overwhelming majority of reptiles that carry *Salmonella* are asymptomatic. Human salmonellosis attributable to reptile exposure was first documented in the 1940s, and a large number of case reports have since described zoonotic transmission of *Salmonella* from reptiles. A substantial number of human salmonellosis cases have been linked to contact with turtles, terrapins, snakes, and lizards (6).

IDENTIFICATION AND SURVEILLANCE

The wide variety of *Salmonella* serovars, coupled with potential confusion among infections with different food-borne pathogens, provides a challenge for characterizing the source of an outbreak. However, a number of genetic differences among serovars can be exploited for precise identification of different *Salmonella* strains. To improve the accurate identification and comparison of food-borne pathogens, the U.S. Centers for Disease Control and Prevention (CDC) developed the International Molecular Subtyping Network for Foodborne Disease Surveillance, dubbed PulseNet (http://www.pulsenetinternational. org). This site presents the six regional networks and different protocols for the molecular subtyping of *Salmonella*. The website, supported by the World Health Organization, contains phenotypic and epidemiological information from the Global Salm-Surv *Salmonella* surveillance program (http://www.who.int/salmsurv/en/), including information on the major *Salmonella* serovars identified globally as well as antimicrobial resistance. The European Union performs *Salmonella* surveillance in all member countries. A description of *Salmonella*, epidemiological information, and related information about the international surveillance network for the enteric infections *Salmonella* and verocytotoxin-producing *Escherichia coli* O157 (Enter-net) can be accessed through the United Kingdom Health Protection Agency website (http://www.hpa.org.uk). Additionally, the

Eurosurveillance journal publishes information on infectious disease, epidemiology, prevention, and control (http://www.eurosurveillance.org/).

The genomes of many *Salmonella* serovars have now been sequenced (a current list and links to related sites are available at https://www.sanger.ac.uk/resources/downloads /bacteria/salmonella.html). Pairwise genome sequence comparisons between each of the serovars indicate that they have >96% DNA sequence identity between shared genes (7). Each serovar has many insertions and deletions (indels) relative to the other serovars, accounting for 500 to 600 kb of unique DNA in each serovar (10 to 15% of their approximately 4.8-Mbp genomes). The unique regions are distributed over many regions of the chromosome and range in size from <1 kb to >50 kb. The success of rapid full-genome sequencing in response to the *E. coli* O104:H4 outbreak in Europe in 2011 (8), coupled with the increased availability and reduced cost of whole-genome sequencing, makes it likely that this approach will become more widely used for the identification of food-borne pathogens in the near future.

Because few cases are sufficiently severe to demand professional medical care, providing information to the public about *Salmonella* infections is essential for accurate reporting of outbreaks. General information about *Salmonella* can be accessed at the website of the CDC (http://www.cdc.gov/Salmonella/). This website describes *Salmonella* in language accessible to the general public. In addition, this site provides links to descriptions of *Salmonella* outbreaks. The website salmonella.org (http://www .salmonella.org/) provides general information about *Salmonella* and links to genome sequencing projects and to researchers working on *Salmonella* around the world, to information on transmission from reptiles, and to strain collections available to the research community.

SALMONELLA HOST SPECIFICITY

The genetic differences between the host-restricted, host-adapted, and generalist serovars provide insights into the bacterial characteristics that determine host range. Broad-host-range pathogens must persist in a wide variety of host niches with a diversity of physiological requirements, and thus are under considerable selective constraints. Even small impacts on fitness may prevent broad-host-range bacteria from competing with other bacteria in one of these niches. In contrast, host-specific pathogens persist in a restricted environmental niche and have fewer selective constraints—a lifestyle that sacrifices fast growth in a wide variety of environments for slower growth and persistence in a more protected environment. The slower growth and more uniform metabolic requirements of host-specific *Salmonella* serovars eliminate the potential impact of genetic changes that invoke a fitness cost in fast-growth conditions with fluctuating metabolic demands (9). The loss of selective pressure for many of these functions allows host-restricted serovars to acquire many more loss-of-function mutations (pseudogenes) than broad-host-range serovars (10, 11). Some of these pseudogenes actually benefit survival in certain hosts by preventing expression of gene products that stimulate an immune response.

In addition to changes in the chromosome of *Salmonella*, mobile genetic elements can also play a key role in determining host specificity (12). One noteworthy difference between host-restricted and generalist *Salmonella* serovars is the presence of the *Salmonella* virulence plasmid (pSV). A small fraction of the *S. enterica* subspecies I serovars contain pSV. This plasmid encodes the *spv* operon, which plays a role in the expression of the virulence of the serovars in their specific hosts (13–17). The nine *S. enterica* serovars in which a pSV has been found are Abortusovis, Abortusequis, Choleraesuis, Dublin, Gallinarum, Paratyphi C, Sendai, Enteritidis, and Typhimurium. With the exception of the broad-host-range serovars *S.* Enteritidis and *S.* Typhimurium, few broad-host-range serovars carry pSV. Moreover, the host-restricted *S.* Typhi lacks pSV. Despite many common properties shared by the pSVs of different serovars, each plasmid seems to be specific to its bacterial host, exemplified by a unique plasmid size in different serovars (18). Numerous virulence determinants involved in modulation of the host immune response to infection, such as *rck*, *rsk*, and *spf*, are carried on pSV. Most of the variation among serovars in the pSV is due to the presence or absence of the conjugal transfer operon (*tra*) and the *pef* or *fae* fimbrial operons (18, 19). The *spv* region is inserted into the chromosome in subspecies II, IIIa, IV, and VII (20).

Loss of the *spv* region abolishes the virulence phenotype of the serovars in their animal hosts, and often in the mouse model (14, 15, 21). On the other hand, the introduction of a pSV to a serovar that is naturally devoid of it does not increase the virulence properties of the strain (22–24), suggesting that other chromosomally encoded factors are responsible for the virulence phenotype. Not all the members of a serovar contain the pSV; often within the population some members carry the plasmid while others do not (23, 24). The prevalence of the pSV in *S.* Typhimurium isolates from pigs in Japan can be illustrative of this point: only 36% carried the pSV, but they were predominantly associated with systemically infected pigs (92%), in contrast to pigs with gastrointestinal symptoms (19%) or healthy pigs (17%) (25). Broad-host-range serovars display more genetic variability than host-adapted or host-restricted serovars, which may account for their abundance of genetic resources to produce diverse clinical outcomes (5).

EVOLUTION OF HOST RANGE OF VARIANTS

S. Typhimurium has been isolated from essentially all warm-blooded animals and reptiles and is the most frequently documented serovar implicated in transmission of salmonellosis from mammals to humans (6). This serovar can infect some animal hosts without producing disease (asymptomatic carriers) while causing acute disease in others (5). Subtyping methods, such as phage typing, macrorestriction mapping via pulsed-field gel electrophoresis, and multilocus sequence typing, have been used to characterize the genetic variability within *S.* Typhimurium strains isolated from a wide range of hosts in different geographic regions, such as a recent study done by us in Mexico (12, 26, 27). These studies have revealed that although *S.* Typhimurium has been regarded as a broad-host-range serovar, some strains have a broad host range while other strains are closely associated with particular hosts.

The definitive phage type 104 (DT104) is an example of a broad-host-range *S.* Typhimurium strain. This clone emerged during the 1980s and rapidly spread around the world, infecting a wide variety of animals, including humans. DT104 acquired a genomic island carrying multidrug resistance determinants, making it a major public health threat (28).

On the other hand, certain *S.* Typhimurium strains have a narrow host range. *S.* Typhimurium DT40 and DT56v are commonly associated with passerine birds. These strains are rarely detected in other animals, but there have been reports of infection of livestock from wild birds and infection of cats that consumed infected birds (29). *Salmonella* can be isolated from birds that show symptoms of salmonellosis, but birds of the same species can also be asymptomatic carriers (29). In addition, Rabsch et al. (30) demonstrated that DT2 and DT99 (variant Copenhagen) were almost exclusively associated with pigeons for many decades and over a wide geographic range. These strains produce fatal systemic disease in pigeons, similar to other highly host-adapted or host-restricted *Salmonella* serovars, although they retain the ability to cause disease in BALB/c mice. Host adaptation is often associated with increased survival in macrophages of the preferred host (31). The pigeon-adapted *Salmonella* strains were tested for virulence in mammals and pigeons (30). The pigeon-adapted strains showed enhanced cytotoxicity in pigeon macrophages and led to the development of typhoid fever-like syndrome with a high mortality rate in pigeons, with higher bacterial counts in the internal organs.

These observations indicate that increased adaptation of a *Salmonella* serovar to a certain host is associated with increased virulence, systemic disease, and asymptomatic carriers that shed the pathogen over extended periods (3). Furthermore, the pigeon-adapted *S.* Typhimurium strain was found in the ovaries of infected pigeons, a characteristic of other known host-adapted and host-restricted *S. enterica* serovars, including Pullorum, Gallinarum, Abortusovis, and Dublin (5). This potential for vertical transmission may facilitate the maintenance of a host-adapted *Salmonella* serovar in the limited available population.

In certain cases the outcome of infection may result from a natural balance in which one serovar competitively excludes other members of the same serogroup. The natural balance may be disrupted by human intervention (4). This scenario was documented by the investigation of the epidemiological consequences of eradication of the avian-adapted *S.* Gallinarum from poultry in the United States and Europe (32). Infections with the two host-restricted strains, *S.* Gallinarum and *S.* Pullorum, cause severe disease with high mortality and considerable economic losses on poultry farms. Adult animals often develop a carrier state, with transovarian transmission to newly hatched chicks (33). Because *S.* Gallinarum and *S.* Pullorum are host restricted, they are not a risk to human health. Like *S.* Gallinarum and *S.* Pullorum infections, infections with *S.* Enteritidis are typically asymptomatic in adult poultry, but transovarian transmission of *S.* Enteritidis results in high mortality of newly hatched chicks. In addition, because *S.* Enteritidis is a broad-host-range serovar, rodents and other vectors can readily facilitate transmission between poultry facilities. National efforts to eliminate *S.* Gallinarum and *S.* Pullorum from poultry farms greatly reduced these serovars in the United States and Europe, but apparently *S.* Enteritidis filled this vacant ecological niche, because the dramatic increase in *S.* Enteritidis in poultry coincided with the eradication of *S.* Gallinarum and *S.* Pullorum (Fig. 1) (32). This example nicely illustrates how a better understanding of host adaptation may provide new insights into the emergence of infectious disease (4).

NONMAMMALIAN VECTORS FOR *SALMONELLA*

Salmonella has been isolated from a large number of vertebrate species, and outbreaks can often be linked to infected animals. Once excreted from an animal host, *Salmonella* faces limited nutrient availability, osmotic stress, large variations in temperature and pH,

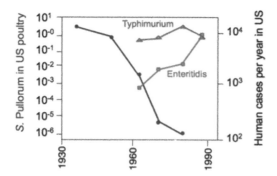

Figure 1. Changes in prevalence of *S. enterica* serovars Pullorum versus Enteritidis and Typhimurium in the United States. As the prevalence of Pullorum in U.S. poultry flocks decreased as a result of a U.S. Department of Agriculture program (blue line), the prevalence of Enteritidis in humans increased (red line). Transmission of Enteritidis to humans from chicken eggs increased coordinately with the increased prevalence in poultry. During the period when the incidence of Enteritidis infections in humans was increasing, the incidence of Typhimurium infections in humans (green line) was relatively unchanged. Figure redrawn from reference 65. See the original reference for precise numbers. doi:10.1128/microbiolspec.OH-0020-2013.f1

and predation (34, 35). The survival of *Salmonella* in the secondary habitat ensures its passage to the next host. *Salmonella* has been detected in several locations within farms and slaughterhouses, and long-term contamination of farms appears to be a widespread phenomenon. Insects and worms have been proposed as disease vectors for *Salmonella* on farms and agricultural fields, in animal feed, and in households. Biting mites have also been shown to efficiently transit *Salmonella* to chickens, and houseflies have been implicated in the transmission of typhoid fever vectors in military camps. Moreover, insects may represent reservoir hosts that play pivotal roles in *Salmonella* persistence. Birds, mice, litter beetles, and flies are important vectors for the rapid dissemination of *Salmonella* in the environment (6, 35, 36). Flies that come in contact with contaminated material, such as manure, food, and water, are capable of transmitting bacteria (37, 38). Association of *Salmonella* with insect vectors may be determined by specific adhesion-receptor interactions. Initial attempts at recovering *S*. Enteritidis from the surface of the houseflies by using an aqueous rinse were largely unsuccessful, but rinsing the flies with 0.5% detergent demonstrated that the flies were contaminated with high levels of bacteria. These results imply that *S*. Enteritidis was tightly associated with houseflies (37).

Salmonella has been collected from soil samples from both agricultural and recreational areas that serve as bacterial reservoirs and may aid transmission between hosts (39). Broad-host-range strains effectively cycle through ecosystems, and there are more environmental reservoirs where they can multiply than previously thought. Semenov et al. (40) designed long-chain experiments to follow bacteria through abiotic habitats (dung and soil), plant habitats (fodder and oats), and animal digestive tracts (snails, mice, and chicken), where the organisms underwent significant shifts in temperature, pH, oxygen, substrate availability, grazing by predators, and exposure to parasites like phages and amebae. They concluded that the population density of the enteric pathogens in these different habitats is sufficiently high (ca. 10^3/g) to cause disease in humans (40).

Salmonella is adapted to survive in host macrophages, so it is not surprising that it can also survive in protozoa in nature. *Salmonella* can survive in the vacuoles of protozoa, providing another niche for *Salmonella* in the environment (41–43). *S.* Thompson is expelled from *Tetrahymena* in vesicles containing a high density of bacteria, and the surrounding membrane may help protect bacteria from desiccation and disinfectants such as chlorine. Furthermore, it has been recently proposed that *Salmonella* organisms from rumen protozoa display a hypervirulent phenotype due to the hyperactivation of virulence gene expression, and that this environment provides a venue for conjugal transfer of antibiotic resistance plasmids (44, 45). Indeed, it has been postulated that protozoan predation may be the selective pressure maintaining O-antigen diversity among *Salmonella* organisms (46, 47).

SALMONELLA-PLANT INTERACTIONS AND THE FOOD CHAIN

Fresh fruit and vegetables are now recognized to be a major route of entry for pathogenic enterobacteria into the food chain. *Salmonella* and *E. coli* are among the most prevalent food-borne bacterial pathogens in the developed world and are able to enter the food chain at any point from farm to table (48). Changes in farming practices, food production, consumer habits, and improved surveillance are all possible factors in the increased prevalence of pathogenic enterobacteria in fresh produce. However, recent studies have demonstrated that *Salmonella* can interact specifically with plants, indicating that plants can serve as alternative hosts for the transmission of disease (49).

A wide range of fresh fruit and vegetable products have been implicated in *Salmonella* infection, most commonly lettuce, sprouted seeds, melons, and tomatoes (50). Plants may experience high concentrations of *Salmonella* when infected animals defecate in farmland or as a result of fertilization of farmland with animal manure. Thus, *Salmonella* transmission from plants was initially thought to be simply due to surface contamination. However, it is now clear that enteric pathogens have acquired mechanisms to enter plants and reproduce inside of plants (51, 52), a discovery that explains the failure of sanitizers to efficiently eradicate food-borne pathogens in produce.

Similar strategies are required for bacteria to colonize both animal and plant hosts. The details of the initial adherence, invasion, and establishment differ depending on the specific interaction, but there are striking parallels between the processes (49, 53). A combination of bioinformatic approaches and molecular techniques has been used to study mechanisms of plant colonization by pathogenic enterobacteria. It was initially thought that the unique factors required for plant infections could be identified by genome comparisons between bacteria that are frequently or exclusively associated with plants and those that are only associated with human or animal hosts (49). However, many factors involved in infection of animals are also required for successful infection of plants, including type 3 secretion systems that modulate host cell responses, and suppression of the host immune response (53, 54).

Bacterial adherence to host tissue is a prerequisite of both animal and plant infection. Bacteria encode a large number of adherence factors with diverse receptor-binding capability. Among the better-known examples are adhesins of the chaperone-usher family, generally located on the ends of long hair-like structures termed fimbriae, and surface-associated afimbrial adhesins. These adhesins often recognize a range of glycosylation patterns that decorate surface proteins of eukaryotic cells. Among enterobacteria, different isolates commonly encode specific sets of adhesin gene clusters that confer tropism to a particular host tissue type. Other fimbriae-like structures contribute to functions in pathogenesis.

Bacterial adherence to biotic and abiotic surfaces is often due to a combination of factors rather than the action of a single adhesin. For example, Barak et al. (55) showed that the pilus curli (encoded by *agfB*), thin, coiled, fimbriae-like fibers that mediate cell-cell interactions in biofilms and binding to animal cell surfaces, play an important role in adhesion of *S*. Enteritidis and *S*. Newport to alfalfa sprouts. However, they also found that deletion of *agfB* did not completely prevent leaf attachment, indicating that other adhesins likely play a role as well. Likewise, the O-antigen capsule and cellulose synthesis play a role in adhesion of *S*. Enteritidis to plants (56). Curli and cellulose also facilitate transfer of *S*. Typhimurium from contaminated water to parsley (57). Curli and cellulose form a cellular matrix that promotes formation of biofilms. *Salmonella* strains that form extensive biofilms were found to have stronger adhesion to romaine lettuce leaves and greater persistence than weak biofilm-producing strains (58). Not surprisingly, curli, cellulose, and capsule are regulated by a common regulatory gene, *agfD*, which may play a major role in environmental fitness of *Salmonella* organisms (59).

In comparison with bacterial attachment to plant surfaces, the internal movement and translocation of *Salmonella* in plants is less well understood. Many animal-pathogenic enterobacteria preferentially invade plant root tissue rather than foliage (49), but recent reports show that *Salmonella* can invade leaves and developing fruit. The ability of *Salmonella* to penetrate plant cells has been demonstrated in *Arabidopsis thaliana* by tracking fluorescently marked *S*. Typhimurium cells. Colonization of foliage was found to be less extensive than root colonization, and bacteria that were artificially internalized into the leaves did not appear to spread systemically from the point of infiltration. However, bacteria could be detected in newly formed leaves 1 month after introduction (60). The initial entry is not a passive process: *S*. Typhimurium invades iceberg lettuce leaves through the stoma during active photosynthesis but not in the dark (61). The results indicate that *Salmonella* undergoes active chemotaxis toward metabolites produced by photosynthesis.

Studies on the invasion of tomato plants have shown that *Salmonella* can colonize developing fruit. When tomato plants were inoculated by injecting stems or brushing flowers with *Salmonella*, the bacteria remained viable during fruit development, surviving within the ripened fruit (62, 63). Not surprisingly, some strains are more effective at infecting plants than others. For example, *S*. Montevideo appeared to be more adapted to survival within tomatoes and was recovered from 90% of the fruit screened, providing a potential explanation of the narrow range of *Salmonella* serovars associated with *Salmonella* outbreaks linked to tomatoes. *Salmonella* can move inside tomato plants and colonize fruits at high levels without inducing any symptoms, except for a slight reduction in plant growth (64). The results indicate that direct transmission of *Salmonella* can occur between plants (49).

The study of the microbial ecology of food-borne pathogens associated with produce may allow the development of evidence-based policies, procedures, and technologies aimed at reducing the risk of contamination of fresh produce. For instance, better understanding of the competitive interactions of enteropathogens with the naturally

Table 1. Some sources of *Salmonella* outbreaks

Animal products	Pets	Plant products
Poultry	Turtles	Alfalfa sprouts
Beef	Reptiles	Bean sprouts
Pork	Dogs	Melons
Fish	Cats	Marijuana
Milk	Birds	Lettuce
Cheese	Ducks	Onions
Chocolate	Hedgehogs	Tomatoes
Eggs	Pet food	Peppers
Ice cream	Pet treats	Cilantro
		Spinach
		Cucumber
		Cereal
		Rice
		Flour
		Nuts (almonds, peanut butter, pistachios, hazelnuts)
		Spices (pepper, celery seed, basil, sesame seeds)

occurring microbiota in the rhizosphere and phyllosphere suggests that there is potential for the naturally occurring microbiota to be used as biocontrol agents to prevent the establishment of enteropathogenic pathogens in plants (50–52).

CONCLUDING REMARKS

Salmonella can be transmitted by a wide variety of food products and environmental sources (Table 1). Thus, transmission of *S. enterica* provides a compelling example of the One Health paradigm, with reservoirs of pathogens in humans, animals, plants, and the environment. Furthermore, the secondary consequences of efforts to eliminate the poultry-restricted *Salmonella* serovars demonstrate that basic ecological principles govern the environmental niches occupied by pathogens, making it impossible to thwart *Salmonella* infections without a clear understanding of One Health.

Acknowledgments. The authors have no conflict of interest in the research described in this article.

Citation. Silva C, Calva E, Maloy S. 2014. One Health and food-borne disease: *Salmonella* transmission between humans, animals, and plants. Microbiol Spectrum 2(1):OH-0020-2013. doi:10.1128/microbiolspec. OH-0020-2013.

REFERENCES

1. **Le Minor L, Popoff MY.** 1987. Designation of *Salmonella enterica* sp. nov., nom. rev., as the type and only species of the genus *Salmonella*. *Int J Syst Bacteriol* **37**:465–468.
2. **Silva C, Wiesner M.** 2009. An introduction to systematics, natural history and population genetics of *Salmonella*, p 1–17. *In* Calva JJ, Calva E (ed.), *Molecular Biology and Molecular Epidemiology of Salmonella Infections*. Research Signpost, Trivandrum, India.

3. **Bäumler AJ, Tsolis RM, Ficht TA, Adams LG.** 1998. Evolution of host adaptation in *Salmonella enterica*. *Infect Immun* **66**:4579–4587.

4. **Kingsley RA, Bäumler AJ.** 2000. Host adaptation and the emergence of infectious disease: the *Salmonella* paradigm. *Mol Microbiol* **36**:1006–1014.

5. **Uzzau S, Brown DJ, Wallis T, Rubino S, Leori G, Bernard S, Casadesús J, Platt DJ, Olsen JE.** 2000. Host adapted serotypes of *Salmonella enterica*. *Epidemiol Infect* **125**:229–255.

6. **Hoelzer K, Moreno Switt AI, Wiedmann M.** 2011. Animal contact as a source of human non-typhoidal salmonellosis. *Vet Res* **42**:34. doi:10.1186/1297-9716-42-34.

7. **Edwards RA, Olsen GJ, Maloy SR.** 2002. Comparative genomics of closely related salmonellae. *Trends Microbiol* **10**:94–99.

8. **Karch H, Denamur E, Dobrindt U, Finlay BB, Hengge R, Johannes L, Ron EZ, Tønjum T, Sansonetti PJ, Vicente M.** 2012. The enemy within us: lessons from the 2011 European *Escherichia coli* O104:H4 outbreak. *EMBO Mol Med* **4**:841–848.

9. **Winter SE, Lopez CA, Bäumler AJ.** 2013. The dynamics of gut-associated microbial communities during inflammation. *EMBO Rep* **14**:319–327.

10. **Maloy S, Mora G.** 2012. Unnecessary baggage, p 93–98. *In* Kolter R, Maloy S (ed), *Microbes and Evolution: The World That Darwin Never Saw*. ASM Press, Washington, DC.

11. **Matthews TD, Maloy SR.** 2011. Genome rearrangements in *Salmonella*, p 41–66. *In* Fratamico P, Liu Y, Kathari S (ed), *Genomes of Foodborne and Waterborne Pathogens*. ASM Press, Washington, DC.

12. **Silva C, Wiesner M, Calva E.** 2012. The importance of mobile genetic elements in the evolution of *Salmonella*: pathogenesis, antibiotic resistance and host adaptation, p 231–254. *In* Kumar Y (ed), *Salmonella: A Diversified Superbug*. InTech, Rijeka, Croatia.

13. **Chu C, Feng Y, Chien AC, Hu S, Chu CH, Chiu CH.** 2008. Evolution of genes on the *Salmonella* virulence plasmid phylogeny revealed from sequencing of the virulence plasmids of *S. enterica* serotype Dublin and comparative analysis. *Genomics* **92**:339–343.

14. **Guiney DG, Fierer J.** 2011. The role of the *spv* genes in *Salmonella* pathogenesis. *Front Microbiol* **2**:129. doi:10.3389/fmicb.2011.00129.

15. **Gulig PA, Curtiss R III.** 1987. Plasmid-associated virulence of *Salmonella typhimurium*. *Infect Immun* **55**:2891–2901.

16. **Gulig PA, Doyle TJ.** 1993. The *Salmonella typhimurium* virulence plasmid increases the growth rate of salmonellae in mice. *Infect Immun* **61**:504–511.

17. **Rychlik I, Gregorova D, Hradecka H.** 2006. Distribution and function of plasmids in *Salmonella enterica*. *Vet Microbiol* **112**:1–10.

18. **Chu C, Hong SF, Tsai C, Lin WS, Liu TP, Ou JT.** 1999. Comparative physical and genetic maps of the virulence plasmids of *Salmonella enterica* serovars Typhimurium, Enteritidis, Choleraesuis, and Dublin. *Infect Immun* **67**:2611–2614.

19. **Feng Y, Liu J, Li YG, Cao FL, Johnston RN, Zhou J, Liu GR, Liu SL.** 2012. Inheritance of the *Salmonella* virulence plasmids: mostly vertical and rarely horizontal. *Infect Genet Evol* **12**:1058–1063.

20. **Boyd EF, Hartl DL.** 1998. *Salmonella* virulence plasmid. Modular acquisition of the *spv* virulence region by an F-plasmid in *Salmonella enterica* subspecies I and insertion into the chromosome of subspecies II, IIIa, IV and VII isolates. *Genetics* **149**:1183–1190.

21. **Jones GW, Rabert DK, Svinarich DM, Whitfield HJ.** 1982. Association of adhesive, invasive, and virulent phenotypes of *Salmonella typhimurium* with autonomous 60-megadalton plasmids. *Infect Immun* **38**:476–486.

22. **Gulig PA, Danbara H, Guiney DG, Lax AJ, Norel F, Rhen M.** 1993. Molecular analysis of *spv* virulence genes of the *Salmonella* virulence plasmids. *Mol Microbiol* **7**:825–830.

23. **Olsen JE, Brown DJ, Thomsen LE, Platt DJ, Chadfield MS.** 2004. Differences in the carriage and the ability to utilize the serotype associated virulence plasmid in strains of *Salmonella enterica* serotype Typhimurium investigated by use of a self-transferable virulence plasmid, pOG669. *Microb Pathog* **36**:337–347.

24. **Ou JT, Baron LS.** 1991. Strain differences in expression of virulence by the 90 kilobase pair virulence plasmid of *Salmonella* serovar Typhimurium. *Microb Pathog* **10**:247–251.

25. **Namimatsu T, Asai T, Osumi T, Imai Y, Sato S.** 2006. Prevalence of the virulence plasmid in *Salmonella* Typhimurium isolates from pigs. *J Vet Med Sci* **68**:187–188.

26. **Wiesner M, Calva E, Fernández-Mora M, Cevallos MA, Campos F, Zaidi MB, Silva C.** 2011.

Salmonella Typhimurium ST213 is associated with two types of IncA/C plasmids carrying multiple resistance determinants. *BMC Microbiol* **11:**9. doi:10.1186/1471-2180-11-9.

27. **Wiesner M, Zaidi MB, Calva E, Fernández-Mora M, Calva JJ, Silva C.** 2009. Association of virulence plasmid and antibiotic resistance determinants with chromosomal multilocus genotypes in Mexican *Salmonella enterica* serovar Typhimurium strains. *BMC Microbiol* **9:**131. doi:10.1186/1471-2180-9-131.

28. **Mulvey MR, Boyd DA, Olson AB, Doublet B, Cloeckaert A.** 2006. The genetics of *Salmonella* genomic island 1. *Microbes Infect* **8:**1915–1922.

29. **Lawson B, Hughes LA, Peters T, de Pinna E, John SK, Macgregor SK, Cunningham AA.** 2011. Pulsed-field gel electrophoresis supports the presence of host-adapted *Salmonella enterica* subsp. *enterica* serovar Typhimurium strains in the British garden bird population. *Appl Environ Microbiol* **77:**8139–8144.

30. **Rabsch W, Andrews HL, Kingsley RA, Prager R, Tschäpe H, Adams LG, Bäumler AJ.** 2002. *Salmonella enterica* serotype Typhimurium and its host-adapted variants. *Infect Immun* **70:**2249–2255.

31. **Xu T, Maloy S, McGuire KL.** 2009. Macrophages influence *Salmonella* host-specificity *in vivo*. *Microb Pathog* **47:**212–222.

32. **Rabsch W, Hargis BM, Tsolis RM, Kingsley RA, Hinz KH, Tschäpe H, Bäumler AJ.** 2000. Competitive exclusion of *Salmonella enteritidis* by *Salmonella gallinarum* in poultry. *Emerg Infect Dis* **6:**443–448.

33. **Anderson LA, Miller DA, Trampel DW.** 2006. Epidemiological investigation, cleanup, and eradication of pullorum disease in adult chickens and ducks in two small-farm flocks. *Avian Dis* **50:**142–147.

34. **Rozen Y, Belkin S.** 2001. Survival of enteric bacteria in seawater. *FEMS Microbiol Rev* **25:**513–529.

35. **Winfield MD, Groisman EA.** 2003. Role of nonhost environments in the lifestyles of *Salmonella* and *Escherichia coli*. *Appl Environ Microbiol* **69:**3687–3694.

36. **Liebana E, Garcia-Migura L, Clouting C, Clifton-Hadley FA, Breslin M, Davies RH.** 2003. Molecular fingerprinting evidence of the contribution of wildlife vectors in the maintenance of *Salmonella* Enteritidis infection in layer farms. *J Appl Microbiol* **94:**1024–1029.

37. **Holt PS, Geden CJ, Moore RW, Gast RK.** 2007. Isolation of *Salmonella enterica* serovar Enteritidis from houseflies (*Musca domestica*) found in rooms containing *Salmonella* serovar Enteritidis-challenged hens. *Appl Environ Microbiol* **73:**6030–6035.

38. **Mian LS, Maag H, Tacal JV.** 2002. Isolation of *Salmonella* from muscoid flies at commercial animal establishments in San Bernardino County, California. *J Vector Ecol* **27:**82–85.

39. **Thomason BM, Biddle JW, Cherry WB.** 1975. Dection of salmonellae in the environment. *Appl Microbiol* **30:**764–767.

40. **Semenov AM, Kuprianov AA, van Bruggen AH.** 2010. Transfer of enteric pathogens to successive habitats as part of microbial cycles. *Microb Ecol* **60:**239–249.

41. **Gaze WH, Burroughs N, Gallagher MP, Wellington EM.** 2003. Interactions between *Salmonella typhimurium* and *Acanthamoeba polyphaga*, and observation of a new mode of intracellular growth within contractile vacuoles. *Microb Ecol* **46:**358–369.

42. **Gourabathini P, Brandl MT, Redding KS, Gunderson JH, Berk SG.** 2008. Interactions between food-borne pathogens and protozoa isolated from lettuce and spinach. *Appl Environ Microbiol* **74:** 2518–2525.

43. **Tezcan-Merdol D, Ljungström M, Winiecka-Krusnell J, Linder E, Engstrand L, Rhen M.** 2004. Uptake and replication of *Salmonella enterica* in *Acanthamoeba rhysodes*. *Appl Environ Microbiol* **70:** 3706–3714.

44. **Brewer MT, Xiong N, Dier JD, Anderson KL, Rasmussen MA, Franklin SK, Carlson SA.** 2011. Comparisons of *Salmonella* conjugation and virulence gene hyperexpression mediated by rumen protozoa from domestic and exotic ruminants. *Vet Microbiol* **151:**301–306.

45. **Rasmussen MA, Carlson SA, Franklin SK, McCuddin ZP, Wu MT, Sharma VK.** 2005. Exposure to rumen protozoa leads to enhancement of pathogenicity of and invasion by multiple-antibiotic-resistant *Salmonella enterica* bearing SGI1. *Infect Immun* **73:**4668–4675.

46. **Wildschutte H, Lawrence JG.** 2007. Differential *Salmonella* survival against communities of intestinal amoebae. *Microbiology* **153:**1781–1789.

47. **Wildschutte H, Wolfe DM, Tamewitz A, Lawrence JG.** 2004. Protozoan predation, diversifying selection, and the evolution of antigenic diversity in *Salmonella*. *Proc Natl Acad Sci USA* **101:**10644–10649.

48. **Fisher IS, Threlfall EJ.** 2005. The Enter-net and Salm-gene databases of foodborne bacterial pathogens that cause human infections in Europe and beyond: an international collaboration in surveillance and the development of intervention strategies. *Epidemiol Infect* **133:**1–7.

49. **Holden N, Pritchard L, Toth I.** 2009. Colonization outwith the colon: plants as an alternative environmental reservoir for human pathogenic enterobacteria. *FEMS Microbiol Rev* **33**:689–703.

50. **Heaton JC, Jones K.** 2008. Microbial contamination of fruit and vegetables and the behaviour of enteropathogens in the phyllosphere: a review. *J Appl Microbiol* **104**:613–626.

51. **Berger CN, Sodha SV, Shaw RK, Griffin PM, Pink D, Hand P, Frankel G.** 2010. Fresh fruit and vegetables as vehicles for the transmission of human pathogens. *Environ Microbiol* **12**:2385–2397.

52. **Critzer FJ, Doyle MP.** 2010. Microbial ecology of foodborne pathogens associated with produce. *Curr Opin Biotechnol* **21**:125–130.

53. **Schikora A, Garcia AV, Hirt H.** 2012. Plants as alternative hosts for *Salmonella*. *Trends Plant Sci* **17**: 245–249.

54. **Schikora A, Virlogeux-Payant I, Bueso E, Garcia AV, Nilau T, Charrier A, Pelletier S, Menanteau P, Baccarini M, Velge P, Hirt H.** 2011. Conservation of *Salmonella* infection mechanisms in plants and animals. *PLoS One* **6**:e24112. doi:10.1371/journal.pone.0024112.

55. **Barak JD, Gorski L, Naraghi-Arani P, Charkowski AO.** 2005. *Salmonella enterica* virulence genes are required for bacterial attachment to plant tissue. *Appl Environ Microbiol* **71**:5685–5691.

56. **Barak JD, Jahn CE, Gibson DL, Charkowski AO.** 2007. The role of cellulose and O-antigen capsule in the colonization of plants by *Salmonella enterica*. *Mol Plant Microbe Interact* **20**:1083–1091.

57. **Lapidot A, Yaron S.** 2009. Transfer of *Salmonella enterica* serovar Typhimurium from contaminated irrigation water to parsley is dependent on curli and cellulose, the biofilm matrix components. *J Food Prot* **72**:618–623.

58. **Kroupitski Y, Pinto R, Brandl MT, Belausov E, Sela S.** 2009. Interactions of *Salmonella enterica* with lettuce leaves. *J Appl Microbiol* **106**:1876–1885.

59. **Gibson DL, White AP, Snyder SD, Martin S, Heiss C, Azadi P, Surette M, Kay WW.** 2006. *Salmonella* produces an O-antigen capsule regulated by AgfD and important for environmental persistence. *J Bacteriol* **188**:7722–7730.

60. **Schikora A, Carreri A, Charpentier E, Hirt H.** 2008. The dark side of the salad: *Salmonella* Typhimurium overcomes the innate immune response of *Arabidopsis thaliana* and shows an endopathogenic lifestyle. *PLoS One* **3**:e2279. doi:10.1371/journal.pone.0002279.

61. **Kroupitski Y, Golberg D, Belausov E, Pinto R, Swartzberg D, Granot D, Sela S.** 2009. Internalization of *Salmonella enterica* in leaves is induced by light and involves chemotaxis and penetration through open stomata. *Appl Environ Microbiol* **75**:6076–6086.

62. **Guo X, Chen J, Brackett RE, Beuchat LR.** 2001. Survival of salmonellae on and in tomato plants from the time of inoculation at flowering and early stages of fruit development through fruit ripening. *Appl Environ Microbiol* **67**:4760–4764.

63. **Shi X, Namvar A, Kostrzynska M, Hora R, Warriner K.** 2007. Persistence and growth of different *Salmonella* serovars on pre- and postharvest tomatoes. *J Food Prot* **70**:2725–2731.

64. **Gu G, Hu J, Cevallos-Cevallos JM, Richardson SM, Bartz JA, van Bruggen AH.** 2011. Internal colonization of *Salmonella enterica* serovar Typhimurium in tomato plants. *PLoS One* **6**:e27340. doi:10.1371/journal.pone.0027340.

65. **Bäumler AJ, Hargis BM, Tsolis RM.** 2000. Tracing the origins of *Salmonella* outbreaks. *Science* **287**: 50–52.

One Health: People, Animals, and the Environment
Edited by Ronald M. Atlas and Stanley Maloy
© 2014 American Society for Microbiology, Washington, DC
doi:10.1128/microbiolspec.OH-0003-2012

Chapter 10

Cholera: Environmental Reservoirs and Impact on Disease Transmission

Salvador Almagro-Moreno[1] and Ronald K. Taylor[1]

INTRODUCTION

Cholera is a severe and sometimes fatal diarrheal disease caused by the comma-shaped bacterium *Vibrio cholerae*. The disease is acquired through the consumption of food or water contaminated by this microorganism. Cholera has virtually disappeared from developed countries due to high hygiene standards and water quality; however, many developing countries that lack the needed infrastructure and have poor sanitation continue to endure the menace of the disease (1). Disease outbreaks are often associated with and accentuated by floods and conflict that allow increased fecal contamination of water supplies.

There are more than 200 known serogroups of *V. cholerae*, yet only 2 of them are known to cause cholera in humans (choleragenic): serogroups O1 and O139 (2). The two major pathogenicity factors of choleragenic *V. cholerae* are the cholera toxin (CT), the enzymatic source of the watery diarrhea; and the toxin-coregulated pilus (TCP), an essential colonization factor (3, 4). Nonetheless, there are several other serogroups of *V. cholerae* that, even though they do not cause cholera, can cause bloody diarrhea, gastroenteritis, and extraintestinal infections (5–8). These strains use an alternative set of virulence factors than those used by choleragenic *V. cholerae*, such as type III and type VI secretion systems (9–11).

V. cholerae belongs to the family *Vibrionaceae*, a highly varied group that encompasses both pathogenic and nonpathogenic bacteria (12). The *Vibrionaceae* are part of the marine and riverine microbiota and can be found both free living and in association with biotic and abiotic surfaces (12). Like other members of the *Vibrionaceae*, *V. cholerae* can be found associated with numerous components of its native ecosystem (Fig. 1). *V. cholerae* has been found associated with invertebrate members of the zooplankton such as crustaceans, dipterae, and shellfish; with vertebrates such as fish and waterfowl; and with other microorganisms such as *Acanthamoeba castellanii* (Fig. 1) (12–18). Also, a handful of studies found *V. cholerae* attached to the mucilaginous sheath of the blue-green algae *Anabaena* sp. (Fig. 1) (19, 20).

The infectious dose of *V. cholerae* required to cause cholera in healthy individuals is quite high; nonetheless, when the low pH of the stomach is buffered with sodium

---

[1]Department of Microbiology and Immunology, Geisel School of Medicine at Dartmouth, Hanover, NH 03755.

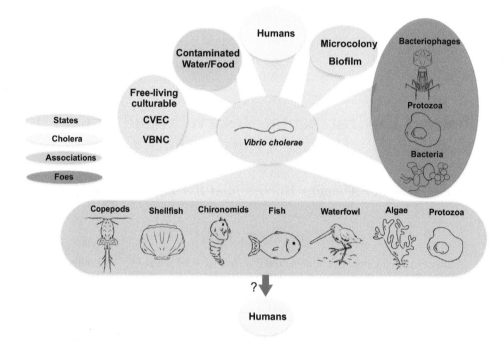

Figure 1. *V. cholerae* life cycle and interactions.The life cycle of *V. cholerae* is complex and includes numerous physiological states and interactions with natural inhabitants of brackish riverine, estuarine, and coastal waters. *V. cholerae* can be directly isolated from the water (free-living culturable) or found in a VBNC state, as CVEC, or in the form of biofilms on diverse surfaces. It has been shown that the stools of patients with cholera still contain microcolonies of pathogenic *V. cholerae*. *V. cholerae* has several known natural predators, such as bacteriophages and protozoa. These predators are thought to play a crucial role in the dynamics of cholera epidemics by thriving on choleragenic *V. cholerae* when their numbers flourish. Also, some bacteria have antagonistic interactions with *V. cholerae*, preventing its growth on solid surfaces. Cholera can be acquired not only through the consumption of contaminated water containing choleragenic *V. cholerae* but also through the ingestion of foods contaminated with the bacterium. *V. cholerae* has been found associated with several sea and riverine dwellers such as algae, shellfish, chironomids and their egg masses, fish, waterfowl, amebae, and crustaceans, most critically copepods. The role of some of these environmental reservoirs of *V. cholerae* in cholera epidemics remains to be clarified. Nonetheless, several novel findings discussed in the text point to *V. cholerae* naturally requiring some of these hosts as vectors to cause cholera in humans, which establishes the disease as a zoonosis. doi:10.1128/microbiolspec.OH-0003-2012.f1

bicarbonate prior to the oral administration, the required dose to elicit the diarrhea decreases several logs (1). These results indicate that it is unlikely for *V. cholerae* in the free-living state to be the major source of epidemic cholera, as the stomach barrier appears to be a major hindrance to its survival. Thus, the association of the bacterium with other organisms and/or abiotic surfaces facilitates the ability of *V. cholerae* to cause the disease. Numerous findings support this hypothesis; for instance, it was found that ingestion of *V. cholerae* with food products decreases the infectious dose required to cause cholera, and the removal of particulate matter through filtration with a sari cloth reduced the incidence of the disease (1, 21–23). Whether *V. cholerae* interacts with other inhabitants of the aquatic environment and some of those interactions are involved in pathogenesis remains to be elucidated. Nonetheless, it is clear that *V. cholerae* can be transmitted through a set of vectors, indicating that cholera is a zoonosis.

What are the ecological factors affecting the life cycle of *V. cholerae* and its interactions with other inhabitants of the aquatic environment? What are the differences between organisms that act as reservoirs of *V. cholerae* and those that act as vectors of the bacterium?

VIBRIONACEAE

The family *Vibrionaceae* encompasses eight genera, of which the best studied are *Vibrio* and *Photobacterium*. The *Vibrionaceae* have an astonishingly wide array of hosts and they range from pathogens to symbionts. Some of the pathogenic members of the *Vibrionaceae* include *Vibrio vulnificus*, which causes fulminant septicemia in humans and is acquired through wounds mainly caused while handling shellfish. *Vibrio parahaemolyticus* causes an acute gastroenteritis in humans and is acquired primarily through the consumption of raw or undercooked seafood. Some members of the *Vibrionaceae* can be pathogenic in species other than humans. Many of those are of particular significance as they sicken and kill species related to aquaculture, causing major economic losses to the industry. For instance, *Vibrio anguillarum* causes vibriosis in farmed salmon, *Vibrio tubiashi* kills Pacific oysters, and *Vibrio harveyi* causes vibriosis in shrimp. Moreover, some members of the *Vibrionaceae* family affect the food industry negatively by establishing a symbiosis with their hosts. This is the case of the pufferfish and its *Vibrio* symbiont. The pufferfish meat is highly toxic to humans with the exception of some parts; however, the edible parts are a delicacy in countries such as Japan, where it is known as fugu. Some pufferfish species are poisonous due to a toxin produced by its *Vibrio* symbiont, which provides protection to its host from predators in its natural environment. Some members of the *Vibrionaceae* also pose ecological risks. This is the case with *Vibrio mediterranei*, *Vibrio shiloi*, and *Vibrio corallilyticus*, which are thought to be major causes of coral bleaching. These vibrios attack the endosymbionts (zooxanthellae) of the coral, and the loss of these pigmented symbionts results in bleaching of the coral. Many species belonging to the *Vibrionaceae* are bioluminescent, such as *V. harveyi* and *Vibrio fischeri*. *V. fischeri* establishes a symbiotic relationship with the Hawaiian squid *Euprymna scolopes*. *V. fischeri* colonizes the light organ of the squid and provides luminescence that is thought to confer protection from predators to its host by negating its shadow from the moon. Other species such as *Photobacterium phosphoreum* are the bioluminescent symbionts of jellyfish. None of these species are either obligate pathogens or obligate symbionts, as they can be found as free living in their natural environment.

V. CHOLERAE AND CHOLERA

Cholera causes death due to dehydration and electrolyte loss. Historically, only strains belonging to serogroups O1 and O139 have been known to cause the disease (1, 24). O1 strains can be subdivided into two biotypes: classical and El Tor. O1 classical was the cause of the first six recorded pandemics of cholera, which lasted from 1817 until 1923 (1, 24). O1 El Tor is the cause of the current seventh pandemic, which started in 1961. Since 1993 El Tor has virtually displaced classical (24). Serogroup O139 emerged in 1992, causing an explosive outbreak. That was first reported in India and Bangladesh. Serogroup O139 was originally thought to be a potential source for the eighth cholera pandemic; however, just a few years after the 1992 outbreak, cholera cases due to strains belonging to serogroup O139 steadily dwindled in number and are now virtually non-existent (24). Recently, a series of El Tor clinical isolates have been identified that possess several classical traits (25–29). These El Tor variants have, among other characteristics, classical cholera toxin genes and increased CT production (25–29). Cholera remains endemic in parts of Africa, Latin America, and southern Asia, where seasonal epidemics occur frequently (1). Cholera still affects hundreds of thousands of people every year; for instance, a recent outbreak of cholera in Haiti killed more than 7,000 Haitians and sickened more than 500,000, affecting approximately 5% of the population (30, 31). Nonetheless, a simple effective treatment for cholera patients is fluid replacement with the appropriate electrolyte composition. To shorten the recovery time, antibiotics can be given to patients with severe cholera symptoms.

How *V. cholerae* regulates its virulence genes has been extensively studied. Briefly, two inner membrane-localized regulators, ToxR and TcpP, are required to transcribe the *toxT* gene, which encodes the master regulator of virulence in choleragenic *V. cholerae* (32, 33). ToxT is a transcriptional regulator required for the expression of the *ctxAB* operon, which encodes the two subunits of CT; and the *tcp* operon, which encodes TCP. Nonetheless, little is known about what role these virulence factors may have in the environment, if any.

NONCHOLERAGENIC, PATHOGENIC *V. CHOLERAE*

Several non-O1, non-O139 strains have been identified as the cause of sporadic cases of gastroenteritis, bloody diarrhea, and extraintestinal infections (5–9, 34, 35). Non-O1, non-O139 strains are very heterogeneous by nature, so it is highly likely that they have developed independent ways of colonizing the intestine and causing disease (36). In particular, the mechanisms of two non-O1, non-O139 strains have recently been eluci-dated. *V. cholerae* V52 belongs to the O37 serogroup and encodes a type VI secretion system that allows it to be virulent toward amebae, mice, and other bacteria such as *Escherichia coli* (37–40). *V. cholerae* AM-19226 is a non-O1, non-O139 strain that belongs to the O39 serogroup (10). In 2005 it was found that AM-19226 encodes a type III secretion system that might confer pathogenic properties to the microorganism (10). Recently, it was shown that *V. cholerae* AM-19226 requires the type III secretion system to produce diarrhea and epithelial damage in rabbits (11, 41). Further research will likely uncover novel mechanisms of pathogenesis for some of the yet unstudied virulent non-O1, non-O139 strains.

EPIDEMIOLOGY AND ECOLOGY OF CHOLERA

The vast majority of *V. cholerae* strains isolated in their natural environment, brackish rivers, estuaries, and coastal areas, are nonpathogenic. In one study of an area of cholera endemicity, only 0.8% of the strains isolated encoded TCP and carried the phage encoding CT, CTXΦ (36). Furthermore, in areas of endemicity such as the Ganges Delta region, cholera is strongly seasonal, with outbreaks occurring twice a year. Typically there is one major outbreak right after the monsoon and another one during the spring. Its marked seasonality and association with a small number of pathogenic strains make the epidemiology of cholera quite puzzling and complex. In the natural environment of *V. cholerae* there are numerous factors that affect its persistence, survival, and pathogenic potential (Fig. 1).

Some studies have shown that *V. cholerae* can be directly cultured from water samples (42). However, in most cases *V. cholerae* has been found to persist in its natural environment mainly in two forms: viable but not culturable (VBNC) and conditionally viable environmental cells (CVEC) (42, 43). VBNC is a dormant state that *V. cholerae* enters in response to nutrient deprivation and other environmental conditions (42). These forms cannot be recovered by culture techniques but are still able to cause infection and under certain conditions can revert to the culturable form (42). It was recently shown that *V. cholerae* can also enter a CVEC state in which it can be recovered after the appropriate enrichment culture techniques are applied (43).

Several physicochemical conditions affect *V. cholerae* populations in the natural environment, such as water temperature, salinity, oxygen tension, sunlight, rainfall, pH, and the availability of trace elements and chemical nutrients (42, 44). Although there are strong correlations between the changes in the physicochemical conditions in the environment of *V. cholerae*, the mechanisms by which some of them affect the population dynamics of *V. cholerae* remain unknown.

The known environmental hosts of *V. cholerae* include algae, shellfish, chironomid egg masses, fish, waterfowl, amebae, and most ubiquitously, copepods (15–18, 42, 45–53). Nonetheless, it is very possible that *V. cholerae* associates with a larger number of dwellers of its natural environment as the field is still young and some of these associations were found recently. Some associations might allow the bacterium to persist during interepidemic periods and act as a reservoir for *V. cholerae*. Nevertheless, there are several instances where *V. cholerae* is transmitted through a vector due to the consumption of fish or shellfish, indicating that cholera can perhaps more accurately be described as a zoonosis (54–60).

Prior to a full epidemic outbreak, several factors have to be met. From the environmental standpoint, there need to be changes in the physicochemical conditions that have been linked with algal blooms, where copepods thrive. Two major drivers of phytoplankton abundance have been found: the upwelling of cold, nutrient-rich deep ocean waters and, more recently, river discharges with terrestrial nutrients (61, 62). *V. cholerae* in turn establishes a commensal association with the copepods by forming biofilms on their chitinous surfaces, thus also multiplying during the algal blooms (13, 42, 44). Since the number of toxigenic strains during interepidemic episodes is very limited, it is thought that there is a period of enrichment for choleragenic strains both in the human host and in the environment prior to an epidemic of cholera (36). Briefly, intestinal passage of a mixed population of *V. cholerae* allows pathogenic clones to colonize and multiply, going through a selective enrichment period. However, due to low initial concentrations of choleragenic *V. cholerae*, the carriers can show no symptoms of the disease. Nonetheless, these asymptomatic carriers will shed pathogenic clones in their stools, further enriching the water sources with virulent bacteria and facilitating the initiation of an epidemic (36). In the early epidemic period a similar process happens; this time the patients will show symptoms of cholera and will shed strongly adapted and highly virulent epidemic clones (36). It is thought that when the number of predators of *V. cholerae* significantly outnumbers the total of toxigenic clones, the epidemics come to a collapse (63, 64). For example, an increase in the number of bacteriophages that thrive on *V. cholerae* in both water and stools is directly correlated with the termination of cholera epidemics (63, 64). Nonetheless, other environmental factors likely also play a role in the self-limiting nature of cholera epidemics, which we will discuss in further sections.

GENOME EVOLUTION OF CHOLERAGENIC *V. CHOLERAE*

Only O1 and O139 isolates of *V. cholerae* have been reported to be choleragenic. Interestingly, their two major virulence factors are encoded within mobile genetic elements that were acquired through horizontal gene transfer (65, 66). CT is encoded within the filamentous phage CTXΦ (65). The CTXΦ phage has been demonstrated to be transferable between *V. cholerae* strains, with TCP acting as the phage receptor (65). Interestingly, the transfer rate was higher within the gastrointestinal tracts of mice than under laboratory conditions (65). These findings place the human gastrointestinal tract of asymptomatic carriers not only as a vehicle for multiplication of toxigenic *V. cholerae* but also as a possible niche where the acquisition of virulence genes might occur. TCP is encoded within the *Vibrio* pathogenicity island-1 (VPI-1) (66). Like CTXΦ, VPI-1 is able to excise from its host chromosome and form circular intermediates (67). This would potentially allow for the transfer of the TCP operon to "naïve" strains of *V. cholerae*.

Other mobile genetic elements have been associated with virulence in choleragenic isolates of *V. cholerae*: the SXT integrative conjugative element, VPI-2, and *Vibrio* seventh pandemic island-1 (VSP-1) and -2 (VSP-2) (68–70). The SXT element is self-transmissible and confers to *V. cholerae* isolates resistance to streptomycin, sulfamethoxazole, and trimethoprim (68). VPI-2 is confined to pathogenic isolates of *V. cholerae* and encodes a cluster of genes involved in the transport and catabolism of sialic acid (71, 72). The ability to utilize sialic acid as a carbon source confers a competitive advantage to choleragenic vibrios in the mouse intestine (71). VSP-1 and VSP-2 were identified a decade ago using microarray technology to identify regions that were unique to El Tor strains; however, not until recently has a putative function for VSP-1 been described (70, 73). VSP-1 encodes a transcription factor, VspR, that is under the control of a ToxT-regulated small RNA (73). VspR modulates the expression of several genes encoded within VSP-1, one of which encodes a new class of dinucleotide cyclase, DncV (73). DncV synthesizes a hybrid cyclic AMP-GMP molecule, which is required for efficient intestinal colonization and downregulates *V. cholerae* chemotaxis, a phenotype that is associated with hyperinfectivity (73, 74). To date, no putative function has been associated with VSP-2. The four pathogenicity islands that choleragenic *V. cholerae* encodes, VPI-1, VPI-2, VSP-1, and VSP-2, can excise from their host's genome and form circular intermediates, which could hypothetically allow the transfer of virulence genes to other nonpathogenic *V. cholerae* strains (67, 75, 76).

The fact that the major pathogenicity factors of *V. cholerae* are encoded within mobile genetic elements suggests that there might be hybrid strains that have acquired only a subset of these elements. Interestingly, it has been repeatedly found that some non-O1, non-O139 environmental strains carry virulence genes (77–80). These strains have the potential of acting as reservoirs of virulence genes for noncholeragenic strains of *V. cholerae*.

It was recently found that the major component of the shell of crustaceans, chitin, induces natural competence of *V. cholerae* (81). *V. cholerae* has been found associated with copepods in its natural environment, where it forms biofilms while attached to their chitinous surface. The remarkable finding that *V. cholerae* becomes naturally competent when thriving on chitin, together with the existence of numerous hybrid strains of *V. cholerae* that encode some of the mobile genetic elements associated with virulence, strongly points to the shell of copepods being a crucial place where exchange of genetic material occurs among *V. cholerae* strains and where novel pathogenic isolates might arise.

INTERACTIONS OF *V. CHOLERAE* WITH ITS MULTIPLE ENVIRONMENTAL HOSTS

V. cholerae establishes complex interactions with a plethora of sea and riverine dwellers (Fig. 1).

Crustaceans

Of the many associations in which *V. cholerae* has been found, the most widely studied and feasibly critical one is that with copepods (13, 42, 44). Copepods, from the Greek for "oar feet," encompass a group of small crustaceans that are natural inhabitants of sea- and freshwater. Copepods feed on microscopic algae and, in turn, critically serve as food for millions of other invertebrates and fish, as they tend to be dominant members of the zooplankton. The population size of copepods is strongly associated with phytoplankton blooms from which they graze.

The exoskeleton of copepods and other crustaceans is composed of chitin. Chitin is a polymer of N-acetylglucosamine and is the most abundant polysaccharide found in aquatic environments. However, chitin is insoluble, and without bacterial activity that returns the polysaccharide into a soluble and thus biologically useful form, seawater would become depleted of carbon (82). *V. cholerae* has been found associated with the exoskeleton of copepods in large numbers (16, 51). *V. cholerae* is able to utilize chitin as a carbon source and has a complex chitin utilization program consisting of three sets of differentially regulated genes (83). The commensal relationship between *V. cholerae* and chitinaceous hosts provides several advantages to the bacterium other than nutrients. It has been found that when attached to copepods *V. cholerae* cells can withstand changes in salinity and pH that are detrimental to the organism in its free-living state (14, 84). *V. cholerae* forms biofilms while associated with copepods; this facilitates its growth, survival, and persistence in aquatic ecosystems. Biofilm formation requires the presence of the mannose-sensitive hemagglutinin type IV pilus and the flagellum (85). The mannose-sensitive hemagglutinin type IV pilus contributes to the attachment of *V. cholerae* to the copepod *Daphnia pulex* (52). The chitin-regulated pilus is also involved in the attachment of *V. cholerae* to chitin (83). Interestingly, one colonization factor, GbpA, mediates attachment to the exoskeleton of *D. pulex*, epithelial intestinal cell lines, and the mouse intestine (86). This finding provides a link between environmental survival and the pathogenesis of *V. cholerae*, indicating that the functions of some pathogenicity factors do not have to be exclusively related to virulence (86). Furthermore, when *V. cholerae* grows on chitin, it becomes naturally competent; that is, it can take up DNA from its environment (81). Therefore, the possibility of horizontal gene transfer, that is, the bacterial acquisition of genes or gene clusters that might confer pathogenic potential, is greater when *V. cholerae* is attached to the chitinous surface of the copepods. It was recently found that *V. cholerae* also enters a hyperinfectious state when growing on biofilms (87). Tamayo et al. showed that the infectious dose required to colonize the mouse intestine was orders of magnitude lower for biofilm-derived *V. cholerae* than for planktonic cells (87).

The association with copepods provides at least four crucial advantages to *V. cholerae*: its exoskeleton can be used as a carbon source; and it provides protection, induces the transfer and acquisition of genes, and promotes *V. cholerae* entry into a hyperinfectious state. Overall, these findings show that the association with copepods is critical in the epidemiology of cholera. Several findings support this hypothesis. First, the infectious dose of *V. cholerae* needed to cause cholera in healthy individuals decreases several logs when the low pH of the stomach is buffered with sodium bicarbonate prior to oral administration or when the bacterium is found associated with food products (1). As aforementioned, the association of *V. cholerae* with copepods confers resistance to low pH and might be a requirement to go through the stomach. This hypothesis seems to be supported by recent findings (21–23). It was found that the removal of particulate matter from drinking water through filtration with a traditional Indian garment termed a sari yielded a 48% reduction in the incidence of cholera in some areas of endemicity in rural Bangladesh (23). A subsequent study showed a sustained decrease in the incidence of cholera in those villages that kept using the sari filtration method (21).

V. cholerae also associates with other crustaceans such as shrimp and blue crab (48, 49, 88). Nonetheless, the direct association between the presence of *V. cholerae* attached to these crustaceans and its survival through the stomach remains to be elucidated.

Shellfish

V. cholerae has recurrently been isolated from raw oysters at a wide variety of locations around the world, including the United States, Australia, Brazil, and India (47, 50, 53, 59, 89–92). The bacterium has also been found associated with clams and other mollusks (93). Strikingly, there are several reported cases of cholera and severe diarrhea due to ingestion of raw oysters harboring *V. cholerae* (58–60). Several of those cases occurred in the United States in places such as Texas, Florida, and Louisiana, where regular inspections occur and hygiene standards are high, stressing the difficulty of detecting *V. cholerae* and preventing it from establishing itself within its host (58, 59). The presence of choleragenic *V. cholerae* poses a potential threat to public health that might be on the rise as waters warm up due to climate change and *V. cholerae* populations migrate to previously inhospitable new niches (94, 95).

Arthropods

In 2001, Broza and Halpern showed that *V. cholerae* also associate with egg masses of the nonbiting midge *Chironomus* sp. (51, 96–99). They found that the egg masses acted as the sole carbon source for *V. cholerae*, allowing the bacterial population to be sustained solely on that substrate. This finding introduced a novel natural reservoir for *V. cholerae*, which is also highly abundant as chironomids are the most widely distributed insect in freshwater (51). Additionally, *V. cholerae* can colonize the fly intestine in a biofilm-dependent manner (100). Overall, these findings clearly reveal that arthropods act as major reservoirs of *V. cholerae*.

Fish

Isolated cases of cholera have been associated with the consumption of sardines, salt fish, and dried fish in places such as Australia, Peru, India, Italy, and Tanzania (54–57, 101). *V. cholerae* was isolated from fish, *Sciaena deliciosa*, that were caught in Peru during a Peruvian epidemic (55). It has even been postulated that the endemicity of *V. cholerae* in areas of India and Bangladesh might be due to its association with hilsa fish (15). Only recently has *V. cholerae* been directly isolated from fish samples (15). Senderovich et al. found that several fish species from different habitats contained *V. cholerae* in their digestive tract, with concentrations as high as 5×10^3 CFU per gram of intestine (15). Among them was *Tilapia* spp., which is known to consume copepods and chironomids, known reservoirs of *V. cholerae* (15, 18). These findings demonstrate that fish act both as a reservoir and vector for the transmission of *V. cholerae*, facilitating colonization of humans and also dispersal of the bacterium and its migration to novel habitats.

Waterfowl

Recently, attention has been directed toward the role that waterfowl have in the dispersal of *V. cholerae* into novel areas (18). Residential and migratory waterfowl thrive on chironomids and copepods, which can survive within the gut of water birds (18, 102). There is also evidence that viable copepods and chironomids can be found associated with the feet and feathers of waterfowl (18). These two findings indicate that waterfowl could potentially disseminate two major reservoirs of *V. cholerae*. As previously mentioned, fish also act as reservoirs of *V. cholerae* (15). *Tilapia* spp., from which *V. cholerae* has been isolated, are regularly consumed by numerous species of waterfowl such as cormorants, pelicans, seagulls, egrets, and herons (103). Waterfowl also consume other potential reservoirs of *V. cholerae* such as shellfish and crustaceans (18).

Both O1 and non-O1, non-O139 strains of *V. cholerae* have been isolated from a wide variety of birds (18). *V. cholerae* was detected in cloacal swabs taken from gulls in England and from the feces of aquatic birds in Colorado and Utah (104, 105). It is noteworthy that the incidence of isolations followed a strong seasonal pattern, with the highest numbers of *V. cholerae* being isolated in spring and fall (105). The seasonality in the isolations of *V. cholerae* from waterfowl follows a similar pattern as that of cholera outbreaks. Overall, these findings strongly support the hypothesis that migratory waterfowl act as disseminators of *V. cholerae* across water bodies.

Protozoa

In its natural environment, *V. cholerae* becomes the prey of several inhabitants of the aquatic ecosystem. *V. cholerae* has been found to establish two kinds of associations with different amebae species: as prey and as a putative symbiont. It was recently shown that *V. cholerae* can survive and multiply intracellularly inside the free-living amebae *A. castellanii* and *Acanthamoeba polyphaga*, which indicates that these protozoa may act as reservoirs of *V. cholerae* in the aquatic environment (17, 106, 107). It is possible that the association of *V. cholerae* with amebae and other protozoa might favor its transmission and survival within the human host, in a similar fashion to how *A. polyphaga* acts not only as a reservoir but also as a vector for *Legionella pneumophila* (108).

Algae and Water Plants

Using immunofluorescence, several studies have found *V. cholerae* associated with a wide variety of algal species and water plants. *V. cholerae* attaches to the mucilaginous sheath of cyanobacteria (*Anabaena variabilis*), diatoms (*Skeletonema costatum*), and phaeophytes (*Ascophyllum nodosum*) and to freshwater vascular aquatic plants such as water hyacinths and duckweed (20, 45, 46, 109, 110). Several studies have found some factors involved in pathogenesis to be expressed or required while *V. cholerae* associates with algae. Islam et al. detected an increase in toxin production when *V. cholerae* is in association with the green alga *Rhizoclonium fontanum* (45). Also, a mucinase (HapA) that is part of the intestinal escape response of *V. cholerae* was found to play an important role in the association of *V. cholerae* O1 with *Anabaena* sp. (109, 111). HapA is additionally involved in the chemotactic response of *V. cholerae* toward the mucilaginous sheath of the green alga (112). These findings not only show that algae and other water plants can act as reservoirs of *V. cholerae* but also that some pathogenicity factors might have an environmental function and are useful for the bacterium outside of the human host.

THE FOES OF *V. CHOLERAE*

In its natural environment *V. cholerae* encounters two main predators: bacteriophages and protozoa. It has also been found that some antagonistic bacteria inhibit the growth of *V. cholerae* (Fig. 1).

Bacteriophages

There are more than 200 identified species of bacteriophages that can infect *V. cholerae*, known as vibriophages (113). Vibriophages can be lytic and/or lysogenic. The best-characterized vibriophage, CTXΦ, is a filamentous lysogenic phage that harbors the CT genes (65). In the last few years, the close relationship between the abundance of vibriophages and the seasonal nature of cholera epidemics has been revealed (63, 64, 114). Faruque et al. found that during a 3-year period (2001 to 2003) in Dhaka, Bangladesh, the number of cholera patients increased whenever the number of lytic vibriophages in water decreased (63). The study also found that the number of patients decreased and the overall cholera epidemics ended at the same time that the population of the vibriophages in the water increased to large numbers (63). Likewise, prior to the peak of the epidemic in Dhaka in 2004 there was high prevalence of *V. cholerae* in the environment, and as the epidemic ended the numbers of the lytic vibriophage JSF4 increased (64). Furthermore, there is a correlation between the peak in the numbers of the vibriophages and an increase in the presence of JSF4 in patients' stools (64). Mathematical models predict that if a cholera outbreak originates through an increase of *V. cholerae* in the environment, then the number of vibriophages will consequently proliferate, eventually leading to the decline and termination of the outbreak (114). It is likely that other factors are also involved in the termination of a cholera outbreak; however, their nature and role remain to be determined.

Protozoa

The relationship between *V. cholerae* and protozoa is puzzling, as some studies have found that *V. cholerae* can kill amebae but also survive and persist inside amebae or be consumed by them (37, 39, 106). The factors that modify and affect the nature of their relationship are beginning to be elucidated. For instance, it was recently found that the virulence regulator ToxR in *V. cholerae* is required for survival inside *A. castellanii*, providing an environmental function for a master regulator that is involved in the virulence of *V. cholerae* (115). This study highlights how just one factor can erase the thin line between being a commensal and becoming prey (115). Amebae such as *Dictyostelium discoideum* thrive on *V. cholerae* O1; however, it was recently found that some non-O1, non-O139 strains encode a mechanism that prevents *D. discoideum* from grazing on them (39). Pukatzki et al. determined that a type VI secretion system was responsible for killing *D. discoideum* in the strain V52, which belongs to the O37 serogroup (39). How grazing by amebae affects epidemics of cholera has yet to be determined; however, it seems likely that they might act synergistically with phages in the termination of cholera epidemics along with other factors such as changes in the environment.

Other Bacteria

Little is known about the relationship of *V. cholerae* with other marine bacteria, in particular regarding antagonistic interactions. Long et al. found that some marine bacteria inhibit the growth of *V. cholerae* on surfaces (116). Interestingly, they found that bacterial isolates derived from the surface of particles made of marine agar show a greater frequency of *V. cholerae* inhibition than free-living bacteria (116). *V. cholerae* is less susceptible to inhibition at higher temperatures, such as those measured during El Niño–Southern Oscillation and other seasonal events such as the monsoon. The mechanism of inhibition was linked to the biosynthesis of andrimid, an antibacterial agent produced by the antagonistic bacteria. The production of andrimid is decreased at higher temperature, which correlates with the lower susceptibility of *V. cholerae* at these temperatures (116). Overall, these findings corroborate the increased competitiveness of *V. cholerae* under warmer conditions and substantiate the hypothesis that many factors act in conjunction during cholera epidemics.

CONCLUDING REMARKS

V. cholerae associates with numerous dwellers of its natural environment, and its relationships with the different hosts vary widely. In this article we have presented a comprehensive description of these diverse associations. As can be gathered from the available data, an important distinction must be made between these associations: reservoirs and vectors of *V. cholerae*. A reservoir is a habitat in which an infectious agent generally lives, grows, and multiplies and can include humans, animals, and environmental niches. From this description we can contend that algae, arthropods, waterfowl, and protozoa act as reservoirs of *V. cholerae*, as the bacterium has been found associated with them but, so far, there is no evidence of cholera cases directly associated with these reservoirs. We argue that there is a distinction between reservoirs of *V. cholerae* and organisms that act as its vector—an epidemiological term that describes any living organism that carries and transmits an infectious pathogen into another living organism. There is significant supporting evidence that fish and shellfish act as vectors of *V. cholerae*, as they can directly transmit the disease. A very interesting association is that of *V. cholerae* with copepods, because those crustaceans may be one of the major vectors of cholera. However, linking the consumption of *V. cholerae* associated with copepods and the appearance of cholera is not trivial, as the crustaceans are microscopic and the patient is often unaware of ingesting them. Nonetheless, from these facts one can propose that cholera is a zoonosis with a diverse group of vectors and reservoirs, since a zoonosis is an infectious disease that can be transmitted from animals to humans by a vector. These advances in the ecoepidemiology of cholera and the subsequent changes in the terminology used to describe the disease will allow us to better understand how *V. cholerae* behaves in its natural environment and, thus, help researchers foresee and eventually prevent cholera outbreaks in areas of endemicity.

Acknowledgments. The authors thank Karen Skorupski for insightful conversations and critical reading of the manuscript. This work was supported by NIH grants AI025096 and AI039654 to RKT.

Citation. Almagro-Moreno S, Taylor RK. 2013. Cholera: environmental reservoirs and impact on disease transmission. Microbiol Spectrum 1(2):OH-0003-2012. doi:10.1128/microbiolspec.OH-0003-2012.

REFERENCES

1. **Kaper JB, Morris JG, Levine MM.** 1995. Cholera. *Clin Microbiol Rev* **8**:48–86.
2. **Faruque SM, Albert MJ, Mekalanos JJ.** 1998. Epidemiology, genetics, and ecology of toxigenic *Vibrio cholerae*. *Microbiol Mol Biol Rev* **62**:1301–1314.
3. **Finkelstein RA, LoSpalluto JJ.** 1969. Pathogenesis of experimental cholera. Preparation and isolation of choleragen and choleragenoid. *J Exp Med* **130**:185–202.
4. **Taylor RK, Miller VL, Furlong DB, Mekalanos JJ.** 1987. Use of *phoA* gene fusions to identify a pilus colonization factor coordinately regulated with cholera toxin. *Proc Natl Acad Sci USA* **84**:2833–2837.
5. **Dalsgaard A, Albert MJ, Taylor DN, Shimada T, Meza R, Serichantalergs O, Echeverria P.** 1995. Characterization of *Vibrio cholerae* non-O1 serogroups obtained from an outbreak of diarrhea in Lima, Peru. *J Clin Microbiol* **33**:2715–2722.
6. **Bagchi K, Echeverria P, Arthur JD, Sethabutr O, Serichantalergs O, Hoge CW.** 1993. Epidemic of diarrhea caused by *Vibrio cholerae* non-O1 that produced heat-stable toxin among Khmers in a camp in Thailand. *J Clin Microbiol* **31**:1315–1317.
7. **Dalsgaard A, Serichantalergs O, Pitarangsi C, Echeverria P.** 1995. Molecular characterization and antibiotic susceptibility of *Vibrio cholerae* non-O1. *Epidemiol Infect* **114**:51–63.
8. **Morris JG, Wilson R, Davis BR, Wachsmuth IK, Riddle CF, Wathen HG, Pollard RA, Blake PA.** 1981. Non-O group 1 *Vibrio cholerae* gastroenteritis in the United States: clinical, epidemiologic, and laboratory characteristics of sporadic cases. *Ann Intern Med* **94**:656–658.
9. **Bag PK, Bhowmik P, Hajra TK, Ramamurthy T, Sarkar P, Majumder M, Chowdhury G, Das SC.** 2008. Putative virulence traits and pathogenicity of *Vibrio cholerae* non-O1, non-O139 isolates from surface waters in Kolkata, India. *Appl Environ Microbiol* **74**:5635–5644.

10. **Dziejman M, Serruto D, Tam VC, Sturtevant D, Diraphat P, Faruque SM, Rahman MH, Heidelberg JF, Decker J, Li L, Montgomery KT, Grills G, Kucherlapati R, Mekalanos JJ.** 2005. Genomic characterization of non-O1, non-O139 *Vibrio cholerae* reveals genes for a type III secretion system. *Proc Natl Acad Sci USA* **102:**3465–3470.

11. **Shin OS, Tam VC, Suzuki M, Ritchie JM, Bronson RT, Waldor MK, Mekalanos JJ.** 2011. Type III secretion is essential for the rapidly fatal diarrheal disease caused by non-O1, non-O139 *Vibrio cholerae*. *MBio* **2:**e00106-11.

12. **Reen FJ, Almagro-Moreno S, Ussery D, Boyd EF.** 2006. The genomic code: inferring Vibrionaceae niche specialization. *Nat Rev Microbiol* **4:**697–704.

13. **de Magny GC, Mozumder PK, Grim CJ, Hasan NA, Naser MN, Alam M, Sack RB, Huq A, Colwell RR.** 2011. Role of zooplankton diversity in *Vibrio cholerae* population dynamics and in the incidence of cholera in the Bangladesh Sundarbans. *Appl Environ Microbiol* **77:**6125–6132.

14. **Huq A, West PA, Small EB, Huq MI, Colwell RR.** 1984. Influence of water temperature, salinity, and pH on survival and growth of toxigenic *Vibrio cholerae* serovar O1 associated with live copepods in laboratory microcosms. *Appl Environ Microbiol* **48:**420–424.

15. **Senderovich Y, Izhaki I, Halpern M.** 2010. Fish as reservoirs and vectors of *Vibrio cholerae*. *PLoS ONE* **5:**e8607.

16. **Tamplin ML, Gauzens AL, Huq A, Sack DA, Colwell RR.** 1990. Attachment of *Vibrio cholerae* serogroup O1 to zooplankton and phytoplankton of Bangladesh waters. *Appl Environ Microbiol* **56:** 1977–1980.

17. **Abd H, Saeed A, Weintraub A, Nair GB, Sandström G.** 2007. *Vibrio cholerae* O1 strains are facultative intracellular bacteria, able to survive and multiply symbiotically inside the aquatic free-living amoeba *Acanthamoeba castellanii*. *FEMS Microbiol Ecol* **60:**33–39.

18. **Halpern M, Senderovich Y, Izhaki I.** 2008. Waterfowl: the missing link in epidemic and pandemic cholera dissemination? *PLoS Pathog* **4:**e1000173.

19. **Islam MS, Drasar BS, Sack RB.** 1994. The aquatic flora and fauna as reservoirs of *Vibrio cholerae*: a review. *J Diarrhoeal Dis Res* **12:**87–96.

20. **Islam MS, Miah MA, Hasan MK, Sack RB, Albert MJ.** 1994. Detection of non-culturable *Vibrio cholerae* O1 associated with a cyanobacterium from an aquatic environment in Bangladesh. *Trans R Soc Trop Med Hyg* **88:**298–299.

21. **Huq A, Yunus M, Sohel SS, Bhuiya A, Emch M, Luby SP, Russek-Cohen E, Nair GB, Sack RB, Colwell RR.** 2010. Simple sari cloth filtration of water is sustainable and continues to protect villagers from cholera in Matlab, Bangladesh. *MBio* **1:**e00034-10.

22. **Huo A, Xu B, Chowdhury MA, Islam MS, Montilla R, Colwell RR.** 1996. A simple filtration method to remove plankton-associated *Vibrio cholerae* in raw water supplies in developing countries. *Appl Environ Microbiol* **62:**2508–2512.

23. **Colwell RR, Huq A, Islam MS, Aziz KMA, Yunus M, Khan NH, Mahmud A, Sack RB, Nair GB, Chakraborty J, Sack DA, Russek-Cohen E.** 2003. Reduction of cholera in Bangladeshi villages by simple filtration. *Proc Natl Acad Sci USA* **100:**1051–1055.

24. **Sack DA, Sack RB, Nair GB, Siddique AK.** 2004. Cholera. *Lancet* **363:**223–233.

25. **Ansaruzzaman M, Bhuiyan NA, Safa A, Sultana M, McUamule A, Mondlane C, Wang XY, Deen JL, von Seidlein L, Clemens JD, Lucas M, Sack DA, Nair GB.** 2007. Genetic diversity of El Tor strains of *Vibrio cholerae* O1 with hybrid traits isolated from Bangladesh and Mozambique. *Int J Med Microbiol* **297:** 443–449.

26. **Nair GB, Faruque SM, Bhuiyan NA, Kamruzzaman M, Siddique AK, Sack DA.** 2002. New variants of *Vibrio cholerae* O1 biotype El Tor with attributes of the classical biotype from hospitalized patients with acute diarrhea in Bangladesh. *J Clin Microbiol* **40:**3296–3299.

27. **Lan R, Reeves PR.** 2002. Pandemic spread of cholera: genetic diversity and relationships within the seventh pandemic clone of *Vibrio cholerae* determined by amplified fragment length polymorphism. *J Clin Microbiol* **40:**172–181.

28. **Safa A, Nair GB, Kong RYC.** 2010. Evolution of new variants of *Vibrio cholerae* O1. *Trends Microbiol* **18:**46–54.

29. **Son MS, Megli CJ, Kovacikova G, Qadri F, Taylor RK.** 2011. Characterization of *Vibrio cholerae* O1 El Tor biotype variant clinical isolates from Bangladesh and Haiti, including a molecular genetic analysis of virulence genes. *J Clin Microbiol* **49:**3739–3749.

30. **World Health Organization.** 2009. *State of the World's Vaccines and Immunization*, 3rd ed. World Health Organization, Geneva, Switzerland. http://whqlibdoc.who.int/publications/2009/9789241563864_eng.pdf (last accessed April 30, 2013).

31. **Sontag D.** 2012. In Haiti, global failures on a cholera epidemic. March 31, 2012. *The New York Times.* http://www.nytimes.com/2012/04/01/world/americas/haitis-cholera-outraced-the-experts-and-tainted-the-un .html?pagewanted=all (last accessed April 30, 2013).

32. **Krukonis ES, DiRita VJ.** 2003. From motility to virulence: sensing and responding to environmental signals in *Vibrio cholerae. Curr Opin Microbiol* **6:**186–190.

33. **Childers BM, Klose KE.** 2007. Regulation of virulence in *Vibrio cholerae*: the ToxR regulon. *Future Microbiol* **2:**335–344.

34. **Chatterjee S, Ghosh K, Raychoudhuri A, Chowdhury G, Bhattacharya MK, Mukhopadhyay AK, Ramamurthy T, Bhattacharya SK, Klose KE, Nandy RK.** 2009. Incidence, virulence factors, and clonality among clinical strains of non-O1, non-O139 *Vibrio cholerae* isolates from hospitalized diarrheal patients in Kolkata, India. *J Clin Microbiol* **47:**1087–1095.

35. **Sharma C, Thungapathra M, Ghosh A, Mukhopadhyay AK, Basu A, Mitra R, Basu I, Bhattacharya SK, Shimada T, Ramamurthy T, Takeda T, Yamasaki S, Takeda Y, Nair GB.** 1998. Molecular analysis of non-O1, non-O139 *Vibrio cholerae* associated with an unusual upsurge in the incidence of cholera-like disease in Calcutta, India. *J Clin Microbiol* **36:**756–763.

36. **Faruque SM, Chowdhury N, Kamruzzaman M, Dziejman M, Rahman MH, Sack DA, Nair GB, Mekalanos JJ.** 2004. Genetic diversity and virulence potential of environmental *Vibrio cholerae* population in a cholera-endemic area. *Proc Natl Acad Sci USA* **101:**2123–2128.

37. **Zheng J, Ho B, Mekalanos JJ.** 2011. Genetic analysis of anti-amoebae and anti-bacterial activities of the type VI secretion system in *Vibrio cholerae. PLoS ONE* **6:**e23876.

38. **MacIntyre DL, Miyata ST, Kitaoka M, Pukatzki S.** 2010. The *Vibrio cholerae* type VI secretion system displays antimicrobial properties. *Proc Natl Acad Sci USA* **107:**19520–19524.

39. **Pukatzki S, Ma AT, Sturtevant D, Krastins B, Sarracino D, Nelson WC, Heidelberg F, Mekalanos JJ.** 2006. Identification of a conserved bacterial protein secretion system in *Vibrio cholerae* using the *Dictyostelium* host model system. *Proc Natl Acad Sci USA* **103:**1528–1533.

40. **Ma AT, Mekalanos JJ.** 2010. In vivo actin cross-linking induced by *Vibrio cholerae* type VI secretion system is associated with intestinal inflammation. *Proc Natl Acad Sci USA* **107:**4365–4370.

41. **Tam VC, Suzuki M, Coughlin M, Saslowsky D, Biswas K, Lencer WI, Faruque SM, Mekalanos JJ.** 2010. Functional analysis of VopF activity required for colonization in *Vibrio cholerae. MBio* **1:** e00289-10.

42. **Colwell RR, Huq A.** 1994. Environmental reservoir of *Vibrio cholerae.* The causative agent of cholera. *Ann N Y Acad Sci* **740:**44–54.

43. **Faruque SM, Islam MJ, Ahmad QS, Biswas K, Faruque ASG, Nair GB, Sack RB, Sack DA, Mekalanos JJ.** 2006. An improved technique for isolation of environmental *Vibrio cholerae* with epidemic potential: monitoring the emergence of a multiple-antibiotic-resistant epidemic strain in Bangladesh. *J Infect Dis* **193:**1029–1036.

44. **de Magny GC, Colwell RR.** 2009. Cholera and climate: a demonstrated relationship. *Trans Am Clin Climatol Assoc* **120:**119–128.

45. **Islam MS.** 1990. Increased toxin production by *Vibrio cholerae* O1 during survival with a green alga, *Rhizoclonium fontanum*, in an artificial aquatic environment. *Microbiol Immunol* **34:**557–563.

46. **Islam MS, Drasar BS, Bradley DJ.** 1990. Long-term persistence of toxigenic *Vibrio cholerae* O1 in the mucilaginous sheath of a blue-green alga, *Anabaena variabilis. J Trop Med Hyg* **93:**133–139.

47. **Morris JG, Acheson D.** 2003. Cholera and other types of vibriosis: a story of human pandemics and oysters on the half shell. *Clin Infect Dis* **37:**272–280.

48. **Nahar S, Sultana M, Naser MN, Nair GB, Watanabe H, Ohnishi M, Yamamoto S, Endtz H, Cravioto A, Sack RB, Hasan NA, Sadique A, Huq A, Colwell RR, Alam M.** 2011. Role of shrimp chitin in the ecology of toxigenic *Vibrio cholerae* and cholera transmission. *Front Microbiol* **2:**260.

49. **Dalsgaard A, Huss HH, H-Kittikun A, Larsen JL.** 1995. Prevalence of *Vibrio cholerae* and *Salmonella* in a major shrimp production area in Thailand. *Int J Food Microbiol* **28:**101–113.

50. **de Sousa OV, Vieira RH, de Menezes FG, dos Reis CM, Hofer E.** 2004. Detection of *Vibrio parahaemolyticus* and *Vibrio cholerae* in oyster, *Crassostrea rhizophorae*, collected from a natural nursery in the Cocó river estuary, Fortaleza, Ceará, Brazil. *Rev Inst Med Trop Sao Paulo* **46:**59–62.

51. **Broza M, Halpern M.** 2001. Pathogen reservoirs. Chironomid egg masses and *Vibrio cholerae*. *Nature* **412**:40.

52. **Huq A, Small EB, West PA, Huq MI, Rahman R, Colwell RR.** 1983. Ecological relationships between *Vibrio cholerae* and planktonic crustacean copepods. *Appl Environ Microbiol* **45**:275–283.

53. **Chiavelli DA, Marsh JW, Taylor RK.** 2001. The mannose-sensitive hemagglutinin of *Vibrio cholerae* promotes adherence to zooplankton. *Appl Environ Microbiol* **67**:3220–3225.

54. **Forssman B, Mannes T, Musto J, Gottlieb T, Robertson G, Natoli JD, Shadbolt C, Biffin B, Gupta L.** 2007. *Vibrio cholerae* O1 El Tor cluster in Sydney linked to imported whitebait. *Med J Aust* **187**:345–347.

55. **Carvajal GH, Sanchez J, Ayala ME, Hase A.** 1998. Differences among marine and hospital strains of *Vibrio cholerae* during Peruvian epidemic. *J Gen Appl Microbiol* **44**:27–33.

56. **McIntyre RC, Tira T, Flood T, Blake PA.** 1979. Modes of transmission of cholera in a newly infected population on an atoll: implications for control measures. *Lancet* **1**:311–314.

57. **Maggi P, Carbonara S, Fico C, Santantonio T, Romanelli C, Sforza E, Pastore G.** 1997. Epidemiological, clinical and therapeutic evaluation of the Italian cholera epidemic in 1994. *Eur J Epidemiol* **13**:95–97.

58. **Klontz KC, Tauxe RV, Cook WL, Riley WH, Wachsmuth IK.** 1987. Cholera after the consumption of raw oysters. A case report. *Ann Intern Med* **107**:846–848.

59. **Twedt RM, Madden JM, Hunt JM, Francis DW, Peeler JT, Duran AP, Hebert WO, McCay SG, Roderick CN, Spite GT, Wazenski TJ.** 1981. Characterization of *Vibrio cholerae* isolated from oysters. *Appl Environ Microbiol* **41**:1475–1478.

60. **Piergentili P, Castellani-Pastoris M, Fellini RD, Farisano G, Bonello C, Rigoli E, Zampieri A.** 1984. Transmission of non O group 1 *Vibrio cholerae* by raw oyster consumption. *Int J Epidemiol* **13**: 340–343.

61. **Jutla AS, Akanda AS, Griffiths JK, Colwell RR, Islam S.** 2011. Warming oceans, phytoplankton, and river discharge: implications for cholera outbreaks. *Am J Trop Med Hyg* **85**:303–308.

62. **Lobitz B, Beck L, Huq A, Wood B, Fuchs G, Faruque AS, Colwell RR.** 2000. Climate and infectious disease: use of remote sensing for detection of *Vibrio cholerae* by indirect measurement. *Proc Natl Acad Sci USA* **97**:1438–1443.

63. **Faruque SM, Naser IB, Islam MJ, Faruque AS, Ghosh AN, Nair GB, Sack DA, Mekalanos JJ.** 2005. Seasonal epidemics of cholera inversely correlate with the prevalence of environmental cholera phages. *Proc Natl Acad Sci USA* **102**:1702–1707.

64. **Faruque SM, Islam MJ, Ahmad QS, Faruque AS, Sack DA, Nair GB, Mekalanos JJ.** 2005. Self-limiting nature of seasonal cholera epidemics: role of host-mediated amplification of phage. *Proc Natl Acad Sci USA* **102**:6119–6124.

65. **Waldor MK, Mekalanos JJ.** 1996. Lysogenic conversion by a filamentous phage encoding cholera toxin. *Science* **272**:1910–1914.

66. **Karaolis DK, Johnson JA, Bailey CC, Boedeker EC, Kaper JB, Reeves PR.** 1998. A *Vibrio cholerae* pathogenicity island associated with epidemic and pandemic strains. *Proc Natl Acad Sci USA* **95**: 3134–3139.

67. **Rajanna C, Wang J, Zhang D, Xu Z, Ali A, Hou YM, Karaolis DK.** 2003. The vibrio pathogenicity island of epidemic *Vibrio cholerae* forms precise extrachromosomal circular excision products. *J Bacteriol* **185**:6893–6901.

68. **Waldor MK, Tschäpe H, Mekalanos JJ.** 1996. A new type of conjugative transposon encodes resistance to sulfamethoxazole, trimethoprim, and streptomycin in *Vibrio cholerae* O139. *J Bacteriol* **178**:4157–4165.

69. **Jermyn WS, Boyd EF.** 2002. Characterization of a novel *Vibrio* pathogenicity island (VPI-2) encoding neuraminidase (*nanH*) among toxigenic *Vibrio cholerae* isolates. *Microbiology* **148**:3681–3693.

70. **Dziejman M, Balon E, Boyd D, Fraser CM, Heidelberg JF, Mekalanos JJ.** 2002. Comparative genomic analysis of *Vibrio cholerae*: genes that correlate with cholera endemic and pandemic disease. *Proc Natl Acad Sci USA* **99**:1556–1561.

71. **Almagro-Moreno S, Boyd EF.** 2009. Sialic acid catabolism confers a competitive advantage to pathogenic *Vibrio cholerae* in the mouse intestine. *Infect Immun* **77**:3807–3816.

72. **Almagro-Moreno S, Boyd EF.** 2009. Insights into the evolution of sialic acid catabolism among bacteria. *BMC Evol Biol* **9**:118.

73. **Davies BW, Bogard RW, Young TS, Mekalanos JJ.** 2012. Coordinated regulation of accessory genetic elements produces cyclic di-nucleotides for *V. cholerae* virulence. *Cell* **149**:358–370.

74. **Merrell DS, Butler SM, Qadri F, Dolganov NA, Alam A, Cohen MB, Calderwood SB, Schoolnik GK, Camilli A.** 2002. Host-induced epidemic spread of the cholera bacterium. *Nature* **417**:642–645.

75. **Almagro-Moreno S, Napolitano MG, Boyd EF.** 2010. Excision dynamics of *Vibrio* pathogenicity island-2 from *Vibrio cholerae*: role of a recombination directionality factor VefA. *BMC Microbiol* **10**:306.

76. **Murphy RA, Boyd EF.** 2008. Three pathogenicity islands of *Vibrio cholerae* can excise from the chromosome and form circular intermediates. *J Bacteriol* **190**:636–647.

77. **Chakraborty S, Mukhopadhyay AK, Bhadra RK, Ghosh AN, Mitra R, Shimada T, Yamasaki S, Faruque SM, Takeda Y, Colwell RR, Nair GB.** 2000. Virulence genes in environmental strains of *Vibrio cholerae*. *Appl Environ Microbiol* **66**:4022–4028.

78. **Rivera IN, Chun J, Huq A, Sack RB, Colwell RR.** 2001. Genotypes associated with virulence in environmental isolates of *Vibrio cholerae*. *Appl Environ Microbiol* **67**:2421–2429.

79. **Mukhopadhyay AK, Chakraborty S, Takeda Y, Nair GB, Berg DE.** 2001. Characterization of VPI pathogenicity island and CTXΦ prophage in environmental strains of *Vibrio cholerae*. *J Bacteriol* **183**: 4737–4746.

80. **Gennari M, Ghidini V, Carburlotto G, Lleo MM.** 2012. Virulence genes and pathogenicity islands in environmental *Vibrio* strains nonpathogenic to humans. *FEMS Microbiol Ecol* **82**:563–573.

81. **Meibom KL, Blokesch M, Dolganov NA, Wu CY, Schoolnik GK.** 2005. Chitin induces natural competence in *Vibrio cholerae*. *Science* **310**:1824–1827.

82. **Yu C, Lee AM, Bassler BL, Roseman S.** 1991. Chitin utilization by marine bacteria. A physiological function for bacterial adhesion to immobilized carbohydrates. *J Biol Chem* **266**:24260–24267.

83. **Meibom KL, Li XB, Nielsen AT, Wu CY, Roseman S, Schoolnik GK.** 2004. The *Vibrio cholerae* chitin utilization program. *Proc Natl Acad Sci USA* **101**:2524–2529.

84. **Nalin DR, Daya V, Reid A, Levine MM, Cisneros L.** 1979. Adsorption and growth of *Vibrio cholerae* on chitin. *Infect Immun* **25**:768–770.

85. **Watnick PI, Fullner KJ, Kolter R.** 1999. A role for the mannose-sensitive hemagglutinin in biofilm formation by *Vibrio cholerae* El Tor. *J Bacteriol* **181**:3606–3609.

86. **Kirn TJ, Jude BA, Taylor RK.** 2005. A colonization factor links *Vibrio cholerae* environmental survival and human infection. *Nature* **438**:863–866.

87. **Tamayo R, Patimalla B, Camilli A.** 2010. Growth in a biofilm induces a hyperinfectious phenotype in *Vibrio cholerae*. *Infect Immun* **78**:3560–3569.

88. **Huq A, Huq SA, Grimes DJ, O'Brien M, Chu KH, Capuzzo JM, Colwell RR.** 1986. Colonization of the gut of the blue crab (*Callinectes sapidus*) by *Vibrio cholerae*. *Appl Environ Microbiol* **52**:586–588.

89. **Eyles MJ, Davey GR.** 1988. *Vibrio cholerae* and enteric bacteria in oyster-producing areas of two urban estuaries in Australia. *Int J Food Microbiol* **6**:207–218.

90. **Tamplin ML, Fisher WS.** 1989. Occurrence and characteristics of agglutination of *Vibrio cholerae* by serum from the eastern oyster, *Crassostrea virginica*. *Appl Environ Microbiol* **55**:2882–2887.

91. **Hood MA, Ness GE, Rodrick GE.** 1981. Isolation of *Vibrio cholerae* serotype O1 from the eastern oyster, *Crassostrea virginica*. *Appl Environ Microbiol* **41**:559–560.

92. **DePaola A, Kaysner CA, McPhearson RM.** 1987. Elevated temperature method for recovery of *Vibrio cholerae* from oysters (*Crassostrea gigas*). *Appl Environ Microbiol* **53**:1181–1182.

93. **Saravanan V, Sanath Kumar H, Karunasagar I, Karunasagar I.** 2007. Putative virulence genes of *Vibrio cholerae* from seafoods and the coastal environment of Southwest India. *Int J Food Microbiol* **119**: 329–333.

94. **Schuster BM, Tyzik AL, Donner RA, Striplin MJ, Almagro-Moreno S, Jones SH, Cooper VS, Whistler CA.** 2011. Ecology and genetic structure of a northern temperate *Vibrio cholerae* population related to toxigenic isolates. *Appl Environ Microbiol* **77**:7568–7575.

95. **Baker-Austin C, Trinanes JA, Taylor NG, Hartnell R, Siitonen A, Martinez-Urtaza J.** 2013. Emerging *Vibrio* risk at high latitudes in response to ocean warming. *Nat Climate Change* **3**:73–77.

96. **Senderovich Y, Gershtein Y, Halewa E, Halpern M.** 2008. *Vibrio cholerae* and *Aeromonas*: do they share a mutual host? *ISME J* **2**:276–283.

97. **Halpern M, Broza YB, Mittler S, Arakawa E, Broza M.** 2004. Chironomid egg masses as a natural reservoir of *Vibrio cholerae* non-O1 and non-O139 in freshwater habitats. *Microb Ecol* **47**: 341–349.

98. **Halpern M, Landsberg O, Raats D, Rosenberg E.** 2007. Culturable and VBNC *Vibrio cholerae*: interactions with chironomid egg masses and their bacterial population. *Microb Ecol* **53**:285–293.

99. **Halpern M, Gancz H, Broza M, Kashi Y.** 2003. *Vibrio cholerae* hemagglutinin/protease degrades chironomid egg masses. *Appl Environ Microbiol* **69:**4200–4204.

100. **Purdy AE, Watnick PI.** 2011. Spatially selective colonization of the arthropod intestine through activation of *Vibrio cholerae* biofilm formation. *Proc Natl Acad Sci USA* **108:**19737–19742.

101. **Acosta CJ, Galindo CM, Kimario J, Senkoro K, Urassa H, Casals C, Corachán M, Eseko N, Tanner M, Mshinda H, Lwilla F, Vila J, Alonso PL.** 2001. Cholera outbreak in southern Tanzania: risk factors and patterns of transmission. *Emerg Infect Dis* **7**(3 Suppl):583–587.

102. **Green AJ, Sánchez MI.** 2006. Passive internal dispersal of insect larvae by migratory birds. *Biol Lett* **2:** 55–57.

103. **Rabbani GH, Greenough WB.** 1999. Food as a vehicle of transmission of cholera. *J Diarrhoeal Dis Res* **17:**1–9.

104. **Lee JV, Bashford DJ, Donovan TJ, Furniss AL, West PA.** 1982. The incidence of *Vibrio cholerae* in water, animals and birds in Kent, England. *J Appl Bacteriol* **52:**281–291.

105. **Ogg JE, Ryder RA, Smith HL.** 1989. Isolation of *Vibrio cholerae* from aquatic birds in Colorado and Utah. *Appl Environ Microbiol* **55:**95–99.

106. **Abd H, Weintraub A, Sandström G.** 2005. Intracellular survival and replication of *Vibrio cholerae* O139 in aquatic free-living amoebae. *Environ Microbiol* **7:**1003–1008.

107. **Sandström G, Saeed A, Abd H.** 2010. *Acanthamoeba polyphaga* is a possible host for *Vibrio cholerae* in aquatic environments. *Exp Parasitol* **126:**65–68.

108. **Newsome AL, Scott TM, Benson RF, Fields BS.** 1998. Isolation of an amoeba naturally harboring a distinctive *Legionella* species. *Appl Environ Microbiol* **64:**1688–1693.

109. **Islam MS, Goldar MM, Morshed MG, Khan MN, Islam MR, Sack RB.** 2002. Involvement of the *hap* gene (mucinase) in the survival of *Vibrio cholerae* O1 in association with the blue-green alga, *Anabaena* sp. *Can J Microbiol* **48:**793–800.

110. **Epstein PR.** 1993. Algal blooms in the spread and persistence of cholera. *BioSystems* **31:**209–221.

111. **Finkelstein RA, Boesman-Filkenstein M, Chang Y, Hase CC.** 1992. *Vibrio cholerae* hemagglutinin/ protease, colonial variation, virulence, and detachment. *Infect Immun* **60:**472–478.

112. **Islam MS, Goldar MM, Morshed MG, Bahkt HB, Islam MS, Sack DA.** 2006. Chemotaxis between *Vibrio cholerae* O1 and a blue-green alga, *Anabaena* sp. *Epidemiol Infect* **134:**645–648.

113. **Nelson EJ, Harris JB, Morris JG, Calderwood SB, Camilli A.** 2009. Cholera transmission: the host, pathogen and bacteriophage dynamic. *Nat Rev Microbiol* **7:**693–702.

114. **Jensen MA, Faruque SM, Mekalanos JJ, Levin BR.** 2006. Modeling the role of bacteriophage in the control of cholera outbreaks. *Proc Natl Acad Sci USA* **103:**4652–4657.

115. **Valeru SP, Wai SN, Saeed A, Sandström G, Abd H.** 2012. ToxR of *Vibrio cholerae* affects biofilm, rugosity and survival with *Acanthamoeba castellanii*. *BMC Res Notes* **5:**33.

116. **Long RA, Rowley DC, Zamora E, Liu EJ, Bartlett DH, Azam F.** 2005. Antagonistic interactions among marine bacteria impede the proliferation of *Vibrio cholerae*. *Appl Environ Microbiol* **71:**8531–8536.

One Health: People, Animals, and the Environment
Edited by Ronald M. Atlas and Stanley Maloy
© 2014 American Society for Microbiology, Washington, DC
doi:10.1128/microbiolspec.OH-0008-2012

Chapter 11

White-Nose Syndrome: Human Activity in the Emergence of an Extirpating Mycosis

Hannah T. Reynolds[1] and Hazel A. Barton[1]

INTRODUCTION

Although One Health is often associated with transmission of disease from animals to humans, white-nose syndrome (WNS) of bats is an example of how humans and environment can influence the transmission of a devastating disease to wildlife. In winter 2006, the bat population in Howe Cave, in central New York State, USA, contained a number of bats displaying an unusual white substance on their muzzles (1). The following year, numerous bats in four surrounding caves displayed unusual winter hibernation behavior, including day flying and entrance roosting. A number of bats were found dead and dying, but all demonstrated a white, powdery substance on their muzzles, ears, and wing membranes, which was later identified as the conidia of a previously undescribed fungal pathogen, *Geomyces destructans* (2). The growth of the conidia gave infected bats the appearance of having dunked their faces into powdered sugar (Fig. 1A). The disease was named white-nose syndrome (WNS) and represents an emerging zoonotic mycosis, likely introduced through human activities, which has led to a precipitous decline in North American bat species (3, 4).

The genus *Geomyces* (teleomorph *Pseudogymnoascus*) consists of 11 described species within the *Ascomycota* (5). Prior to the emergence of WNS, we knew very little about this fungal genus other than its general role as a soil saprobe (5). *Geomyces* spp. have been isolated from a number of diverse environments across a wide geographic region, from the Arctic to the Antarctic (5–9). The association of *Geomyces* with temperate and low-temperature (as low as –11°C) environments has suggested that members of the genus are either psychrotolerant or psychrophilic, while their close association with keratinaceous materials (10) and old wood (11, 12) suggests that the genus contains important keratin and cellulose degraders (5).

Despite the histological observation of an invasive fungal mycosis in infected bats, initial attempts to isolate the WNS pathogen were difficult due to overgrowth by commensal fungal species (D. S. Blehert, personal communication, 2008). Nonetheless, the pathogen was successfully cultured from the guard hairs of infected bats by growth at low temperatures (3 to 6°C). This new species, named *Geomyces destructans*, is closely

[1]Department of Biology, University of Akron, Akron, OH 44325.

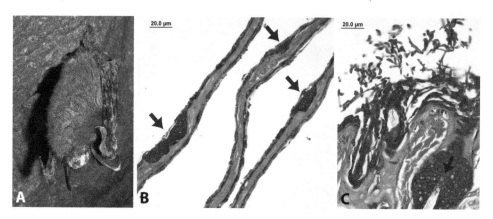

Figure 1. The pathology of WNS. (**A**) A little brown bat (*M. lucifugus*) displaying the characteristic white powder on the muzzle and wings from the production of *G. destructans* conidia. (**B**) Pathology of *G. destructans* on the wing membrane of *M. lucifugus* (bat tissues stain blue, while fungal material stains pink), demonstrating the characteristic devascularization and breakdown of connective tissues, including the characteristic cupping lesions (arrows). (**C**) Invasive pathology of *G. destructans* on the muzzle of *M. lucifugus*. Once colonization occurs, the invasion of hair follicles (arrow) and sweat glands is characteristic of WNS. Images B and C would both be considered WNS positive based on histology. Image A courtesy of U.S. Fish & Wildlife Service; B and C courtesy of Kevin Keel. doi:10.1128/microbiolspec.OH-0008-2012.f1

related to *Geomyces pannorum* var. *pannorum* (2), a fungal species that has been associated with superficial infections of the skin, nails, and hair in humans and other mammals, including both immunocompetent and immunocompromised patients (13–16). Infections with *G. pannorum* are extremely rare and are generally confined to superficial mycoses, although an inflammatory response can lead to irritation for the patient. Treatment of *G. pannorum* is difficult and often involves systemic treatment with antifungals (itraconazole) for extended periods of time (>6 months) (13, 14). Unlike *G. pannorum*, *G. destructans* is unable to cause disease in endothermic mammals due to its temperature restriction (<19°C); however, bats become susceptible due to their drop in body temperature during torpor.

Torpor in hibernating mammals is a period of unconsciousness in which the animal enters a hypometabolic state, allowing its body temperature to drop to ambient conditions (generally <12°C). This cooling is associated with a drop in the metabolic rate, with the breathing and heart rates falling to <1% of normal (17) and a suppression of the innate and adaptive immune responses, including a drop in complement, phagocytic, cytokine, and lymphocyte activities (18). Arousal naturally occurs in hibernating bats, in which bouts of torpor are punctuated with short periods (<8 hours) of activity every 6 to 14 days, depending on the bat species (19). The role of arousal in bats is still contested, with some investigators suggesting that it allows the individual to urinate/defecate, change roost position, mate, and even sleep (20). Other researchers have postulated that arousal plays a critical role in immune avoidance, allowing reactivation of B- and T-cell populations to screen for disease, a hypothesis supported by the rapid mobilization of lymphocyte populations from secondary lymphoid organs in arousing mammals (21). Whatever the physiological driver, arousal comes at a significant energetic cost: during arousal the bat must increase its body temperature from ambient to euthermic (36°C), which can consume critical fat reserves stored for hibernation. In a small bat, such as the little brown bat (*Myotis lucifugus*), arousal consumes 108 mg of fat—an amount that could support a bat in torpor for 67 days (17).

WNS

During hibernation, keratinophilic *G. destructans* targets the keratin-rich areas of the bat, including the muzzle, ears, and wing membranes (Fig. 1A). Initially infection is superficial with no inflammatory response, presumably due to immune suppression during torpor (1). The continued superficial growth of the fungus on the skin and wing membranes results in the production of curved, nonmelanotic, aerial conidia (Fig. 1B), which give the animal the characteristic appearance of having been dipped in powdered sugar (Fig. 1A).

It is unclear how this comparatively superficial *G. destructans* infection kills the bat; however, during an experimental infection with *G. destructans*, Warnecke et al. (2012) observed that infected bats roused from torpor more frequently than uninfected bats, with an arousal rate 3 to 4 times greater than control animals (22). This increase in arousal could lead to the acute inflammatory response observed in infected bats, as well as the depletion of essential fat reserves before the end of the winter; starvation is an important arousal trigger in bats, causing the animals to wake in search of food (22). An alternative WNS pathology has also been proposed, based on observed changes in the structure of the bat's wing membrane (23). The wing membranes of bats are remarkably elastic, allowing them to balloon out and contract, increasing flight efficiency and providing the remarkable maneuverability that enables a bat to capture insects in flight (24). The wing membranes also play an import role in physiology, being responsible for up to 10% of total gas exchange (both O_2 and CO_2) during flight and providing an important mechanism for water adsorption during hibernation (25, 26). Hydration during hibernation is critical to survival and an important arousal trigger: even reducing the humidity of the hibernacula by 15% (from 97 to 82%) can lead to a 20% mortality rate in *M. lucifugus* populations (22). Cryan et al. (2010) observed dramatic structural changes in wing membranes from *G. destructans* infection: previously malleable and elastic tissue became brittle and dry, with the consistency of tissue paper (23). As *G. destructans* infection causes such gross structural changes to the wing membrane, including the loss of internal vasculature (Fig. 1B) (23), it is possible that wing damage prevents water homeostasis during torpor in these animals.

The unusual behavior often seen during winter in bats with WNS, including entrance roosting and day flying, could therefore be indicative of starvation or dehydration, prompting arousal. The bats then emerge onto the winter landscape in search of food and water; in the midst of a northeastern U.S. winter, the frozen water, lack of food, and frigid temperatures quickly lead to death. Indeed, WNS produces greater declines in bat populations at higher latitudes, where the hibernation season is longer and winter temperatures are colder (cave-hibernating *M. lucifugus* bats demonstrate a much higher mortality rate in New York [91%] than in Virginia [79%] [27]). In southern states such as Tennessee, the observed high rates of WNS morbidity do not correlate with high mortality, suggesting that the length of the hibernation season is critical to the outcome of disease (22). Thus, while *G. destructans* itself is not directly fatal, the physiological changes induced by the pathogen ultimately lead to its host's death.

DETECTION

Although gross diagnostic identification of WNS is possible, the aerial conidia of *G. destructans* are easily damaged during handling of infected bats and confirmatory analyses are necessary (28). Due to the invasive nature of *G. destructans* in the pathogenesis of WNS, histology remains the gold standard for differentiating WNS infections from other, more generic mycoses. As WNS develops, *G. destructans* hyphae invade the hair follicles and associated sweat glands of infected bats (2), breaching the basement membrane and invading the regional tissue (Fig. 1C). This leads to gross morphological changes in the wing membranes that are characteristic of WNS, including devascularization, loss of connective tissue, and ulceration (Fig. 1B and C) (23). The fungus also creates a characteristic cupping: cup-like lesions in the wing membrane that are often filled with conidia (Fig. 1B) (23, 28). PCR methods have been developed to detect *G. destructans* on suspect animals, with a detection limit of ~100 conidia (29); however, the presence of PCR-detectable *G. destructans* on an animal does not confirm the development of the WNS pathology, but simply the presence of the fungus. It is therefore necessary to confirm all PCR-based findings with histology before a diagnosis of progression to WNS can be made (29). These same PCR methods have also been used to successfully detect *G. destructans* in contaminated hibernacula, although such methods find the fungus only in sediments closely associated with WNS-infected bats (30).

EPIDEMIC WNS

Upon the first detection of WNS, it was unclear whether this emerging infectious disease was the result of a mutation in an endemic organism or the introduction of a foreign pathogen to a susceptible community. Nonetheless, as long ago as the 1970s, bat biologists in Europe had been describing a white substance on the muzzles of hibernating bats (31), although these bats did not display any signs of infection, wing damage, behavioral change, or increased mortality (32). Following the identification of WNS in the United States, a comprehensive microscopic and PCR analysis of this substance on European bats led to the identification of *G. destructans* in numerous European countries, including the Czech Republic, France, Germany, Hungary, Slovakia, Switzerland, and Romania (32, 33). Genetic comparisons of the European *G. destructans* across a large geographic range suggest that *G. destructans* is endemic to Europe and closely related to North American *G. destructans* (34), although the vast mortalities in North American bat populations could not provide a more dramatic contrast between the two strains. The differences in mortality rate may stem from the pattern of European bats hibernating as solitary individuals or in small (two to three animals) groups, rather than as thousands of animals clustering together as in North America (35), suggesting that alternative hibernation patterns in the European bat population may reflect an adaptation to past epidemics.

Warnecke et al. demonstrated that both European *G. destructans* and North American *G. destructans* are able to cause morbidity and mortality in North American bat species, suggesting that the survival of European bats includes an intrinsic resistance to the pathogen (22). Of particular interest in this study was the finding that European *G. destructans* was more pathogenic in bats than North American *G. destructans*, indicating that despite its short history in North America, North American *G. destructans* has already become less virulent (22). This supports an origin for WNS in the European bat population (22, 34); with mortality rates in infected bat populations reaching 100% in North America, North American *G. destructans* must adapt to allow the host to survive long enough to be transmitted to new susceptible individuals.

After the initial identification of 18 infected bats in New York in February 2006, the winter of 2007–2008 saw the infection zone increase to >100 miles, with bat mortality rates exceeding 75% and an estimated 500,000 animals dead (Fig. 2) (A. C. Hicks, personal communication, 2008). This rapid expansion has continued, with the epidemic appearing to follow bat migration patterns along the Appalachian Mountains in the United States (Fig. 2). Currently the Great Plains of the central United States, which extend from Montana down through northern Texas, serve as a natural barrier to the westerly movement of WNS by migrating bat species; however, the early detection by PCR assay of *G. destructans* in a cave bat (*Myotis velifer*) (D. S. Blehert, personal communication, 2010) confounded this pattern (Fig. 2). The significance of this case is important, as *M. velifer*'s range extends to the southwestern United States and down through Mexico into Central America. Infection in *M. velifer* would greatly increase the potential spread of *G. destructans* into the cooler climates of the western United States, which is home to the highest diversity of hibernating bat species in the Americas (19). Nonetheless, in the 2 years since the detection of *G. destructans* in Oklahoma, WNS has not been detected at or around the original site. This suggests that either *M. velifer* is resistant to a progressive WNS infection or that the *G. destructans* detected did not constitute a minimum infectious dose.

ROLE OF HUMANS IN TRANSMISSION

The identification of European *G. destructans* raises the question of how the pathogen arrived in North America. There have been numerous hypotheses as to the transport of *G. destructans*, with human activities central to all of them (3). The human-vectored transport of Old World mycoses to North America has an inglorious past and includes import of chestnut blight from invasive *Cryphonectria parasitica*; Dutch elm disease caused by three species of *Ophiostoma*; and *Batracochytrium* in amphibians, which has spread rapidly and is threatening numerous species globally (3). Similar human activities are likely responsible for the movement of *G. destructans*, although our currently limited understanding of *G. destructans* transmission and infectious dose makes it difficult to distinguish whether it was moved through human travel or the movement of bats via trade. To dissect the differences between the two, and hence the likelihood of the transmission of *G. destructans* elsewhere, it is important to understand the survival and environmental resistance of the pathogen as well as potential vectors, fomites, and reservoirs.

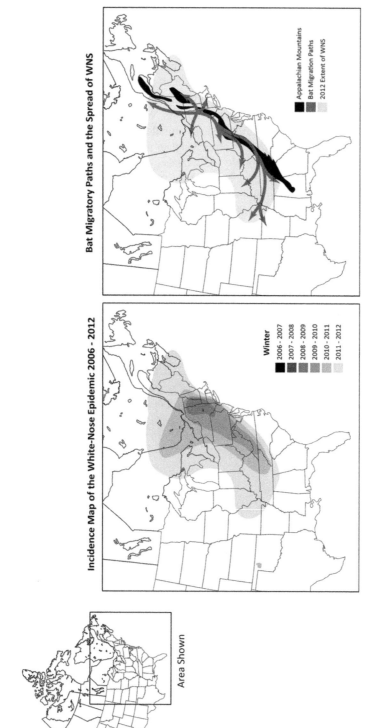

Figure 2. Incidence and spread of WNS. (**A**) The regional spread of infected hibernacula based on the winter observation of WNS-infected bats. The winter 2006–2007 data represent a single cave, with just a few infected individuals, while the winter 2011–2012 data represent hundreds of hibernacula and millions of infected bats. (**B**) The epidemic spread of WNS overlaid by the location of the Appalachian Mountains and significant bat migration routes in North America. Both maps are based on a map provided by Cal Butchkoski and the Pennsylvania Game Commission. doi:10.1128/microbiolspec.OH-0008-2012.f2

The activity of bats within the hibernacula covered with *G. destructans* spores likely spreads the fungus on air currents, bringing it into contact with surfaces, water, or other animals in this environment. Although we have little information on the propagation of *G. destructans* on surfaces, we do have some clues based on the physiology and survivability of the *Geomyces*. It is known that *G. destructans* can be detected both in the sediments and on the walls of WNS-impacted hibernacula (30, 34), and members of the *Geomyces* appear to be common residents of cave environments, being found on speleothems, in guano, and in the air (36). These data suggest that *Geomyces* may have a saprophytic lifestyle within caves, feeding on cellulose-rich organic detritus or the keratinaceous remnants of decaying arthropods. *G. destructans* itself has a narrow growth temperature range (from 0 to 19°C) (2) and requires high humidity, making it ideally suited for growth in caves (19). Anecdotal evidence suggests that once contaminated, an infected hibernaculum can serve as a reservoir for WNS: 2 years following the loss of all bat species from a WNS-impacted mine, the reintroduction of naïve bats to the same location led to a 100% mortality from WNS (Fig. 3) (A. C. Hicks, personal communication, 2010). The ability of infected hibernacula to serve as reservoirs for *G. destructans* will have a profound impact on the recovery and/or reintroduction of bat species following the WNS epidemic: while the ability of *G. destructans* to grow as a saprotroph within hibernacula can increase the overall virulence of the pathogen, freedom from the constraints imposed by reliance on a host for continued survival may allow *G. destructans* to drive its host species to extinction (3).

Subterranean hibernacula are often shared with other animals, including trogloxenes (cave visitors) and troglobites (obligate cave residents) (37). If bats disperse *G. destructans*

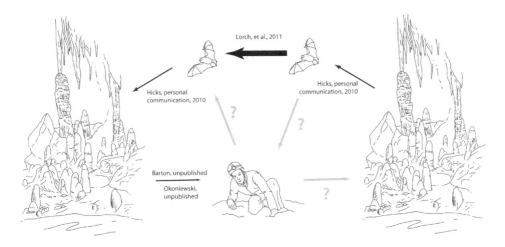

Figure 3. Known and postulated mechanisms of *G. destructans* transmission and WNS establishment. Bat-to-bat transmission has been demonstrated in laboratory experiments and based on epidemiology. Cave-to-bat and bat-to-cave transmission has been shown anecdotally. Fungal spores can be picked up by human activities in caves, while the ability of humans to pick up spores and serve as vectors for *G. destructans* transmission remains speculative. Black arrows demonstrate known fungal transport, with the thickness of the arrow indicative of the known significance of transfer. Gray arrows indicate as yet unknown mechanisms. doi:10.1128/microbiolspec.OH-0008-2012.f3

through their in-cave activities, it is likely that cave-inhabiting species would also come into contact with the pathogen, although to date no other animals have demonstrated the ability to develop a progressive *G. destructans* infection. Further, trogloxenes and troglobites are generally restricted to one or a group of closely related caves, making it unlikely that they could serve as vectors to spread the pathogen over long distances (37). The potential to transmit the fungus via water is possible, and water does flow through WNS-impacted caves; however, cave conduits often form part of regional groundwater flow, flowing toward the regional aquifer or watershed rather than to other caves and susceptible populations (38). This again limits the potential of water to play a role in transmission.

The only other potential vectors of *G. destructans* in hibernacula are humans (Fig. 3). After visiting a tourist cave, humans pick up $>1 \times 10^6$ fungal spores on their feet (H. A. Barton, unpublished data), while cave explorers (cavers) visiting a WNS-infected site can pick up *G. destructans* spores on their equipment (J. C. Okoniewski, personal communication, 2010). This suggests that human clothing and equipment can serve as fomites for the movement of *G. destructans*. The question remains as to whether these fomites can in turn serve as sources of *G. destructans* infection of bats or seed *G. destructans* into caves to create new reservoirs (Fig. 3).

The successful introduction of any xenobiotic species into an ecosystem is generally limited by resource competition, nutrient availability, and in the case of *G. destructans*, the nonconducive geochemistry of cave and mine environments (39). Therefore, the ability of a human to serve as a vector for WNS depends on a number of currently unknown factors, such as the survivability of the fungus/spores during transport, the minimum infectious dose for bats, and the inoculum size that is permissive of the establishment of *G. destructans* in a new site (Fig. 3). At this time, much of this information is lacking, other than the known susceptibility of *G. destructans* to heat (40) and the general tolerances of the *Geomyces* to cold and freezing (6).

Recreational cave exploration is common throughout North America and Europe and is particularly popular in many of the countries where European *G. destructans* is endemic, including France, Germany, Romania, and the Czech Republic. Indeed, cavers have been visiting North America from these countries since the 1940s. The first detected site of WNS is within 200 feet of Howe Caverns, a commercial cave open to both tourists and cavers since 1843 and receiving upwards of 200,000 visitors a year. While it is not surprising that such a site could serve for the introduction of an invasive species, other commercial caves in North America have been open for as long and receive much larger numbers of international visitors (~8% of total visitation) (National Caves Association, personal communication, 2012). Wind Cave (South Dakota, opened 1891) receives >600,000 visitors/year, Mammoth Cave (Kentucky, opened 1838) >500,000 visitors/year, and Carlsbad Caverns (New Mexico, opened 1915) >400,000 visitors/year. WNS has not been seen in any of these caves, despite their significant bat populations and long history of international visitation. These data may suggest that while the human-vectored transport of *G. destructans* is possible, disease establishment itself must be quite rare.

Bats are obvious vectors of *G. destructans*, and bat-to-bat transmission of WNS is well established and demonstrable under laboratory conditions (Fig. 3) (41). The fungus produces abundant conidia on the wings and fur of infected bats (Fig. 1A), which routinely come into contact with other bats through swarming, grooming, and mating events prior to and during hibernation. Indeed, bats routinely change roost positions and even hibernacula during arousal periods (19), thus providing a mechanism of *G. destructans* movement from both bat to bat and cave to cave. Given that *G. destructans* is unable to infect naïve bats segregated from WNS-infected bats by a wire mesh (allowing airborne movement of the fungus) and that laboratory infection studies require 1×10^5 spores, it is possible that the minimum infectious dose of *G. destructans* is high (41). This, along with the epidemic spread of WNS along bat migration paths (Fig. 2), opens up the possibility that bats themselves moved *G. destructans* from Europe to North America. While bats are not capable of transoceanic flight, bats migrating across bodies of water have occasionally been blown off course during storms and forced to seek refuge on any object they find, including ships (42). These bats then ride along on the vessel to its final destination. Such travel has been recorded in cases of North American bats ending up in Europe and Russia (42). Bats are also known to roost in shipping containers, only to become trapped on an oceangoing vessel and transplanted to the final port of call. The translocation of bats in this way has been documented from Asia and Europe to North America and vice versa (42). Given that Howe Caverns is within 40 miles of Albany, NY, one of the busiest shipping ports in North America, this opens the possibility that *G. destructans* may have been transported by a European *G. destructans*-infected bat.

IMPACT

Whatever the mechanism of transfer, *G. destructans* is now in North America and is having a profound impact on bats and the environment. Bats have a remarkable environmental distribution and range of potential food sources, including vegetarian, omnivorous, insectivorous, and nectarivorous diets (very few species are hematophagic), allowing them to colonize virtually every available habitat, from desert to coastal and tropical to the Arctic Circle (19). With such a wide distribution and variety of foodstuffs, it is not surprising that bats play an important role in the ecosystem, including in pest control, the pollination of plants (including agaves, mangoes, guavas, and bananas), and seed dispersal. Adaptive behavioral patterns also allow insectivorous bats to migrate during the winter when food is unavailable (Mexican free-tailed bats, *Tadarida brasiliensis*, can migrate as far as 2,000 km) or hibernate in situ until favorable conditions return (19). Of bats that hibernate, those that choose subterranean (mines and caves) sites are susceptible to WNS. Of the 47 bat species in North America, 12 species are currently found within the WNS epidemic range, including the little brown bat (*M. lucifugus*), Indiana bat (*Myotis sodalis*), gray bat (*Myotis grisescens*), northern long-eared bat (*Myotis septentrionalis*), southeastern bat (*Myotis austroriparius*), eastern small-footed bat (*Myotis leibii*), big brown bat (*Eptesicus fuscus*), tricolored bat (*Perimyotis subflavus*), Virginia big-eared bat (*Corynorhinus townsendii virginianus*), eastern red bat (*Lasiurus borealis*), and Rafinesque's big-eared bat (*Corynorhinus rafinesquii*). Of these, *L. borealis* and *C. rafinesquii* do not hibernate in caves and mines, limiting their exposure to the fungus. Of the remaining 10 species, all except *C. townsendii virginianus* are experiencing population declines from the WNS epidemic (27).

Insectivorous bats are voracious hunters, able to feed on a diverse range of insects, from small midges (*Chironomidae* at ~2 mm) up to large beetles (*Coleoptera* at ≤5 cm); a nursing female *M. lucifugus* can consume up to 30% of her body weight during one evening, catching up to 520 insects/hour (43). The insects consumed by WNS-impacted bat species include members of the *Diptera* (true flies), *Trichoptera* (aquatic caddisflies), *Lepidoptera* (moths), and *Homoptera* (including cicadas and aphids) (43). These are important agricultural pests that lay eggs on crops, which hatch into caterpillars and other larval forms with ravenous appetites. With the current loss of 6.7 million bats translating into an additional 5,000 to 10,000 metric tons of insects per year, the potential agricultural impacts are staggering. Boyles et al. (55) estimated in 2011 that current declines in the bat population would result in more than $3.7 billion per year in crop losses and increased costs of pesticide application.

The other commercial impacts of WNS have yet to be calculated. In the United States, there are 142 commercial caves and 14 national parks containing caves, with an annual visitation of >32 million people/year generating local revenues of more than $549 million and employing an estimated 10,000 people directly or indirectly (National Caves Association, personal communication, 2012; K. Castle, personal communication, 2012). While no show caves have been closed during the WNS epidemic, increasing pressure has been placed on these businesses to limit the potential human spread of *G. destructans*. In addition, the perception by the general public that caves are closed or that *G. destructans* itself poses a danger to human health has severely affected the operations of these caves (P. Youngbaer, personal communication, 2012). Income is also generated by the activities of recreational cave explorers. With an estimated 50,000 active recreational cavers spending more than $50 million annually on cave exploration (through travel and equipment), as well as >1 million cave visits by youth groups including Boy Scouts, church groups, etc., annual losses from the WNS epidemic in cave-rich areas could be as high as $700 million.

The WNS epidemic can also affect humans beyond simple economics. The diet of *M. lucifugus* consists of 10 to 20% mosquitoes (*Culicidae*), with a daily intake of 200 to 800 (43). This means that the current losses of *M. lucifugus* alone correspond to an extra 200 billion mosquitoes/year. West Nile virus, an introduced viral pathogen vectored by mosquitoes, has been responsible for >1 million human infections since its introduction in 1999, including >1,300 deaths (44). With a significant increase in the mosquito population, there may also be a dramatic increase in the incidence of and morbidity from West Nile virus, which could be particularly significant in states such as New York, which has been heavily affected by both West Nile virus and WNS (44).

RESPONSE

The ability of a superficial mycosis to cause a fatal infection in an immunocompetent, endothermic mammal is rare (3). As a result, WNS was originally thought to be caused by an underlying regional or environmental factor, such as an immunosuppressive virus or unidentified pesticide (45). This problem was compounded by the difficulty in culturing the pathogen and establishing the environmental conditions necessary for both fungal growth and bat hibernation. Because of this, it took 4 years beyond the emergence of WNS before Koch's postulates were satisfied for *G. destructans* (41). Nonetheless, Chaturvedi et al. used random amplified polymorphic DNA analyses to demonstrate that *G. destructans* isolates from WNS-infected bats had shared genetic loci over a geographically wide area (46). This identity, demonstrated using five different random amplified polymorphic DNA primer sets, indicated that a single source organism was responsible for all WNS cases and argued for the epidemic spread of a single etiologic agent (46). At this point, biologists realized they were witnessing an emerging zoonosis on an epidemic scale, and the questions immediately focused on controlling the epidemic.

While humans have been unable to constrain or eradicate a single epidemic mycosis (3), the pressure from business stakeholders and the general public in the face of such a devastating epidemic required action on the part of federal and state agencies. But there are limited options available to wildlife and land managers in the face of such devastating epidemics, and the response to WNS has mirrored that to other infectious mycoses: research results are often outpaced by population declines, with the result that some type of action has to be perceived to be happening (3). Initial efforts were directed toward limiting transport of the pathogen. While it is impossible to control bat movement and migration, it is possible to limit human activities that could transport the fungus. In states affected by WNS, caves were closed to visitation, while a nationally adopted disinfection protocol against the fungus was developed (40). Initial indications show that these measures may have contributed to the absence of new disease epicenters, particularly in the more vulnerable western United States.

Other intervention options are limited. As a superficial mycosis, *G. destructans* does not generate a strong adaptive immune response, so vaccination may have limited impact (1). Antifungal agents are often deleterious to bats themselves, through both toxic and endocrine effects, limiting the usefulness of treatment. If an antifungal agent that did not harm bats was found, bat activity during hibernation, such as grooming, would remove any superficial application, while repeated administration would lead to a WNS-like disturbance mortality. Therefore, any effective treatments would require a long-lasting antifungal agent, which would have to be administered directly to each bat. As bats hibernate in nooks and crevices, often high in the ceiling, with colonies that can exceed thousands of individuals, such direct administration efforts are extremely difficult on an environmental scale. Remaining options that have been tried are even more dramatic, including the culling of infected individuals, particularly in newly identified WNS sites. Modeling of such action has shown that, given the difficulty in identifying all infected organisms, culling would not prevent the spread of WNS and would actually prevent the emergence of naturally resistant communities (47, 48).

With the impending extirpation of certain bat species, biologists are working toward methods of maintaining genetic diversity, including the establishment of "Ark" communities: colonies of individuals that are maintained until the WNS epidemic has passed. A similar approach has been developed for threatened amphibians in the face of the chytrid fungus (49). The establishment of such colonies would allow the reintroduction of bats post-WNS; however, if *G. destructans* can survive in a saprophytic lifestyle in hibernacula, even this approach may be limited in its effectiveness. Further, a preliminary attempt to maintain a small, exploratory community of *C. townsendii virginianus* in captivity resulted in the complete loss of the colony, reflecting the difficulty in maintaining healthy bats in nonnative environments.

Some researchers have pushed for the disinfection of hibernacula to break the chain of transmission and to prevent reinfection of bats. This approach is fraught with problems, the primary being the as yet unknown impact of biocides on the subterranean ecosystem: caves represent intricate ecosystems, including a great diversity of cave-adapted and endemic species (37), of which fungi play an important role in nutrient mobilization (50). Indeed, the use of disinfectants to limit the spread of xenobiotic species has a dire history, and such attempts have been devastating (51). Lascaux Cave, France, is a culturally important cave due to its extensive Neolithic paintings. In 2000, an invasive fungus, *Fusarium solani*, began to colonize surfaces within the cave. In an attempt to control this fungus, biocides including quaternary ammonium compounds were applied in the cave. Unfortunately, the use of these disinfectants destroyed the native microbial flora of the cave, selecting for disinfectant-resistant entomophilous fungi that were previously contained by the endemic microbial community (52, 53). The results were disastrous for both the cave ecosystem and, through the increased and rapid growth of these introduced fungi, the paintings themselves (51). Antifungals therefore have the potential to collapse the cave ecosystem, a difficult problem given the other threatened and endangered species that share this environment (37).

FUTURE

The fate of bats in North America currently hangs in the balance. The rapid rate of spread and the high mortality of WNS have led to a dramatic decline in cave- and mine-hibernating bat species. At the time of this review, WNS has spread to 22 U.S. states and four Canadian provinces, spreading as far south as Alabama and as far north as Ontario, Canada (Fig. 2). The most recent estimates have put bat mortality at >6.7 million animals, although with the difficulties in accurate counting, this number could be significantly higher (54). At the current rate of decline, it is almost certain that the once common *M. lucifugus* may go extinct within the northeastern United States (4). Other species already on the endangered species list have their entire populations within the WNS epidemic area, including *M. sodalis*, *M. grisescens*, and *C. townsendii virginianus*. These species may well go extinct without human intervention.

But still, there is reason for hope. The high mortality in states such as New York, where WNS was first discovered, has led to the almost complete loss of hibernating bat species. However, in certain hibernacula, remnant populations of bats have been observed to return to the site year after year despite the presence of WNS. This includes *M. lucifugus*, one of the populations hardest hit by WNS, and suggests the emergence of a resistant population (48). Some species, such as *C. townsendii virginianus* and *E. fuscus*, hibernate in caves in which other species have experienced dramatic declines from WNS. Yet members of these species demonstrate little to no observable signs of the disease (G. G. Turner, personal communication, 2011), suggesting that natural resistance to *G. destructans* is present.While this is encouraging news for the persistence of these species, healthy individuals from WNS-impacted sites may act as superspreaders, carrying the disease to uninfected caves and promoting the infection of vulnerable species.

A hindrance in mobilizing resources to combat the WNS epidemic has been the misconceptions of the general public about the importance of bats and bat behavior: the common notion that bats are blood-sucking, flying rodents that get caught in your hair could not be further from the truth. Bats are members of the *Chiroptera*, which share an evolutionary lineage with primates and represent >20% of all known mammalian species. With >1,100 bat species identified, bats are second only to rodents in diversity (19). Their excellent spatial awareness through echolocation, acrobatic flight capabilities, and good eyesight make them the least likely to accidentally land on anyone's head. Bats play an important part in our ecosystem, and the education of the public on the importance of these mammals is critical to their continued survival.

CONCLUDING REMARKS

Perhaps more than any other recent epidemic, WNS exemplifies the impact that infectious agents can have on animals, our environment, and human health. The response to this epidemic demonstrates the necessity of collaboration across a wide range of disciplines, including bat biologists, wildlife managers, veterinary researchers and pathologists, medical mycologists, and environmental microbiologists—together emphasizing the importance of a functioning, holistic approach to emerging diseases and the demonstration of a functioning One Health initiative. The outstanding questions in WNS and *G. destructans* pathology similarly cannot be answered by one discipline alone, but require the shared resources and integrative tools of the medical, veterinary, and environmental sciences.

Whatever the source of WNS or the future of bats in North America, *G. destructans* is here to stay. As we move forward, an integrative approach may allow for the protection or conservation of bat species, but perhaps more importantly, help us to understand the transfer of such devastating mycoses and how future epidemics can be prevented.

Citation. Reynolds HT, Barton HA. 2013. White-nose syndrome: human activity in the emergence of an extirpating mycosis. Microbiol Spectrum 1(2):OH-0008-2012. doi:10.1128/microbiolspec.OH-0008-2012.

REFERENCES

1. **Blehert DS, Hicks AC, Behr M, Meteyer CU, Berlowski-Zier BM, Buckles EL, Coleman JT, Darling SR, Gargas A, Niver R, Okoniewski JC, Rudd RJ, Stone WB.** 2009. Bat white-nose syndrome: an emerging fungal pathogen? *Science* **323:**227.

2. **Gargas A, Trest MT, Christensen M, Volk TJ, Blehert DS.** 2009. *Geomyces destructans* sp. nov. associated with bat white-nose syndrome. *Mycotaxon* **108:**147–154.

3. **Fisher MC, Henk DA, Briggs CJ, Brownstein JS, Madoff LC, McCraw SL, Gurr SJ.** 2012. Emerging fungal threats to animal, plant and ecosystem health. *Nature* **484:**186–194.

4. **Frick WF, Pollock JF, Hicks AC, Langwig KE, Reynolds S, Turner GG, Butchkoski CM, Kunz TH.** 2010. An emerging disease causes regional population collapse of a common North American bat species. *Science* **329:**679–682.

5. **Rice AV, Currah RS.** 2006. Two new species of *Pseudogymnoascus* with *Geomyces* anamorphs and their phylogenetic relationship with *Gymnostellatospora*. *Mycologia* **98:**307–318.

6. **Hughes KA, Lawley B, Newsham KK.** 2003. Solar UV-B radiation inhibits the growth of Antarctic terrestrial fungi. *Appl Environ Microbiol* **69:**1488–1491.

7. **Taylor DL, Herriott IC, Long J, O'Neill K.** 2007. TOPO TA is A-OK: a test of phylogenetic bias in fungal environmental clone library construction. *Environ Microbiol* **9:**1329–1334.

8. **Kochkina GA, Ivanushkina NE, Akimov VN, Gilichinskii DA, Ozerskaya SM.** 2007. Halo- and psychrotolerant *Geomyces* fungi from arctic cryopegs and marine deposits. *Mikrobiologiia* **76:**39–47 (In Russian).

9. **Marshall WA.** 1998. Aerial transport of keratinaceous substrate and distribution of the fungus *Geomyces pannorum* in Antarctic soils. *Microb Ecol* **36:**212–219.

10. **Anbu P, Hilda A, Gopinath SC.** 2004. Keratinophilic fungi of poultry farm and feather dumping soil in Tamil Nadu, India. *Mycopathologia* **158:**303–309.

11. **Blanchette RA, Held BW, Arenz BE, Jurgens JA, Baltes NJ, Duncan SM, Farrell RL.** 2010. An Antarctic hot spot for fungi at Shackleton's historic hut on Cape Royds. *Microb Ecol* **60:**29–38.

12. **Schabereiter-Gurtner C, Piñar G, Lubitz W, Rölleke S.** 2001. Analysis of fungal communities on historical church window glass by denaturing gradient gel electrophoresis and phylogenetic 18S rDNA sequence analysis. *J Microbiol Methods* **47**:345–354.

13. **Christen-Zaech S, Patel S, Mancini AJ.** 2008. Recurrent cutaneous *Geomyces pannorum* infection in three brothers with ichthyosis. *J Am Acad Dermatol* **58**(5 Suppl 1):S112–S113.

14. **Erne JB, Walker MC, Strik N, Alleman AR.** 2007. Systemic infection with *Geomyces* organisms in a dog with lytic bone lesions. *J Am Vet Med Assoc* **230**:537–540.

15. **Gianni C, Caretta G, Romano C.** 2003. Skin infection due to *Geomyces pannorum* var. *pannorum*. *Mycoses* **46**:430–432.

16. **Zelenkova H.** 2006. *Geomyces pannorum* as a possible causative agent of dermatomycosis and onychomycosis in two patients. *Acta Dermatovenerol Croat* **14**:21–25.

17. **Speakman JR, Thomas DW.** 2003. Physiological ecology and energetics of bats, p 430–492. *In* Kunz TH, Fenton MB (ed), *Bat Ecology*. University of Chicago Press, Chicago, IL.

18. **Bouma HR, Carey HV, Kroese FG.** 2010. Hibernation: the immune system at rest? *J Leukoc Biol* **88**: 619–624.

19. **Kunz TH, Fenton MB (ed).** 2003. *Bat Ecology*. University of Chicago Press, Chicago, IL.

20. **Park KJ, Jones G, Ransome RD.** 2000. Torpor, arousal and activity of hibernating greater horseshoe bats (*Rhinolophus ferrumequinum*). *Funct Ecol* **14**:580–588.

21. **Bouma HR, Kroese FG, Kok JW, Talaei F, Boerema AS, Herwig A, Draghiciu O, van Buiten A, Epema AH, van Dam A, Strijkstra AM, Henning RH.** 2011. Low body temperature governs the decline of circulating lymphocytes during hibernation through spingosine-1-phosphate. *Proc Natl Acad Sci USA* **108**:2052–2057.

22. **Warnecke L, Turner JM, Bollinger TK, Lorch JM, Misra V, Cryan PM, Wibbelt G, Blehert DS, Willis CK.** 2012. Inoculation of bats with European *Geomyces destructans* supports the novel pathogen hypothesis for the origin of white-nose syndrome. *Proc Natl Acad Sci USA* **109**:6999–7003.

23. **Cryan PM, Meteyer CU, Boyles JG, Blehert DS.** 2010. Wing pathology of white-nose syndrome in bats suggests life-threatening disruption of physiology. *BMC Biol* **8**:135–143.

24. **Song A, Tian X, Israeli E, Galvao R, Bishop R, Bishop K, Swartz S, Breuer K.** 2008. Aeromechanics of membrane wings with implications for animal flight. *AIAA J* **46**:2096–2106.

25. **Makanya AN, Mortola JP.** 2007. The structural design of the bat wing web and its possible role in gas exchange. *J Anat* **211**:687–697.

26. **Thomas DW, Geiser F.** 1997. Periodic arousals in hibernating mammals: is evaporative water loss involved? *Funct Ecol* **11**:585–591.

27. **Turner GG, Reeder DM, Coleman JT.** 2011. A five-year assessment of mortality and geographic spread of white-nose syndrome in North American bats and a look at the future. *Bat Res News* **52**:13–27.

28. **Meteyer CU, Buckles EL, Blehert DS, Hicks AC, Green DE, Shearn-Bochsler V, Thomas NJ, Gargas A, Behr MJ.** 2009. Histopathologic criteria to confirm white-nose syndrome in bats. *J Vet Diagn Invest* **21**: 411–414.

29. **Lorch JM, Gargas A, Meteyer CU, Berlowski-Zier BM, Green DE, Shearn-Bochsler V, Thomas NJ, Blehert DS.** 2010. Rapid polymerase chain reaction diagnosis of white-nose syndrome in bats. *J Vet Diagn Invest* **22**:224–230.

30. **Lindner DL, Gargas A, Lorch JM, Banik MT, Glaeser J, Kunz TH, Blehert DS.** 2011. DNA-based detection of the fungal pathogen *Geomyces destructans* in soils from bat hibernacula. *Mycologia* **103**: 241–246.

31. **Feldmann R.** 1984. Teichfledermaus—*Myotis dasycneme* (Boie, 1825), p 107–111. *In* Schröpfer R, Feldmann R, Vierhaus H (ed), *Die Säugetiere Westfalens*. Westfalisches Museum fur Naturkunde, Münster, Germany.

32. **Wibbelt G, Kurth A, Hellmann D, Weishaar M, Barlow A, Veith M, Prüger J, Görföl T, Grosche L, Bontadina F, Zöphel U, Seidl HP, Cryan PM, Blehert DS.** 2010. White-nose syndrome fungus (*Geomyces destructans*) in bats, Europe. *Emerg Infect Dis* **16**:1237–1243.

33. **Puechmaille SJ, Verdeyroux P, Fuller H, Gouilh MA, Bekaert M, Teeling EC.** 2010. White-nose syndrome fungus (*Geomyces destructans*) in bat, France. *Emerg Infect Dis* **16**:290–293.

34. **Puechmaille SJ, Wibbelt G, Korn V, Fuller H, Forget F, Mühldorfer K, Kurth A, Bogdanowicz W, Borel C, Bosch T, Cherezy T, Drebet M, Görföl T, Haarsma AJ, Herhaus F, Hallart G, Hammer M, Jungmann C, Le Bris Y, Lutsar L, Masing M, Mulkens B, Passior K, Starrach M, Wojtaszewski A,**

Zöphel U, Teeling EC. 2011. Pan-European distribution of white-nose syndrome (*Geomyces destructans*) not associated with mass mortality. *PLoS ONE* **6**:e19167.

35. **Masing M, Lutsar L.** 2007. Hibernation temperatures in seven species of sedentary bats (*Chiroptera*) in northeastern Europe. *Acta Zool Lituanica* **17**:47–55.
36. **Nováková A.** 2009. Microscopic fungi isolated from the Domica Cave system (Slovak Karst National Park, Slovakia). A review. *Int J Speleology* **38**:71–82.
37. **Culver DC.** 1982. *Cave Life: Evolution and Ecology.* Harvard University Press, Cambridge, MA.
38. **Klimchouk AB, Ford DC, Palmer AN, Dreybrodt W.** 2000. *Speleogenesis: Evolution of Karstic Aquifers.* National Speleological Society, Huntsville, AL.
39. **Barton HA, Jurado V.** 2007. What's up down there: microbial diversity in starved cave environments. *Microbe* **2**:132–138.
40. **Shelley V, Kaiser S, Shelley E, Williams T, Kramer M, Haman K, Keel K, Barton HA.** 2013. Evaluation of strategies for the decontamination of equipment for *Geomyces destructans*, the causative agent of white-nose syndrome (WNS). *J Cave Karst Stud* **75**:1–10.
41. **Lorch JM, Meteyer CU, Behr MJ, Boyles JG, Cryan PM, Hicks AC, Ballmann AE, Coleman JT, Redell DN, Reeder DM, Blehert DS.** 2011. Experimental infection of bats with *Geomyces destructans* causes white-nose syndrome. *Nature* **480**:376–378.
42. **Constantine DG.** 2003. Geographic translocation of bats: known and potential problems. *Emerg Infect Dis* **9**:17–21.
43. **Anthony EL, Kunz TH.** 1977. Feeding strategies of the little brown bat, *Myotis lucifugus*, in southern New Hampshire. *Ecology* **58**:775–786.
44. **Kilpatrick AM.** 2011. Globalization, land use, and the invasion of West Nile virus. *Science* **334**:323–327.
45. **Blehert DS, Lorch JM, Ballmann AE, Cryan PM, Meteyer CU.** 2011. Bat white-nose syndrome in North America. *Microbe* **6**:267–273.
46. **Chaturvedi V, Springer DJ, Behr MJ, Ramani R, Li X, Peck MK, Ren P, Bopp DJ, Wood B, Samsonoff WA, Butchkoski CM, Hicks AC, Stone WB, Rudd RJ, Chaturvedi S.** 2010. Morphological and molecular characterizations of psychrophilic fungus *Geomyces destructans* from New York bats with white-nose syndrome (WNS). *PloS ONE* **5**:e10783.
47. **Hallen TG, McCracken GF.** 2010. Management of the panzootic white-nose syndrome through culling of bats. *Conserv Biol* **25**:189–194.
48. **Dobony CA, Hicks AC, Langwig KE, von Linden RI, Okoniewski JC, Rainbolt RE.** 2011. Little brown *Myotis* persist despite exposure to white-nose syndrome. *J Fish Wildl Manage* **2**:190–195.
49. **Gewin V.** 2008. Riders of a modern-day Ark. *PLoS Biol* **6**:e24.
50. **Sterflinger K.** 2000. Fungi as geologic agents. *Geomicrobiol J* **17**:97–124.
51. **Di Piazza M.** 2007. The crisis in Lascaux: update March 2007. *Rock Art Res* **24**:136–137.
52. **Dupont J, Jacquet C, Dennetière B, Lacoste S, Bousta F, Orial G, Cruaud C, Couloux A, Roquebert MF.** 2007. Invasion of the French Paleolithic painted cave of Lascaux by members of the *Fusarium solani* species complex. *Mycologia* **99**:135–162.
53. **Fox JL.** 2008. Some say Lascaux Cave paintings are in microbial "crisis" mode. *Microbe* **3**:110–112.
54. **U.S. Fish & Wildlife Service.** 2012. *North American bat death toll exceeds 5.5 million from white-nose syndrome.* U.S. Fish & Wildlife Service Office of Communications, Arlington, VA. http://static.whitenosesyndrome.org/sites/default/files/files/wns_mortality_2012_nr_final_0.pdf (last accessed May 19, 2013).
55. **Boyles JG, Cryan PM, McCracken GF, Kunz TH.** 2011. Economic importance of bats in agriculture. *Science* **6025**:41–42.

One Health and Antibiotic Resistance

One Health: People, Animals, and the Environment
Edited by Ronald M. Atlas and Stanley Maloy
© 2014 American Society for Microbiology, Washington, DC
doi:10.1128/microbiolspec.OH-0005-2012

Chapter 12

Antibiotic Resistance in and from Nature

Julian Davies[1]

INTRODUCTION

Nothing quite exemplifies the concept of One Health better than the fact that many aspects of human, animal, and plant health and function are dependent on the presence of bacteria and their metabolic products: they are harbingers of disease, sources of disease treatment, and the origins of genetic determinants of resistance to these treatments. Bacterial pathogens have been present since early evolution, coexisting with all living organisms, and have probably been responsible for a number of species extinctions.

The rational chemotherapy of microbial diseases dates to 1917 with Ehrlich's discovery of arsenicals for the treatment of parasitic diseases such as trypanosomiasis. Not surprisingly, this was often accompanied by resistance development. Ehrlich later developed the organic mercury antisyphilis drug salvarsan based on his concepts of chemoreceptors. This fearsome molecule had horrible side effects but did effect cures. There were also reports of drug-fastness (resistance) to salvarsan; mercury resistance is quite common in bacteria. Some 20 years later followed the development of sulfonamides, which were (and remain) effective antibacterial agents. Although resistance to this latter class of drugs was identified in the late 1930s, they are still widely used (1).

The introductions of penicillin in the mid-1940s and streptomycin shortly thereafter heralded the antibiotic era, both in terms of use and production. Antibiotics became the foundation for the treatment of infectious diseases, and the pharmaceutical companies flourished. Other applications of antibiotics followed as the industry and numbers of products expanded very rapidly. There are now more than 10 major classes of antibiotics, with hundreds of different derivatives that have been generated as "improvements."

Today it is well known that antibiotic resistance is widespread, and it is now accepted as a sequela of antibiotic use. It is of interest to recount a few early experiences with antibiotic resistance before it became so widespread. A dramatic description from the early 1950s, when antibiotics were first available for general use (previously they were reserved for military personnel), was provided by the well-known infectious disease

[1]Department of Microbiology and Immunology, Life Science Centre, University of British Columbia, Vancouver, BC V6T 1Z3, Canada.

physician Maxwell Finland (at Boston City Hospital). In a review published in 1971, Finland (2) stated the following:

> Our first report on coagulase-positive staphylococci (in 1950) revealed a wide range of susceptibility to penicillin among strains, the MIC ranging from 0.002 to more than 250mg/ml. When MICs of strains isolated before 1946 were compared with those isolated in the subsequent 4 years, it was shown that about 82% of the former were inhibited by 0.04μg/ml or less of penicillin, the remaining strains being susceptible to less than 5μg/ml. Only 25% of strains isolated from 1946 to 1947 and 21% of those isolated in 1948-49 were susceptible within this range of concentrations: the remainder varied in MIC over the entire range of concentrations to more than 250μg/ml.

Similar reports on the development of resistance to erythromycin came from another U.S. hospital. In this case, all staphylococci in the hospital were inhibited by <1.0 μg/ml erythromycin when it was introduced for the treatment of all staphylococcal infections. At the end of a 5-month period, 70% of the *Staphylococcus aureus* isolates from patients and hospital personnel were resistant to 100 μg/ml erythromycin.

EMERGING ANTIBIOTIC RESISTANCE: THE WRITING WAS ON THE WALL

Resistance to antibiotics was already present in the environment when the era of antibiotic use for treating infectious diseases began. But recognition that the ability to resist the toxic effects of antibiotics already existed raises several questions: Where in the environment? What are putative antibiotic resistance genes doing in the environment? How did they spread to humans? Are there other pressures that select for putative resistance genes? (See reference 3 for a discussion of these topics.) Metagenomic analyses of bacterial populations from multiple environmental sources, including the human gut, have demonstrated that genes with DNA sequences closely related to known antibiotic resistance genes are ubiquitous (4, 5). Of course, it is not known if they determine resistance in their natural habitat. Is antibiotic production and activity also widespread in nature? Are microbial populations in nature in constant conflict?

The biosynthetic gene clusters for antibiotic production are complex. These clusters were once thought to be associated mainly with fungi and the actinomycetes, principally the streptomycetes. However, this has been shown not to be the case: it is highly probable that most microbes have the capacity to make a diversity of bioactive small molecules and often possess identifiable biosynthetic clusters. The two major classes of antibiotics are the polyketides and the nonribosomal peptides (as well as their hybrids); the corresponding biosynthetic clusters are the polyketide synthases and the nonribosomal peptide synthases. Such gene clusters are widespread, and their small-molecule products exhibit many different bioactivities, such as antibiotics, virulence factors, and regulatory processes; all these naturally occurring compounds probably play a multitude of different roles in the biological interactions of the microbial world. It is clear that we need to rethink the prevailing notions (largely anthropogenic) of the functions of these exciting low-molecular-weight molecules, ancient and ubiquitous in living organisms. However, this is not the place to undertake this topic, exciting as it may be.

An important finding in 1974 showed that *Streptomyces* strains that produce antibiotics (and many that do not!) carry genes that encode resistance mechanisms against the major classes of antibiotics. Since that time many such combinations have been identified, and Cundliffe and Demain (6) have assembled a complete review of so-called self-protection mechanisms. Is there a good reason to assume this function? Detailed studies of the roles of putative resistance genes in nature have not been done; what if the gene(s) encoding one of the supposed self-protection mechanisms is inactivated in the antibiotic-producing host? Does it die? Or does it simply stop making the antibiotic?

RESISTANCE GENES ARE EVERYWHERE

With the power of high-throughput sequencing, many predicted or suspected biosynthetic clusters for production of small molecules have been identified in microbial genomes (bacteria and fungi), and in many cases putative resistance genes have been identified.

What is the environment? Albert Einstein defined the environment as "anything that is not me." Independently of studies of producing organisms, DNA extracted directly from numerous environments has been scanned for resistance genes using metagenomic analyses. These include organisms in marine environments, in permafrost, deep below the Earth's surface, and in other sites. Intriguingly, a diverse collection of resistance genes has been identified in the human gastrointestinal tract (7). The resistance genes are not only in the environment, but also in us. In addition, resistance genes have been found in ancient soils (8). The prediction is that putative resistance genes are present everywhere and for any natural product in the biosphere, but one can only guess at their real functions.

In addition, modern sequencing technology has permitted searches for putative (potential?) resistance genes, from bacteria associated with birds, insects, fish, humans, and even inanimate objects. Their presence is to be expected in domestic animals associated with human lifestyles and throughout modern society. However, resistance genes (transferable at that) are also found in aboriginal people and their surroundings, despite no known contact with modern civilization (9). One can conclude that antibiotics and antibiotic resistance genes both are ancient. Did they evolve together? Which came first? Certainly they were present in the biosphere before the evolution of pathogens. For more detailed information on these topics, several thorough reviews are available (10–12).

MECHANISMS OF ANTIBIOTIC RESISTANCE

An important question is the relationships between supposed resistance genes in the environment and the real thing in the clinic. One of the most interesting concerns inhibition of cell wall function in gram-positive bacteria, specifically for the important peptide antibiotics vancomycin and daptomycin. The first is widely used in the clinic, and the resistance gene operon is present in many gram-positive bacteria (13). It was presumably acquired when the antibiotic was used extensively for animal growth promotion. It is transferable between certain *Firmicutes*. The vancomycin resistance gene cluster has also been detected in staphylococci, but is less stable or not fully functional in this host compared with the enterococci.

Daptomycin is of more recent introduction as a therapeutic agent, and although genes encoding potential hydrolytic enzymes are found in resistomes (14), no corresponding resistance mechanism has been detected in clinical isolates; in addition, no transferable daptomycin resistance has been identified. One can only speculate as to why such an "ideal" resistance function has not been "picked up" and transferred to pathogens. It is worth noting that daptomycin has not been employed as an animal growth promotant.

Resistance gene clusters involving reconstruction of the bacterial cell wall are unique to the *Firmicutes* and have several possible origins. The vancomycin cluster is present in the genome in members of the paenibacilli ("almost bacilli"), common soil bacteria that inhabit the rhizosphere (15, 16). Certain members of this genus are important plant pathogens, and engineered versions have been used in plant protection against insect infestations. The presence of VanR-like clusters in these organisms is intriguing. What useful function(s) do they provide for the host in the plant environment—perhaps as protective agents against antibiotic action or as signal-quenching agents? Are vancomycin-type molecules involved? Incidentally, some paenibacilli produce lipopeptide antibiotics related to daptomycin and are resistant to daptomycin.

HORIZONTAL GENE TRANSFER AND THE SPREAD OF RESISTANCE

With virtually uncontrolled use of antibiotics and the constant introduction of newer compounds in medical, veterinary, and agricultural practice, the unremitting antibiotic selection pressure on a worldwide basis has led to increasing antibiotic resistance in hospitals and in the community. By the early 1960s, 70% of staphylococci were resistant to penicillin derivatives, and as the β-lactam antibiotics were used more frequently for gram-negative infections, the incidence of resistance expanded due to the growing family of transferable β-lactamases. Horizontal gene transfer is the primary source of multiple-drug resistance in almost all pathogens (although it is still unclear as to the roles of bacteriophages and other transfer agents in this process), and combined with modern intercontinental travel and commerce has successfully disseminated novel resistance genes on a worldwide basis. The mechanisms of the process are mostly understood and have been reviewed ad nauseam, unfortunately with relatively little influence on the outcome. Like other aspects of antibiotic resistance, resistance gene transfer has been rediscovered many times by the popular press (in bold headlines), to little effect, however, and physicians, pharmaceutical companies, and international agencies seem powerless to prevent international traffic in antibiotic resistance genes.

THE WHITE PLAGUE

The case of tuberculosis (TB) is historically and medically interesting. As evidenced from the skeletal abnormalities found in ancient graves from many sites, *Mycobacterium tuberculosis* is probably the oldest human pathogen. TB (the white plague) has killed more humans than the totality of all other plagues and wars in human history. The first effective treatment for TB was streptomycin, discovered in 1945 by Schatz and Waksman; this was a major milestone in human medicine, and the importance of this discovery of a treatment for a disease that had been the cause of such death and suffering for thousands of years is hard to imagine. Albeit, the treatment came with a cost in side effects, notably deafness due to the surprising affinity of streptomycin (and other aminoglycosides) for nerve tissue in the inner ear. There was also the rapid onset of resistance, via mutation to high-level streptomycin resistance during the course of treatment. Streptomycin is no longer the front-line drug for TB treatment, having been replaced by cocktails of inhibitors, but its early success, together with that of penicillin (introduced around the same time), signaled the genesis of the antibiotic era. It is important to note that in the case of TB, resistance to antibiotic treatment develops sequentially, as a result of mutations in different target sites in concert with the use of different drugs and their combinations. Fortunately, no transferable resistance has ever been described for any drug used in the treatment of *M. tuberculosis* or other mycobacteria.

Interestingly, these first antibiotics, penicillin and streptomycin, are still used in many countries for a variety of infections. In addition to TB, streptomycin is used for some enterococcal infections and for the treatment of plague. Penicillin is inexpensive, readily available, and provides relatively nontoxic treatment for a variety of infections in developing countries. In both cases, treatment failures due to resistance development are common (as described above), and the drugs are used mostly for short-term treatment. Resistance to both antibiotics occurs by mutation and also by horizontal gene transfer, depending on the infectious agent. At first, depending on the regimen, mutations reducing antibiotic uptake into the cell occur. Subsequently, in the case of streptomycin, mutations in the antibiotic target prevent binding of the antibiotic to the 30S subunit of the bacterial ribosome. These mutations cause amino acid changes in a single ribosomal protein and engender resistance to very high levels of the drug. In the case of penicillin, a variety of mutations may be responsible, but eventually the pathogens acquire genes for penicillinases that hydrolyze the essential β-lactam ring and so destroy drug activity.

THE BIG MISTAKE

An ominous event happened in the late 1940s. Soon after the introduction of antibiotics such as the tetracyclines and chloramphenicol for human clinical use, it was found that the crude fermentation and purification residues from antibiotic production promoted the growth of chickens. The residues contained vitamin B_{12} plus another component that was subsequently shown to be the antibiotic (17). Many supporting studies were carried out and the FDA eventually approved the use of low concentrations of antibiotics as growth promotants for a variety of animals. Extensive losses due to "shipping fever," a serious problem encountered in the transport of animals, were reduced when the animal feed was supplemented with antibiotics. In addition, antibiotic-supplemented feeds enhanced animal growth such that shorter times were required before sacrifice. Antibiotic-resistant bacteria were detectable in the animals and their excreta, but this warning sign was not appreciated. It should be noted that transferable antibiotic resistance had not yet been identified. The phenomenon of horizontal gene transfer was first reported in Japan in the mid-1950s but was almost certainly active before this time.

The early success led to the extensive use of antibiotics for agriculture and in livestock worldwide. In Japan, antibiotic use in fish farming was adopted. Industrial use (as distinct from therapeutic use) rapidly became the most intensive use of antibiotics, and it has been a significant factor in the selection of antibiotic-resistant bacteria. In addition, huge amounts of fermentation materials have been discarded into the environment: antibiotic production processes involve the use of large fermentation vessels, often 30,000 gallons or more. In addition, antibiotic-contaminated waste (human included) is dumped without too much concern for human and environmental health. Sadly, reports of extreme abuse are frequent (18). The combined selection pressures of extensive human and animal use of antibiotics and antibiotic derivatives have meant that no antibiotic has escaped. However, the representative contributions of the two to the overall problem of resistance cannot be reliably assessed.

Given the fact that putative resistance genes in the environment (resistomes) are everywhere, what roles do they play in the development of clinically significant resistance, especially under such constant selection pressure? Where does antibiotic resistance come from? Are the environmental resistomes the *immediate* sources of the resistance genes in bacterial pathogens, in which case one has to explain their transfer and establishment in human and animal pathogens? Or they are *not* precursors of clinically significant resistance determinants and we have to find an explanation as to where the latter come from!

ORIGINS OF CLINICALLY SIGNIFICANT RESISTANCE

In most studies of resistomes, the putative resistance genes originate in members of the family *Actinobacteria* (streptomycetes, etc.), a widely distributed group of bacteria with relatively high G+C composition (>60%). This is not optimal for translation in the most common pathogens (*Enterobacteriacae*: ~50% G+C; *Firmicutes*: ~35% G+C). Harmonizing or amelioration (19) of the gene sequences for efficient expression in most human pathogens would involve a number of mutational steps, and it is difficult to reconstruct this process except when closely related bacterial species are involved. Interestingly, the opportunistic human pathogen *Pseudomonas* (~60% G+C) might be a tractable host. It can be engineered in the laboratory using recombinant techniques with engineered vectors, and high-GC gene sequences can be transcribed and translated in *Escherichia coli* hosts; definitive evidence for natural transfer and expression of such heterologous genes has not been found. It must be remembered that there would be strong positive selection for resistance in the presence of (even) low concentrations of antibiotics, conditions that could increase spontaneous mutation rates.

Extensive phylogenetic studies of the common resistance determinants of pathogens and antibiotic-producing organisms demonstrate significant levels of similarity/homology in many instances. Some of the protein relationships show surprising cross-kingdom similarities, but definitive origins are difficult to establish. For example, the bacterial aminoglycoside phosphotransferases show striking three-dimensional domain identities with eukaryotic protein kinases as shown by X-ray crystallographic studies (20). The same is true with aminoglycoside acetyltransferases and the GCN5 family of *N*-acetyltransferases. As another example of a putative cross-kingdom transfer, one mechanism of resistance to the bacterial protein synthesis inhibitor mupirocin is the (apparent) inheritance of a gene encoding a eukaryotic isoleucyl-tRNA synthetase (21). Do these similarities identify origins? Which came first?

TOOLS

Antibiotics and their cognate resistance derivatives have been much used in "classic" experiments of molecular genetics and subsequently in recombinant DNA studies and biotechnology. Luria and Delbruck used streptomycin in their seminal studies of mutation; later Hayes used crosses between streptomycin-sensitive and streptomycin-resistant mutants to demonstrate the polarity of gene transfer in bacterial conjugation and identified donor (Hfr) and recipient (F–) cells. The β-lactam antibiotics (penicillin and ampicillin) are widely used for selecting recipients in gram-negative crosses, and the aminoglycoside geneticin (a member of the gentamicin class) can be used to select for recombinant recipients in the engineering of a wide range of eukaryotic cells.

Of course, the use of these antibiotics in biological research and development is yet another source of environmental contamination: many are quite stable and remain active unless specific chemical degradation processes are used. All contribute to the selection and maintenance of antibiotic-resistant strains, especially given that municipal wastewater treatment does not necessarily remove antibiotics. It is evident that directly or indirectly, human civilization continues to contribute maximally to the contamination of the biosphere.

The development of a functional resistance state through mutation is not a simple process. As has been oft described, pathogens have a number of responses to antibiotic exposure. For one thing, mutations to resistance may come at considerable cost in energy and interfere with interactions within microbial communities: a resistant pathogen is often at a disadvantage in the absence of antibiotic (22). This may seem like a state of quasi-dependence, and antibiotic contamination contributes to the maintenance of the organism(s).

WHAT NEXT?

Finally, the burning question: what can be done to control/prevent antibiotic resistance development? There have been countless meeting resolutions, proposals, recommendations, workshops, government statements, and occasionally laws to reduce the threat of antibiotic resistance over the last half century. As an example, see reference 23. The threat is recognized with continuing urgency but diminishing resolve, and the problem is still growing; a return to a pre-antibiotic state is not just a bad dream. From the standpoint of microbes this is not surprising; we are inhabiting "their" planet. As the late Joshua Lederberg said, "In this conflict there is no guarantee that humans will be the survivors." Determined actions should (must?) be taken, but they are hard to implement given our dependence on antibiotics and related drugs.

1. The use of antibiotics must be strictly controlled using all legal steps necessary. They should be restricted to prescription-only use with absolutely no over-the-counter sales anywhere. Their use should be exclusively human (this applies to closely related compounds). This is a near impossible demand and will almost certainly lead to a black

market situation. The international community puts a lot of effort into controlling nuclear weapons; why not antibiotics?

2. Novel antimicrobial agents must be sought and found by increasing discovery research at all levels, supported by governmental policies. There is an enormous wealth of bioactive small molecules waiting to be discovered (24). The giants of the pharmaceutical industry should not be held responsible for this effort; they have already opted out. They are bound by profit making, and antibiotics do not meet their market requirements. More importantly, small companies and academic research institutes should be encouraged and supported, together with the development of a more flexible system of drug approvals.

3. Antibiotics are toxic. If the current FDA drug approval regulations had been in place since the beginning of the antibiotic era, today's most successful antibiotics would not have been approved for human use. However, the use of more-toxic antibiotics should be approved, especially as combination therapies in life-threatening situations. And why not? This is approved practice in the treatment of cancer.

4. The characterization of human and animal microbiomes should be vigorously explored as the basis for new approaches to infectious disease prevention and treatment. It will be important to carry out detailed studies of the effects of various treatments on microbiota in a variety of situations (25). The science of probiotics should be expanded. It is well-known that *Clostridium difficile* infections (the result of antibiotic use) are deadly and expensive, costing more than $3 billion a year in the United States. This is one result of a lack of understanding of the complexities of the human microbiome. Even after the significant accomplishments of the Human Microbiome Project (United States) and MetaHit (Europe), knowledge of microbiome function in health and disease is still primitive.

CONCLUDING REMARKS

There are several matters of concern with respect to our understanding of the biology of antibiotics and antibiotic resistance.

1. Are antibiotics *really* antibiotics as defined by their use as anti-infective agents?

2. Are antibiotics produced and released naturally in the environment? At present there is no evidence for the presence of antibiotics in soils.

3. It has been shown definitively that natural resistomes are common and exist in different environmental niches. Recent studies of soil resistomes show that many of the antibiotic resistance genes present are identical in sequence to the corresponding genes found in bacterial pathogens in hospitals and in animals (26), indicating that the connection between the two lies in the process of mobilization. In principle, the environmental sources comprise *putative* resistance genes for every antibiotic class known. Given points 1 and 2, do the components of environmental resistomes function as antibiotic resistance genes in the organisms that make them, or do they play other metabolic roles? Might they be pleiotropic? This would suggest that all environments have similar collections of pro or putative resistance genes. Do resistome-negative sites exist anywhere?

4. Most resistance enzymes possess binding sites for antibiotics. Might there be alternative biological functions of these interactions yet to be recognized? If we knew more

about the relationship between environmental preresistance and clinical resistance determinants, would it help in controlling the transition?

One last comment. Antibiotics are grossly misused throughout the world, in both application and quantity! Dosing ourselves, our domestic and farm animals, and plants with vast quantities of antibiotics leads to drastic changes in the complex microbial physiology of the organisms exposed to these compounds (27). This is not just any old detritus, but tons of bioactive molecules. Their activities may take years to be reversed (and may never be). The use and disposal of antibiotics on the scale tolerated in the past 60 or so years has proven to be a major evolutionary force in the history of the biosphere. We cannot effectively treat certain diseases without them, but their use as currently practiced may prove to have had more negative than positive consequences. The antibiotic era is a remarkable—and horrific—chapter in the book of life.

Finally, it is interesting to consider how the development and use of antibiotics would have been different if we had approached their use from a One Health perspective. Perhaps we would not have the problem of antibiotic resistance.

Acknowledgments. I wish to thank the U.S. National Institutes of Health and National Science Foundation for their generous financial support during the years 1968 to 1980.

Citation. Davies J. 2013. Antibiotic resistance in and from nature. Microbiol Spectrum 1(1):OH-0005-2012. doi:10.1128/microbiolspec.OH-0005-2012.

REFERENCES

1. **Kirby WM, Rantz LA.** 1943. Quantitative studies of sulfonamide resistance. *J Exp Med* **77:**29–39.
2. **Finland M.** 1971. Changes in susceptibility of selected pathogenic bacteria to widely used antibiotics. *Ann N Y Acad Sci* **182:**5–20.
3. **Keen PL, Montforts MHMM (ed).** 2012. *Antimicrobial Resistance in the Environment.* Wiley-Blackwell, Hoboken, NJ.
4. **D'Costa VM, McGrann KM, Hughes DW, Wright GD.** 2006. Sampling the antibiotic resistome. *Science* **311:**374–377.
5. **Sommer MO, Dantas G, Church GM.** 2009. Functional characterization of the antibiotic resistance reservoir in the human microflora. *Science* **325:**1128–1131.
6. **Cundliffe E, Demain AL.** 2010. Avoidance of suicide in antibiotic-producing microbes. *J Ind Microbiol Biotechnol* **37:**643–672.
7. **Sommer MO, Church GM, Dantas G.** 2010. The human microbiome harbors a diverse reservoir of antibiotic resistance genes. *Virulence* **1:**299–303.
8. **D'Costa VM, King CE, Kalan L, Morar M, Sung WW, Schwarz C, Froese D, Zazula G, Calmels F, Debruyne R, Golding GB, Poinar HN, Wright GD.** 2011. Antibiotic resistance is ancient. *Nature* **477:** 457–461.
9. **Pallecchi L, Lucchetti C, Bartoloni A, Bartalesi F, Mantella A, Gamboa H, Carattoli A, Paradisi F, Rossolini GM.** 2007. Population structure and resistance genes in antibiotic-resistant bacteria from a remote community with minimal antibiotic exposure. *Antimicrob Agents Chemother* **51:**1179–1184.
10. **Martinez JL.** 2009. The role of natural environments in the evolution of resistance traits in pathogenic bacteria. *Proc Soc Biol* **276:**2521–2530.
11. **Asimov A, Mackie RI.** 2007. Evolution and ecology of antibiotic resistance genes. *FEMS Microbiol Lett* **271:**147–161.
12. **Allen HK, Donato J, Wang HH, Cloud-Hansen KA, Davies J, Handelsman J.** 2010. Call of the wild: antibiotic resistance genes in natural environments. *Nat Rev Microbiol* **8:**251–259.
13. **Courvalin P.** 2006. Vancomycin resistance in gram-positive cocci. *Clin Infect Dis* **42**(Suppl 1)**:**S25–S34.
14. **D'Costa VM, Tariq A, Mukhtar TA, Patel T, Koteva K, Waglechner N, Hughes DW, Wright GD, De

Pascale G. 2012. Inactivation of the lipopeptide antibiotic daptomycin by hydrolytic mechanisms. *Antimicrob Agents Chemother* **56**:757–764.

15. **Patel R, Piper K, Cockerill FR III, Steckelberg JM, Yousten AA.** 2000. The biopesticide *Paenibacillus popilliae* has a vancomycin resistance gene cluster homologous to the enterococcal VanA vancomycin resistance gene cluster. *Antimicrob Agents Chemother* **44**:705–709.

16. **Guardabassi L, Perichon B, van Heijenoort J, Blanot D, Courvalin P.** 2005. Glycopeptide resistance *vanA* operons in *Paenibacillus* strains isolated from soil. *Antimicrob Agents Chemother* **49**:4227–4233.

17. **Jukes TH.** 1973. Public health significance of feeding low levels of antibiotics to animals. *Adv Appl Microbiol* **16**:1–54.

18. **Kristiansson E, Fick J, Janzon A, Grabic R, Rutgersson C, Weijdegard B, Soderstrom H, Larsson DG.** 2011. Pyrosequencing of antibiotic-contaminated river sediments reveals high levels of resistance and gene transfer elements. *PLoS ONE* **6**:e17038.

19. **Lawrence JG, Ochman H.** 1997. Amelioration of bacterial genomes: rates of change and exchange. *J Mol Evol* **44**:383–397.

20. **Hon WC, McKay GA, Thompson PR, Sweet RM, Yang DS, Wright GD, Berghuis AM.** 1997. Structure of an enzyme required for aminoglycoside antibiotic resistance reveals homology to eukaryotic protein kinases. *Cell* **89**:887–895.

21. **Yanagisawa T, Kawakami M.** 2003. How does *Pseudomonas fluorescens* avoid suicide from its antibiotic pseudomonic acid? Evidence for two evolutionarily distinct isoleucyl-tRNA synthetases conferring self-defense. *J Biol Chem* **278**:25887–25894.

22. **Andersson DI, Hughes DH.** 2010. Antibiotic resistance and its cost: is it possible to reverse resistance? *Nat Rev Microbiol* **8**:260–271.

23. **Bush K, Courvalin P, Dantas G, Davies J, Eisenstein B, Huovinen P, Jacoby GA, Kishony R, Kreiswirth BN, Kutter E, Lerner S, Levy S, Lewis K, Lomovskaya O, Miller JH, Mobashery S, Piddock LJ, Projan S, Thomas CM, Tomasz A, Tulkens PM, Walsh TR, Watson JD, Witkowski J, Witte W, Wright G, Yeh P, Zgurskaya HI.** 2011. Tackling antibiotic resistance. *Nat Rev Microbiol* **9**: 894–896.

24. **Davies J, Ryan KS.** 2012. Introducing the parvome: bioactive compounds in the microbial world. *ACS Chem Biol* **7**:252–259.

25. **Relman DA.** 2011. Microbial genomics and infectious diseases. *N Engl J Med* **365**:347–357.

26. **Forsberg KJ, Reyes A, Wang B, Selleck EM, Sommer MO, Dantas G.** 2012. The shared antibiotic resistome of soil bacteria and human pathogens. *Science* **337**:1107–1111.

27. **Dethlefsen L, Relman DA.** 2011. Incomplete recovery and individualized responses of the human distal gut microbiota to repeated antibiotic perturbation. *Proc Natl Acad Sci USA* **108**:4554–4561.

Disease Surveillance

One Health: People, Animals, and the Environment
Edited by Ronald M. Atlas and Stanley Maloy
© 2014 American Society for Microbiology, Washington, DC
doi:10.1128/microbiolspec.OH-0002-2012

Chapter 13

Public Health Disease Surveillance Networks

Stephen S. Morse[1]

INTRODUCTION

Zoonotic infections are important sources of human disease. The great majority of emerging infections identified to date (including HIV, Ebola virus, severe acute respiratory syndrome [SARS], Nipah virus, and enteropathogenic *Escherichia coli*) are zoonotic (48). These diseases originate as natural infections of other species that are given opportunities to cross the animal-human interface and come in contact with humans (1–4, 49). Wildlife constitutes a particularly important source (2).

Infectious disease emergence and spread are likely to continue and increase, as drivers such as agriculture, land use change, urbanization, and globalization proceed apace (3). Surveillance is considered the first line of defense for public health (5, 6), and the zoonotic origin of many human infections argues strongly for the synergistic value of a One Health approach (7) to surveillance, which provides the capability to identify pathogens crossing animal-human interfaces and can provide earlier warning of new epidemics waiting in the wings (3). Such knowledge can be used to focus efforts to prevent microbial traffic across animal-human interfaces and thereby reduce the risk of emerging infections. This article gives an overview of public health surveillance and some major existing surveillance networks and reviews progress toward implementing a One Health framework.

WHAT IS PUBLIC HEALTH SURVEILLANCE?

Today, we take for granted the idea of disease surveillance, but the concept as we now know it was formulated in the mid-20th century by Alexander Langmuir at the CDC (the agency was then called the Communicable Disease Center; it is now the Centers for Disease Control and Prevention). Previously, surveillance usually meant observing individuals clinically for disease. Langmuir redefined it to mean identifying and enumerating diseases in populations, as a public health tool (8). Stephen Thacker and Ruth Berkelman at the CDC subsequently suggested the term "public health surveillance" for greater clarity (9). The formal definition currently used by the CDC (10) is widely accepted and often quoted: "Public health surveillance is the ongoing, systematic

---

[1]Department of Epidemiology, Mailman School of Public Health, Columbia University, New York, NY 10032.

collection, analysis, interpretation, and dissemination of data regarding a health-related event for use in public health action to reduce morbidity and mortality and to improve health." A similar definition is used by the World Health Organization (WHO): "Public health surveillance is the continuous, systematic collection, analysis and interpretation of health-related data needed for the planning, implementation, and evaluation of public health practice" (http://www.who.int/topics/public_health_surveillance/en/).

While the purpose of surveillance is often thought of as early warning, and it will be used primarily in this sense in this review, surveillance has many other uses, including evaluating the effectiveness of preventive measures or interventions and providing data for setting disease control priorities. The United States government's recently released *National Strategy for Biosurveillance* (11) reinforces the importance of biosurveillance as an essential tool to inform decision makers and maintain a global health perspective.

Perhaps surprisingly, there is no comprehensive list of surveillance systems around the world. However, many of the existing surveillance systems have been well described in several reviews, which are recommended for more detailed information (9, 12, 13).

Most surveillance systems are disease specific. International public health surveillance systems include those for influenza, polio, HIV, food-borne diseases, and a number of others. Traditionally, surveillance systems are often classified as "active" and "passive." Most systems are passive, requiring a clinician to notice a possible disease of interest (usually based primarily on a list of notifiable diseases) or unusual clinical presentation and to report cases to appropriate authorities and provide access to the patients and suitable specimens. By contrast, in active surveillance systems the interested agencies (such as health departments) make intensive outreach efforts to find cases. Active surveillance is especially resource and labor intensive, and therefore less common.

The majority of current surveillance systems are also hierarchical and relatively simple in structure: ideally, a clinician (the proverbial "astute clinician") notices a sick individual or animal (more often, a sufficiently large cluster to be noticed) and reports the finding to local health authorities. If deemed warranted, the health authorities (ideally) then conduct epidemiological investigation to identify the source, means of transmission, and additional cases, while following up with laboratory investigation. For human diseases, the responsible governmental body will be the public health agency or (nationally) the ministry of health; for most animal diseases, the cognizant agency will be the agriculture ministry. Wildlife diseases often fall between the cracks. In some countries, if there is a responsible agency, it may be the agriculture ministry, while in other countries it could be the environment ministry. Some countries do have specialized agencies for wildlife. Uganda, for example, has a Wildlife Authority, and Malaysia a Department of Wildlife and National Parks.

The influenza network is a good illustration of a classical surveillance system and is one of the most elaborate. The WHO Global Influenza Surveillance and Response System (GISRS) (known as the Global Influenza Surveillance Network, or GISN, until 2011) is a laboratory-based network established in 1952; it currently has 138 National Influenza Centers in 107 member states, 6 WHO Collaborating Centers, and other components (http://www.who.int/gho/epidemic_diseases/influenza/virological_surveillance/en/). National Influenza Centers are hospital or public health laboratories that are likely to receive specimens from suspected cases of influenza and can identify and subtype influenza (viral surveillance), while the Collaborating Centers are reference or research laboratories.

Many illnesses other than influenza can cause influenza-like illness, so laboratory confirmation is essential for accurate diagnosis. As with almost all surveillance systems, because many affected individuals are not sick enough to warrant seeing a clinician, many cases are likely to be missed; others may be overrepresented in areas where there is very intensive surveillance (in epidemiological parlance, ascertainment bias). More recently, recognizing the threat potential of H5N1 avian influenza for human disease (although so far most often occupational), the network has added laboratories for H5N1 and other animal influenzas, an unusual feature for most human disease surveillance systems (but a welcome addition).

This structure is generally mirrored at the national level, although some of the components may differ depending on national capacity and priorities, and may be much more limited in many countries (especially in the developing world). In the United States, there are five nationally dispersed components coordinated by the CDC (http://www.cdc.gov /flu/weekly/overview.htm): viral surveillance by a laboratory network (a number of which feed into the WHO system through the CDC); outpatient surveillance for influenza-like illness by volunteer health care providers (a network of "sentinel physicians"); weekly reports of pneumonia and influenza deaths, in both adults and children, from vital statistics offices in 122 U.S. cities; in selected locations, intensified hospital surveillance for laboratory-confirmed influenza-related hospitalizations in children and adults; and weekly reports from state health departments on estimated level of spread of influenza activity in their state. Some of these components are also part of a state system, and the state forwards the data to the CDC.

Even for influenza, however, there are many gaps in the global system, both geographically and for surveillance of such important animal hosts as pigs, poultry, and waterfowl, as was demonstrated by the last influenza pandemic in 2009—the virus is now known officially as influenza A(H1N1)pdm09—which apparently originated in pigs in Mexico (14, 15).

INTERNATIONAL REPORTING SYSTEMS

Surveillance for many common diseases is fairly routine, and the reports are often just tabulated and filed. However, some have the potential to spread internationally or are of special global concern. As a function of its national sovereignty, each country can decide whether and when to report such an outbreak. In the past, criteria for international reporting were ad hoc, based on the judgment of national governments. The delays in initial reporting of early cases of SARS in China are indicative of the shortcomings of this approach (16, 17). In recent years, there have been increasing efforts to encourage governments to report more systematically and rapidly. For human public health surveillance, the revised, legally binding WHO International Health Regulations, known as IHR(2005), were adopted by the World Health Assembly (the governing body of the WHO) in May 2005 and went into effect in 2007. The revised IHR represent an important paradigm shift (18). They replace the old list of three specific diseases (cholera, yellow fever, and plague) with a broader, syndrome-oriented approach that encourages surveillance for both known and previously unknown infectious diseases. The concept of a public health emergency of international concern, requiring reporting to the WHO within 24 hours of assessment, is introduced and defined. For the first time, a decision tree has been developed to specify criteria for assessing a potential public health emergency of international concern. This may be an unusual disease event based on the clinical presentation; a known disease of concern such as polio, yellow fever, or pneumonic plague; or a novel influenza strain or new antibiotic-resistant pathogen. In another important innovation, the revised regulations specify national core capacity requirements for surveillance and response. Although there is a need for further development of decision criteria and triggers for response, these innovations are a major advance that will require each nation to have a real-time event-monitoring system and strengthened surveillance capabilities.

For animal health, the criteria for surveillance and response are delineated in the Terrestrial Animal Health Code of the World Organisation for Animal Health (Office International des Épizooties, or OIE) (19) and are roughly analogous to those in the IHR (the criteria have actually been in effect longer than the revised IHR). International reports to the OIE are usually submitted by the chief veterinary officer of the reporting country on behalf of the government. Some diseases (currently called listed diseases) are considered to be of particular concern, and countries are expected to notify the OIE of outbreaks within 24 hours; the list currently comprises 116 diseases of various species, mostly of livestock but also some diseases of bees, fish, mollusks and crustaceans, and amphibians (http://www.oie.int/en/animal-health-in-the-world/oie-listed-diseases-2012/). The list includes both infectious diseases of concern for agriculture (e.g., foot-and-mouth disease, bluetongue, and African swine fever) as well as zoonotic diseases such as anthrax, brucellosis, bovine spongiform encephalopathy, Nipah, rabies, and Japanese encephalitis, among others. The OIE maintains a publicly available database and Web interface, the World Animal Health Information Database (WAHID) (http://www. oie.int/wahis_2/public/wahid.php/Wahidhome/Home), which also has a secure portal for reporting from national veterinary authorities.

Within the United Nations system, the agency analogous to the WHO in human health is the Food and Agriculture Organization (FAO), whose mission is food security and animal health. The FAO also maintains a global database of animal disease reports, EMPRES Global Animal Disease Information System (EMPRES-i) (http://empres-i.fao. org/eipws3g/#h=0).

FIRST STEPS TOWARD GLOBAL NETWORKS

In an attempt to alleviate what many saw as the fragmentation of disease surveillance capabilities and the lack of global capacity, in 1993 ProMED (the Program for Monitoring Emerging Diseases) was formed by a group of scientists under the auspices of the Federation of American Scientists. ProMED was intended as an international follow-up to earlier meetings, especially a 1989 National Institutes of Health meeting on emerging viruses (20) and the 1992 Institute of Medicine report (5). At a series of meetings in Geneva and elsewhere, the ProMED Steering Committee, consisting of some 60 prominent scientists and public health experts from around the world, recommended forming a network of regional centers to identify and respond to unusual disease outbreaks (21). This could be seen as also elaborating on the system D. A. Henderson originally proposed at the 1989 National Institutes of Health meeting on emerging viruses (6).

The original ProMED concept of the 1990s was for a surveillance network that could both provide early warning of emerging (previously unknown or unanticipated) infections as well as be able to identify the most common infections. The strategy developed was vigilance for unusual clinical presentations of special concern based on particular case definitions (such as encephalitis, or acute respiratory distress with fever in adults); a set of minimum microbiology capabilities at each site, to identify common diseases; and a system to refer unidentifiable samples to successively more sophisticated reference laboratories, through the network, for possible identification (or recognition as a previously unknown pathogen) (21). The plan also included epidemiological capacity, which could be provided rapidly through the network if needed. While the original ProMED network and plan were largely oriented toward outbreaks of human disease, it was recognized that many of these emerging diseases might be zoonotic, and the Steering Committee and working groups included experts in animal and plant diseases as well as human public health and clinical microbiology.

A few words seem warranted on the origin of ProMED-mail, the Internet service that began as a spinoff from the original ProMED and has taken on a vigorous independent life of its own (50). Its origin was serendipitous. To provide the globally dispersed ProMED Steering Committee members a consistent means to communicate with one another, in 1994 we connected all members by e-mail. The e-mail system, originally envisioned as a direct scientist-to-scientist network, rapidly developed into a prototype outbreak reporting and discussion list. The decision was made almost immediately to make it publicly available to all at no charge (it remains nonprofit and noncommercial). ProMED-mail is One Health by design, covering reports of human, animal (including wildlife), and plant diseases, including disease crossover events. Fortuitously, its inception preceded by a few years the explosive growth of the Internet, which further extended its reach. Ironically, since then, although significant strides have been made toward the original goal of a network of periurban centers with clinical, epidemiological, and diagnostic capacity for surveillance, there is still no fully functional global network of regional centers of the sort envisioned by D. A. Henderson (6) or the original ProMED plan (21).

However, in recent years there have been promising advances in developing networks to build more complete surveillance capacity. Several of these networks are discussed below and in the following sections, including the WHO's Global Outbreak Alert and Response Network (GOARN); Global Early Warning System for Major Animal Diseases, Including Zoonoses (GLEWS), a joint network developed by the FAO, OIE, and WHO; the CDC's Global Disease Detection (GDD) network; the U.S. Department of Defense's Global Emerging Infections Surveillance and Response System (GEIS); regional or subregional networks, such as the Mekong Basin Disease Surveillance (MBDS) system; and the U.S. Agency for International Development's (USAID) Emerging Pandemic Threats (EPT) program and its surveillance component, PREDICT.

Coordinating data from different surveillance systems has always been challenging (in fact, attempting to overcome this fragmentation was one of the original reasons for forming ProMED). As most conventional surveillance systems are disease specific (for a disease or category of diseases), many valuable reports might be discarded simply because they are outside the scope of the system, even though they may be of intense interest to someone else (here, there is no substitute for a well-trained and alert human brain). Countries may also have political concerns about reporting, as with SARS in China in late 2002. The WHO responded to some of these limitations by developing GOARN (now part of WHO Global Alert and Response, or GAR) in 2000 (http://www.who.int/csr /outbreaknetwork/en/). Initially, GOARN was designed as a "network of networks" for human disease surveillance, with a wide variety of inputs from official surveillance systems; other formal surveillance networks (such as the WHO regional and country offices, and military and subregional systems like those to be discussed below); and unofficial systems, including nongovernmental organizations and electronic systems like ProMED-mail and the Global Public Health Intelligence Network (GPHIN), developed by the Canadian government in 1998 to search for relevant news reports on the Web. The initial GOARN meeting summary (22) is a useful source of information on the development of the WHO strategy, and also includes interesting snapshots of several surveillance systems not discussed in this review. In the last few years, GOARN has expanded the network to include outbreak response, using e-mail and other mechanisms to inform partners of emergencies and to request technical or field assistance.

CATALYZING ONE HEALTH: H5N1 AND THE TRIPARTITE

H5N1 highly pathogenic avian influenza, which appeared catastrophically in Asia in late 2003, had a galvanizing effect on the implementation of One Health. The effect was reinforced by the experience with SARS earlier that year, and probably by Nipah on farms several years previously, but H5N1 propelled implementation of the One Health approach to the fore. Although human infections with H5N1 were not frequent and were often occupational, they were associated with severe disease and high case-fatality ratios. It became clear that the disease could only be understood and controlled by following the entire transmission chain, from the migratory waterfowl that carried it to the poultry farms and from poultry to human workers and consumers: a One Health approach.

One outcome of these experiences was the accelerated development of GLEWS, a combined surveillance system by the FAO, OIE, and WHO initiated in 2006 (23; additional information available at: http://www.glews.net/). In addition to combining surveillance information, GLEWS has been developing response criteria based on the IHR (2005) and the OIE Terrestrial Animal Health Code and conducting pilot projects on risk assessment. One of the project's stated goals is monitoring of wildlife disease to support One Health.

The United Nations System Influenza Coordination (UNSIC) has strongly advocated the One Health approach, and the USAID funded an avian influenza program with a number of demonstration projects emphasizing biosecurity at the production level to prevent occupational infections, reduction of high-risk behaviors, market incentives for safer poultry, community-level surveillance for sick poultry, and tracking of H5N1 and other influenza viruses in migratory fowl. Experience with H5N1 as a zoonotic infection crossing species barriers also led USAID to recognize that the origins of most emerging infectious diseases are similar to H5N1, and that this concept could be extended. This led USAID to develop its EPT program, discussed below.

The impact of H5N1 led to a series of ministerial meetings, and at the 2010 International Ministerial Conference on Animal and Pandemic Influenza in Hanoi, Vietnam, representatives of some 70 countries approved a concept note jointly presented by the WHO, FAO, and OIE to work together on H5N1 (the Hanoi Declaration) (24). This triad of the FAO, OIE, and WHO is often referred to as the "tripartite." The tripartite agreement was a great step forward in officially committing these three key intergovernmental organizations to develop joint systems and combine their efforts. Although these are relatively new efforts, the agreement sets an encouraging precedent for cooperation among these agencies in support of better-coordinated infectious disease surveillance and in appreciating the value of One Health.

SURVEILLANCE NETWORKS: FROM GLOBAL TO REGIONAL

The CDC has a long history of international activities, both ad hoc and with established research or surveillance sites in a number of countries. Following the SARS outbreak, Congress provided funds to strengthen the CDC's global capacity to rapidly identify and contain disease outbreaks. The major new initiative developed by the CDC for this purpose was the GDD program, under the Center for Global Health, Division of Global Disease Detection and Emergency Response. GDD began in 2004 with Regional Centers in Kenya and Thailand, and now encompasses 10 GDD Centers, with an ultimate goal of 18 centers. In addition to Thailand and Kenya, there are currently GDD Centers in Bangladesh, China, Egypt, the Republic of Georgia, Guatemala, Kazakhstan, India, and South Africa. The centers, overseen by CDC headquarters in Atlanta, GA, are intended to serve as regional platforms, or hubs, for coordinating CDC and partner activities. Programs at each center include a Field Epidemiology and Laboratory Training Program, an International Emerging Infections Program (health care-based surveillance), projects to strengthen laboratory capacity, pandemic influenza surveillance, and in some of the centers, zoonotic investigation and control and risk communication. In addition to serving as the CDC's primary global platform for surveillance, research, and capacity building, GDD was designated by the WHO to help member states acquire the IHR(2005) core capacities in surveillance and response (http://www.cdc.gov/globalhealth/gdder/gdd/).

An analogous network in the U.S. Department of Defense is GEIS. The Department of Defense has for many years maintained overseas laboratories and surveillance capabilities. This was consolidated several years ago into GEIS, now a division of the Armed Forces Health Surveillance Center (AFHSC) in Silver Spring, MD. AFHSC was formed, in the words of its mission statement, to be the central epidemiological resource and a global health surveillance proponent for the U.S. Armed Forces. The best-known GEIS surveillance centers are the well-established Department of Defense overseas laboratories, currently in Kenya (United States Army Medical Research Unit-Kenya), Egypt (Naval Medical Research Unit 3), Europe, Thailand (Armed Forces Research Institute of Medical Sciences, or AFRIMS), and Peru (Naval Medical Research Unit 6), as well as a number of similar facilities and military medical units in the United States and Asia (25). Most of the centers work regionally, are cooperative efforts between the United States and host country military or research institutes, and often have special research emphasis on regionally important diseases, as well as surveillance for both local and cosmopolitan diseases (such as influenza) and emerging infections. AFRIMS in Bangkok, Thailand, for example, also conducts work in Nepal and has been a center for dengue surveillance and vaccine research, among other projects.

In addition, there are a number of parallel networks in some developing countries sponsored by other governments or organizations, including the Institut Pasteur International Network, with 32 institutes worldwide (http://www.pasteur-international.org /ip/easysite/pasteur-international-en/institut-pasteur-international-network/the-network) and the Rodolphe Mérieux Laboratories of the Mérieux Foundation, begun in 2007 (http://www.fondation-merieux.org/rodolphe-merieux-laboratories-strengthening-health-structures).

A very interesting innovation has been the development of regional disease surveillance networks that have assembled voluntarily, many including both human and animal disease (and in some cases wildlife). The history of these initiatives reflects the changing nature of global health governance. While cooperative public health programs might once have been exclusively bilateral arrangements between governments (and this is still true of many government programs, including GDD and GEIS), newer initiatives increasingly are voluntary multilateral efforts by neighboring countries, often involving public-private partnerships. Several recent reviews discuss the regional networks in detail (26–28). Brief descriptions of these regional networks and others (such as OHASA, the One Health Alliance of South Asia, initiated by EcoHealth Alliance in 2009) are also on the One Health Commission website (http://www.onehealthcommission.org/en/resources/).

These regional or subregional networks include the MBDS, which includes six countries in Southeast Asia (Cambodia, China, Lao PDR, Myanmar/Burma, Thailand, and Vietnam) (27, 29); the Middle East Consortium on Infectious Disease Surveillance (MECIDS), with Israel, Jordan, and the Palestinian Authority; the East Africa Integrated Disease Surveillance Network (EAIDSNet); and the Southern African Centre for Infectious Disease Surveillance (SACIDS). SACIDS includes institutions in Tanzania, Democratic Republic of the Congo, Mozambique, Zambia, and South Africa, as well as other partnerships outside the region, and is explicitly organized on a One Health framework (30).

MBDS, the first, began informally in 1999 at a regional meeting at which health ministers of the six countries agreed to share information and provide mutual assistance on infectious disease events. After a few years of this informal arrangement, the ministers agreed to sign a memorandum of understanding, which was renewed, with expanded goals, in 2007. Commitment occurred at the working and ministerial levels, where common needs and goals were recognized, and was never formalized at the highest levels of government. Another essential element was funding. For MBDS, funding came initially from the Rockefeller Foundation, joined by other funders such as the Nuclear Threat Initiative and its Global Health and Security Initiative, and the Gates Foundation, underscoring the increasingly important role of nongovernmental players. With infectious disease surveillance, one country's success in controlling an infectious disease protects both that country and others (and, conversely, a country's inability to do it endangers its vulnerable neighbors), so the goal of reducing transboundary infectious disease movement was recognized by all the participants as being in their self-interest and served as a strong starting point.

It is too soon to judge the effectiveness and longevity of the regional networks, but the initiative seems promising. Although some have been more successful than others, all have made significant progress. Of the three initiatives, MBDS is the longest running and arguably the most successful, while MECIDS has had some successes and shows promise in a region with little history of trust, and EAIDSNet has yet to reach its potential (28).

All the apparently successful efforts share common features. They began informally, but with ministerial buy-in, and started relatively small, with a pilot project or single goal. MECIDS, for example, started with investigating food-borne disease outbreaks. As the participants began to build trust and learned to work together, the network expanded to take on additional tasks. Long (28) identifies the necessary minimum as "shared interest in a transnational public good," "membership that includes all and only relevant actors," and "creation of a new group identity and building trust through personal, protracted, positive contact," as well as "congruence with international norms and activities of IGOs [intergovernmental organizations]," strengthening core capacities of the members, and "committed founding donors or multiple revenue streams." The WHO's revised IHR have made a fundamental contribution to strengthening the norms, by requiring the 194 signatory countries (the entire membership of the WHO) to report "public health events of international concern," including unusual disease outbreaks. In the long term, sustainability is essential and depends on continuity of efforts and personnel to build trust and human capital. For all these networks, stable funding is no less critical (27, 28).

The Connecting Organizations for Regional Disease Surveillance (CORDS) initiative was developed in 2009 to help tie together the regional networks and encourage networks to share best practices, and is an interesting model for scaling up globally (http://www.nti.org/about/projects/CORDS/).

DETECTING EMERGING INFECTIOUS DISEASES

Despite improvements in recent years, most existing surveillance systems are still unable to identify emerging infectious diseases, which by definition are unexpected and usually previously unknown (1, 3). Although numerous expert groups have long advocated global surveillance (5, 21, 31, 32), there has not been any global program to develop a framework for surveillance of emerging infections before they reach the human population. This would require a One Health framework, following pathogens across species and across the animal-human interfaces. Part of the reason may well be the relative lack of attention to wildlife until very recently (2, 32).

In 2009, USAID rose to this challenge by initiating its EPT program, which includes PREDICT as the surveillance component. EPT builds on USAID's earlier programs in avian influenza, which increased the agency's awareness of the importance of the One Health approach. In fact, one of the EPT program's stated objectives is "institutionalizing One Health."

The general goal of PREDICT, in its own words, is "to build an early warning system for emerging diseases that move between wildlife and people" in order to preempt pandemics at their source. Many of the risk factors, or drivers, of infectious disease emergence increase pathogen transfer across interfaces between humans and other animals (or between animal species) (1–3). Human activities that can facilitate this process often involve changes in land use or population patterns. These include, among others, farming, hunting, live-animal markets, and urbanization. Because many of the most severe zoonotic diseases cause little or no apparent disease in their natural hosts, it is often necessary to test apparently healthy animals, but random testing is likely to have a low success rate. To target the most promising locations for wildlife testing, PREDICT uses risk modeling to identify high-risk sites and interfaces where cross-species transmission appears most likely to occur, and concentrates on host taxa that have historically most often been associated with zoonotic transfers (especially bats, rodents, nonhuman primates, and some birds).

Activities are ongoing in almost two dozen developing countries. An essential part is capacity building, to enable countries to enhance their own surveillance and diagnostic capabilities. Conducted in partnership with national and local governments and in-country scientists and other local personnel, the project brings together workers in a number of disciplines, including field biologists, wildlife veterinarians, epidemiologists, ecological modelers, and laboratory scientists. Activities include field observation and sample collection, reporting, and both broad viral testing (pathogen discovery, discussed further below) and conventional laboratory microbiology. To date, the project has identified over 200 novel viruses spanning a number of viral families, most from bats, rodents, and nonhuman primates.

A digital data system is being used for storing and correlating the data obtained from these diverse sources, which will subsequently be made publicly available on HealthMap (http://www.healthmap.org/predict/). More information on PREDICT can be found at its website (http://www.vetmed.ucdavis.edu/ohi/predict/index.cfm).

SYNDROMIC SURVEILLANCE: ANOTHER PATH TO ONE HEALTH NETWORKS?

With the advent of widespread and relatively inexpensive computing power, many of the distinctions between databases and surveillance systems have blurred. While some surveillance systems are still paper based, and reports often originate and are maintained as paper-based documents, surveillance information is now increasingly reported, collected, and aggregated electronically into computerized databases, especially at the international level, or at least stored electronically. Databases like the OIE's WAHID are an example. Much more is also being done through Web-based or electronic data collection systems.

This convergence of informatics and public health surveillance is clearly illustrated by the development of "syndromic surveillance" as a complement to conventional surveillance. This approach has garnered increasing interest, especially since 2001. Although there are many definitions of syndromic surveillance, most highlight the use of "nondiagnostic" data—that is, information on possible health events before, or without, definitive laboratory identification of the pathogen—using electronic networks.

Unfortunately, there is some confusion about the terminology, as the term had already been used to refer to surveillance based on clinical presentation. Clinical case definitions have long been used in surveillance (33), particularly for newly recognized diseases before laboratory tests have been developed (e.g., Ebola in 1976 or SARS in early 2003), and they are used to some extent in the revised IHR. This strategy has been used successfully in the smallpox and polio eradication programs and proposed for surveillance of emerging infections in the original ProMED plan (21). This strategy using clinical presentation is now often called "symptomatic" or "case-based" surveillance to distinguish it from the newer meaning of syndromic surveillance.

As the term is currently used, syndromic surveillance includes a wide variety of data sources, including nontraditional ones. Although there is some general agreement about the data sources and methods that fall under the rubric of syndromic surveillance, clear definitions are lacking (34). One widely cited definition comes from the CDC's document for evaluating public health surveillance systems for early detection of outbreaks: "Syndromic surveillance for early outbreak detection is an investigational approach where health department staff, assisted by automated data acquisition and generation of statistical signals, monitor disease indicators continually (real-time) or at least daily (near real-time) to detect outbreaks of diseases earlier and more completely than might otherwise be possible with traditional public health methods (e.g., by reportable disease surveillance and telephone consultation). The distinguishing characteristic of syndromic surveillance is the use of indicator data types" (35). One advantage of syndromic surveillance is the flexibility to add new data sources or locations fairly easily. Veterinary reports and animal disease outbreak information, and even environmental data if desired, can be included to begin building a One Health system.

Many localities and agencies have piloted syndromic surveillance systems, with a variety of data sources, including hospital emergency department data, sales of prescription or over-the-counter pharmaceuticals, employee absenteeism, hospital admissions, medical billing or laboratory records, and many others, limited only by ingenuity and data availability (36–38). The Electronic Surveillance System for the Early Notification of Community-Based Epidemics (ESSENCE II) in the Washington, DC, metropolitan area, and several other networks, include veterinary reports in addition to traditional indicators (39).

Syndromic surveillance understandably has a number of skeptics, who accurately note, among other valid criticisms, that between 2001 and 2012 this approach had not provided advance warning of an outbreak (40). While syndromic surveillance provides opportunities to build larger and more inclusive networks, it is still largely experimental. There is a need to identify the most useful data sources and understand how best to analyze and interpret the results. However, it can be a useful complement to existing surveillance systems and shows great promise for the future.

CONCLUDING REMARKS

Despite the fact that global surveillance has been a primary recommendation of every expert group (5, 6, 21, 31, 32), many gaps remain (41, 42). Capabilities remain fragmented at every level. The very uneven geographic distribution of surveillance capacity in the world is also a major cause for concern. While these reporting mechanisms, and the databases that now support them, are enormous improvements over the capabilities of 2 decades ago, systems remain parallel and largely unconnected. Information sharing (in the jargon of the field, data fusion and interoperability) is still often severely limited or nonexistent. The description of the numerous—and mostly independent—surveillance networks above is symptomatic of the current degree of fragmentation. The "network of networks" approach, combining data from a variety of sources, is one feasible solution, although this can present challenges for analysis and interpretation. At the very least, all these networks should have the capability to share information seamlessly and "talk" to each other. Many official networks are also reluctant to share information beyond a relatively small circle.

The importance of zoonotic diseases clearly indicates that effective surveillance requires a One Health approach if we wish to preempt future epidemics upstream, before they reach humans (32). Animal surveillance and disease control systems were originally developed for economic and trade reasons, to prevent the spread of agriculturally important diseases, and only secondarily for zoonotic disease or emerging infections surveillance, and therefore need to be expanded to address these threats (43). Even worse, as mentioned above, surveillance of wildlife, an important source of infectious diseases in humans and other animal species (2, 32), is far less systematic, although the OIE has been developing some welcome efforts in wildlife surveillance, which had largely fallen between the cracks before. Clearly, these are areas in need of the type of cross integration that the One Health concept provides.

There are some promising signs. More is being done now than ever before to consider how to develop effective combined and more comprehensive systems, including wildlife. USAID's vision is forward looking and innovative. Systems covering broad or previously underrepresented geographic areas are beginning to fill in some of the dark areas on the map. Networks that combine data from many different sources or target species, such as GOARN and GLEWS, should be able to take advantage of the recent revolutionary advances in informatics and computer technology to identify the common threads in the data reports. GLEWS and the other tripartite efforts show salutary evidence of interagency cooperation and of broader thinking, more realistically based on how infections emerge and spread.

This integration is being replicated on the ground, although only recently begun. When an Ebola outbreak occurred in Kibaale, in western Uganda, in late July 2012, Uganda formed a national task force that included a wide variety of partners, including senior leaders from the ministries of health and agriculture, the Uganda Wildlife Authority, appropriate laboratories, and other partners such as academic centers in Uganda, the CDC, the WHO, Médecins Sans Frontières/Doctors Without Borders, International Federation of Red Cross and Red Crescent Societies, EPT/PREDICT, and others, in functional working groups with specific objectives for each group. Uganda had used a similar approach during a hemorrhagic fever outbreak in 2010 (now attributed to yellow fever). Other countries are also beginning to use the national task force approach to constructively engage the necessary broad range of expertise and improve regular team communication.

The technologies of diagnostics and communications, both of which are essential for surveillance, have made revolutionary advances in the last 2 decades. Perhaps most notably, now mobile phones can send and receive data almost anywhere in the world, enabling more extensive networks with minimal infrastructure needs, and encouraging what has been dubbed "participatory epidemiology" (44). These technological leaps have led to increasing appreciation of (and increased ability to utilize) the power of networks. This is very timely: it will take all our networking power and technological abilities if we hope to have even a chance to outrun the microbes, which could spread at the speed of an airplane.

Laboratory capacity remains in critically short supply, but here too there is some basis for hope. Diagnostic tools that were unimaginable a decade or two ago, such as PCR-based assays and methods for molecular identification of unknown pathogens by conserved sequences, have now become feasible, even for the better research or diagnostic laboratories in developing countries. The latter (finding and identifying previously unknown and unidentifiable pathogens in nature) is now often referred to as "pathogen discovery" (45, 46). In more advanced laboratories, genome sequencing of pathogens and metagenomics (identifying putative pathogen nucleic acid sequences in crude extracts from biological or environmental samples) has begun to enrich pathogen discovery. In one recent study, as an example of the possible shape of things to come, whole-genome DNA sequencing was used to trace an antibiotic-resistant *Klebsiella pneumoniae* infection in a hospital, in the process yielding some surprising results that will inform future epidemiological investigations (47).

Of course, these capabilities are not yet widely available. But if history is a guide, there is potential for great improvement in the foreseeable future. Field laboratory stations are doing assays that were impossible 2 decades ago except in the most advanced facilities. In the future, one hopes that there will be more point-of-care diagnostics at the local or district level, perhaps reported through mobile telephones in more remote areas. These are hopeful signs for the technical and reporting arenas, as more capability is being developed at increasingly local levels.

But political will and sustained funding are also the lifeblood of global surveillance. There is also, at this moment, some recognition of the urgency of accomplishing these objectives, with some degree of political will, but history has shown this to be too often fleeting. Human capital is essential, but developing it takes time, resources, and stability. Sustainability of capacity, funding, and political will between crises remains a major challenge in the face of the repeated tendency to become complacent until the next crisis galvanizes action once more. Remedying this challenge calls for better advocacy and a clear demonstration of value in economic and development terms, as well as in lives saved or crises averted. With several recent crises and near misses, effective surveillance networks are a wise and critical investment in preventing future disasters.

Acknowledgments. This work was made possible by the generous support of the American people through the USAID EPT PREDICT project (USAID Cooperative Agreement GHN-A-009-00010-00), and by the Arts and Letters Foundation and the Alfred P. Sloan Foundation.

In the interests of full disclosure, the author is global Co-Director of PREDICT and was the Founding Chair of ProMED. The author declares no conflict of interest as a result of association with these nonprofit efforts.

Citation. Morse SS. 2014. Public health disease surveillance networks. Microbiol Spectrum 2(1):OH-0002-2012. doi:10.1128/microbiolspec.OH-0002-2012.

REFERENCES

1. **Morse SS.** 1990. Regulating viral traffic. *Issues Sci Technol* **7**:81–84.
2. **Daszak P, Cunningham AA, Hyatt AD.** 2000. Emerging infectious diseases of wildlife—threats to biodiversity and human health. *Science* **287**:443–449.
3. **Morse SS.** 1995. Factors in the emergence of infectious disease. *Emerg Infect Dis* **1**:7–15.
4. **Wolfe ND, Dunavan CP, Diamond J.** 2007. Origins of major human infectious diseases. *Nature* **447:** 279–283.
5. **Lederberg J, Shope RE, Oaks SC Jr (ed).** 1992. *Emerging Infections: Microbial Threats to Health in the United States.* National Academies Press, Washington, DC.
6. **Henderson DA.** 1993. Surveillance systems and intergovernmental cooperation, p 283–289. *In* Morse SS (ed), *Emerging Viruses.* Oxford University Press, New York, NY.

7. **Karesh WB, Cook RA.** 2009. One world—one health. *Clin Med* **9:**259–260.

8. **Langmuir AD.** 1963. The surveillance of communicable diseases of national importance. *N Engl J Med* **1268:**182–192.

9. **Thacker SB, Berkelman RL.** 1988. Public heath surveillance in the United States. *Epidemiol Rev* **10:** 164–190.

10. **German RR, Lee LM, Horan JM, Milstein RL, Pertowski CA, Waller MN; Guidelines Working Group Centers for Disease Control and Prevention (CDC).** 2001. Updated guidelines for evaluating public health surveillance systems: recommendations from the Guidelines Working Group. *MMWR Recomm Rep* **50:**1–35.

11. **Executive Office of the President, United States Government.** 2012. *National Strategy for Biosurveillance.* http://www.whitehouse.gov/sites/default/files/National_Strategy_for_Biosurveillance_trf: wdr July_2012.pdf (last accessed June 26, 2013).

12. **Hitchcock P, Chamberlain A, Van Wagoner M, Inglesby TV, O'Toole T.** 2007. Challenges to global surveillance and response to infectious disease outbreaks of international importance. *Biosecur Bioterror* **5:** 206–227.

13. **Castillo-Salgado C.** 2010. Trends and directions of global public health surveillance. *Epidemiol Rev* **32:** 93–109.

14. **Butler D.** 2012. Flu surveillance lacking. *Nature* **483:**520–522.

15. **Peiris JS, Poon LL, Guan Y.** 2012. Surveillance of animal influenza for pandemic preparedness. *Science* **335:**1173–1174.

16. **Zhong NS, Zheng BJ, Li YM, Poon LL, Xie ZH, Chan KH.** 2003. Epidemiology and cause of severe acute respiratory syndrome (SARS) in Guangdong, People's Republic of China, in February, 2003. *Lancet* **362:**1353–1358.

17. **Heymann D, Rodier G.** 2004. Global surveillance, national surveillance, and SARS. *Emerg Infect Dis* **10:** 173–175.

18. **World Health Organization.** 2005. *International Health Regulations (2005),* 2nd ed. World Health Organization, Geneva, Switzerland. http://whqlibdoc.who.int/publications/2008/9789241580410_eng.pdf (last accessed June 26, 2013).

19. **OIE (World Organisation for Animal Health).** 2012. *Terrestrial Animal Health Code (2012).* OIE, Paris, France. http://www.oie.int/en/international-standard-setting/terrestrial-code/access-online/ (last accessed June 26, 2013).

20. **Morse SS, Schluederberg A.** 1990. Emerging viruses: the evolution of viruses and viral diseases. *J Infect Dis* **162:**1–7.

21. **Morse SS, Rosenberg BH, Woodall J.** 1996. ProMED global monitoring of emerging diseases: design for a demonstration program. *Health Policy* **38:**135–153.

22. **World Health Organization (WHO).** 2000. *Global Outbreak Alert and Response. Report of a WHO Meeting.* WHO, Geneva, Switzerland. WHO/CDS/CSR/2000.3. http://www.who.int/csr/resources/ publications/surveillance/whocdscsr2003.pdf (last accessed June 26, 2013).

23. **The FAO-OIE-WHO Collaboration.** 2006. Global Early Warning and Response System for major animal diseases, including zoonoses (GLEWS). www.oie.int/fileadmin/Home/eng/Animal_Health_in_the_World/ docs/pdf/GLEWS_Tripartite-Finalversion010206.pdf (last accessed June 26, 2013).

24. **The FAO-OIE-WHO Collaboration.** 2010. Sharing responsibilities and coordinating global activities to address health risks at the animal-human-ecosystems interfaces (A Tripartite Concept Note). http://www. who.int/foodsafety/zoonoses/final_concept_note_Hanoi.pdf (last accessed June 26, 2013).

25. **Russell KL, Rubenstein J, Burke RL, Vest KG, Johns MC, Sanchez JL, Meyer W, Fukuda MM, Blazes DL.** 2011. The Global Emerging Infection Surveillance and Response System (GEIS), a U.S. government tool for improved global biosurveillance: a review of 2009. *BMC Public Health* **11**(Suppl 2): S2. doi:10.1186/1471-2458-11-S2-S2.

26. **Kimball AM, Moore M, French HM, Arima Y, Ungchusak K, Wibulpolprasert S, Taylor T, Touch S, Leventhal A.** 2008. Regional infectious disease surveillance networks and their potential to facilitate the implementation of the International Health Regulations. *Med Clin N Am* **92:**1459–1471.

27. **Moore M, Dausey DJ, Phommasack B, Touch S, Guoping L, Nyein SL, Ungchusak K, Vung ND, Oo MK.** 2012. Sustainability of sub-regional disease surveillance networks. *Global Health Governance* **5:**1–43. http://blogs.shu.edu/ghg/?s=moore.

28. **Long WJ.** 2011. *Pandemics and Peace: Public Health Cooperation in Zones of Conflict.* United States Institute of Peace Press, Washington, DC.

29. **Yong E.** 2011. Disease trackers. *BMJ* **343:**d4117. doi:10.1136/bmj.d4117.

30. **Coker R, Rushton J, Mounier-Jack S, Karimuribo E, Lutumba P, Kambarage D, Pfeiffer DU, Stärk K, Rweyemamu M.** 2011. Towards a conceptual framework to support one-health research for policy on emerging zoonoses. *Lancet Infect Dis* **11:**326–331.

31. **Smolinski MS, Hamburg MA, Lederberg J (ed).** 2003. *Microbial Threats to Health: Emergence, Detection, and Response.* National Academies Press, Washington, DC.

32. **Keusch GT, Pappaioanou M, Gonzalez MC, Scott KA, Tsai P (ed).** 2009. *Sustaining Global Surveillance and Response to Emerging Zoonotic Diseases.* National Academies Press, Washington, DC.

33. **Centers for Disease Control and Prevention.** 1997. Case definitions for infectious conditions under public health surveillance. *MMWR Recomm Rep* **46:**1–55.

34. **Henning KJ.** 2004. What is syndromic surveillance? *MMWR Morb Mortal Wkly Rep* **53**(Suppl):7–11.

35. **Buehler JW, Hopkins RS, Overhage JM, Sosin DM, Tong V; CDC Working Group.** 2004. Framework for evaluating public health surveillance systems for early detection of outbreaks: recommendations from the CDC Working Group. *MMWR Recomm Rep* **53:**1–11.

36. **Centers for Disease Control and Prevention (CDC).** 2004. Syndromic surveillance. Reports from a national conference, 2003. *MMWR Morb Mortal Wkly Rep* **53**(Suppl):1–264.

37. **Mostashari F, Hartman J.** 2003. Syndromic surveillance: a local perspective. *J Urban Health* **80**(2 Suppl 1):i1–i7.

38. **Das D, Weiss D, Mostashari F, Treadwell T, McQuiston J, Hutwagner L, Karpati A, Bornschlegel K, Seeman M, Turcios R, Terebuh P, Curtis R, Heffernan R, Balter S.** 2003. Enhanced drop-in syndromic surveillance in NYC following September 11, 2001. *J Urban Health* **80**(2 Suppl 1):i76–i88.

39. **Lombardo J, Burkom H, Elbert E, Magruder S, Lewis SH, Loschen W, Sari J, Sniegoski C, Wojcik R, Pavlin J.** 2003. A systems overview of the Electronic Surveillance System for the Early Notification of Community-Based Epidemics (ESSENCE II). *J Urban Health* **80**(2 Suppl 1):i32–i42.

40. **Reingold A.** 2003. If syndromic surveillance is the answer, what is the question? *Biosecur Bioterror* **1:** 77–81.

41. **United States Government Accountability Office (GAO).** 2001. *Global Health: Challenges in Improving Infectious Disease Surveillance Systems.* Report GAO-01-722. GAO, Washington, DC. http://www.gao.gov/assets/240/232631.pdf (last accessed June 26, 2013).

42. **Feng Z, Li W, Varma JK.** 2011. Gaps remain in China's ability to detect emerging infectious diseases despite advances since the onset of SARS and avian flu. *Health Aff (Millwood)* **30:**127–135.

43. **Kuiken T, Leighton FA, Fouchier RA, LeDuc JW, Peiris JS, Schudel A, Stöhr K, Osterhaus AD.** 2005. Pathogen surveillance in animals. *Science* **309:**1680–1681.

44. **Freifeld CC, Chunara R, Mekaru SR, Chan EH, Kass-Hout T, Ayala Iacucci A, Brownstein JS.** 2010. Participatory epidemiology: use of mobile phones for community-based health reporting. *PLoS Med* **7:** e1000376. doi:10.1371/journal.pmed.1000376.

45. **Lipkin WI.** 2010. Microbe hunting. *Microbiol Mol Biol Rev* **74:**363–377.

46. **Relman DA.** 2011. Microbial genomics and infectious diseases. *N Engl J Med* **365:**347–357.

47. **Snitkin ES, Zelazny AM, Thomas PJ, Stock F, NISC Comparative Sequencing Program, Henderson DK, Palmore TN, Segre JA.** 2012. Tracking a hospital outbreak of carbapenem-resistant *Klebsiella pneumoniae* with whole-genome sequencing. *Sci Transl Med* **4:**148ra116. doi:10.1126/scitranslmed.3004129.

48. **Woolhouse MEJ, Adair K, Brierley L.** 2013. RNA viruses: a case study of the biology of emerging infectious diseases. *Microbiol Spectrum* **1**(2):OH-0001-2012. doi:10.1128/microbiolspec.OH-0001-2012.

49. **Reperant LA, Osterhaus ADME.** 2013. The human-animal interface. *Microbiol Spectrum* **1**(1): OH-0013-2012. doi:10.1128/microbiolspec.OH-0013-2012.

50. **Madoff LC, Li A.** 2013. Web-based surveillance systems for human, animal, and plant diseases. *Microbiol Spectrum* **1**(3):OH-0015-2012. doi:10.1128/microbiolspec.OH-0015-2012.

One Health: People, Animals, and the Environment
Edited by Ronald M. Atlas and Stanley Maloy
© 2014 American Society for Microbiology, Washington, DC
doi:10.1128/microbiolspec.OH-0015-2012

Chapter 14

Web-Based Surveillance Systems for Human, Animal, and Plant Diseases

Lawrence C. Madoff[1] and Annie Li[2]

INTRODUCTION

The early detection of infectious diseases is critical for early response and control of disease outbreaks. If outbreaks can be detected early, public health interventions may be able to reduce the size of the outbreak and mitigate its consequences. With more than 75% of emerging infectious diseases estimated to be zoonotic (1), the One Health concept can be applied to the surveillance of disease outbreaks that affect human, animal, and plant species. Traditional surveillance systems often rely on time-consuming, labor-intensive, and expensive methods (such as laboratory data or clinician case-report forms) to collect outbreak data, which then pass through multiple levels of health professionals before being confirmed and announced. This conventional system can delay public health responses that would otherwise prevent the spread of disease. However, current information technology allows the use of computers, mobile phones, remote sensing, and Internet searches to globally communicate and share information on disease outbreaks (2, 3). This information is often free to the general public, with access to valuable information from websites and Internet-based applications.

In comparison with traditional surveillance systems, Web-based surveillance systems enable health professionals to identify and disseminate disease outbreak information more rapidly. Many of these systems are automated and search for outbreak information from Web-accessible resources that include official reports (e.g., World Health Organization [WHO], World Organisation for Animal Health [Office International des Épizooties, or OIE], Food and Agriculture Organization [FAO], and Centers for Disease Control and Prevention [CDC] reports) and unofficial reports (e.g., news outlets, blogs, social networks, websites, mailing lists, and discussion sites). By aggregating a plethora of disparate outbreak information, users can visit a Web-based surveillance site to seek information instead of searching through multiple websites. They may also instantly receive alerts through e-mail via unrestricted subscriptions (4, 5).

[1]ProMED-mail, University of Massachusetts Medical School, Massachusetts Department of Public Health, Jamaica Plain, MA 02130; [2]City University of Hong Kong, Department of Biology and Chemistry, Kowloon Tong, Kowloon, Hong Kong.

One of the first examples of early recognition of a disease outbreak occurred in 2002 when a severe acute respiratory syndrome outbreak occurred in Guangdong Province, China. The International Society for Infectious Diseases' (ISID) Program for Monitoring Emerging Diseases (ProMED) and the Global Public Health Intelligence Network (GPHIN) played an important role in detecting the outbreak at an early stage (6, 7). Cases could be found as early as November 2002 from Guangdong Province (7, 8), at least 2 months prior to the WHO's officially declaring cases of a novel respiratory disease.

ProMED-mail, which began operation in 1994 as a mailing list serving about 40 members, explored the ability of informal Internet-based reports from clinician reports, news media, and other sources distributed to a rapidly expanding user base. ProMED stresses transparency and in many ways functioned as a social network, since users interacted with one another, seeking clarification regarding outbreaks and finding expertise among its participants. ProMED has always been available to any interested user and free of charge. Subject area and regional experts screen each report and provide commentary and context (6).

GPHIN, which debuted in 1997, pioneered the use of automatic Web crawling of media sites to discover potential outbreaks. The software searches and reads numerous media sites in multiple languages for stories that might relate to infectious disease outbreaks. It distributes reports to a network comprising largely official public health agencies that subscribe to the service. A team of specialists analyzes reports for subscribers (7).

Since the development of ProMED-mail in 1994 and GPHIN in 1997, many other Internet-based surveillance systems have been developed. HealthMap, for example, which began in 2006, automatically mines a wide variety of public sources and aggregates outbreak reports geospatially. Other systems include Argus, MedISys, and EpiSPIDER. Internet users of these surveillance systems include public health officials, clinicians, and international travelers (4). Public health agencies, such as the WHO, also rely on these sources of information as early evidence of an outbreak and communicate findings via the WHO's Global Outbreak Alert and Response Network (GOARN) (9).

The use of Web-based surveillance systems offers a technologically advanced means of recognizing disease outbreaks in reduced time (5) so that actions can be taken to control diseases that may affect multiple species, food resources, and the environment. Health affects not only an individual or even an individual species, but also other species in a global population. Zoonotic diseases, those that can be transmitted from animals to humans, continue to emerge. Plant diseases plague crops that animal and human populations depend on for their nutrition and health. Plant diseases may have profound effects on human and animal populations (a frequently cited example is the potato blight that affected Europe in the 19th century and led to mass mortality and population movements, particularly in Ireland). In addition, food crops have been considered a target of bioterrorism, since crop loss could lead to human and animal mortality and social disruption. Moreover, transboundary diseases are capable of crossing geographic barriers and political borders through movements, trade, and transportation. These examples are evidence that it is necessary to improve communication, build collaborations, and apply epidemiological intelligence for the promotion of global health. In this article, different digital surveillance systems and their functional capabilities are discussed.

OVERVIEW OF SURVEILLANCE SYSTEMS

Surveillance can be defined as the "ongoing systematic and timely collection, analysis, interpretation, and dissemination of information about the occurrence, distribution, and determinants of diseases" (2). By providing an effective surveillance system, one can monitor diseases to recognize outbreaks so that public health measures can be taken in a timely manner.

In a traditional surveillance system, official reports are often used to count the number of confirmed cases. The process involves a person becoming ill, seeking care, having proper diagnostic testing, and being reported as a confirmed case to the health department or government agency. However, official reports can be slow to receive if reported at all, with the possibility of every line within the surveillance system being breached during the process. For example, official reports depend highly on people—the patient and/or health care provider—to recognize the illness and report it to the appropriate entity. If the patient fails to seek medical care or the health care provider fails to make the correct diagnosis or properly submit a report, the case can be missed by the existing surveillance system. In addition, if a laboratory improperly runs a diagnostic test to confirm the etiological agent or fails to report confirmed results to the appropriate authorities, the case is also lost before it reaches the health ministry. In the traditional surveillance system, underreporting of cases can be problematic because of the possibility of losing cases within the traditional process.

This is especially true for novel infectious diseases, which are difficult to detect because the etiological agent is often unknown and the diagnostic test and health expertise not present. Moreover, resource-limited settings especially face difficulties in detecting newly emerged infectious diseases due to the lack of proper expertise and facilities. Yet they are more threatened by infectious diseases (10). Detecting diseases may therefore depend on other sources of information, since their surveillance systems are limited in scope if available at all.

Over the years, surveillance systems have grown in capacity as early warning systems and have evolved by utilizing today's advancements in technology from computers to phones to the Internet (2). Web-based surveillance systems are becoming more powerful tools for reaching Internet users globally. Systems can be automated to collect articles on a 24/7 basis by using search queries to aggregate data. Alternatively, users who may be eyewitnesses to an outbreak can report cases to the Web-based surveillance system via e-mail, an online submission, or a smartphone application. Analysis and organization of data may also be made by machine learning and verified by health experts. Finally, information may be displayed on the Internet through a website or periodic reports or e-mailed to subscribers (4, 5).

TYPES OF INFORMATION SOURCES FOR DATA COLLECTION

Two main types of data sources exist for Web-based surveillance systems: formal sources of information and informal sources of information (Table 1).

Data from formal sources have traditionally been collected to monitor infectious disease levels. Confirmed case reports are collected by government and academic institutions, including the U.S. CDC, French Institut Pasteur, public health universities,

Table 1. Formal versus informal information sources

Parameter	Formal information	Informal information
Types of surveillance	Passive and active surveillance, traditional and Web-based surveillance	Passive and active surveillance, Web-based surveillance
Examples of resources	Health ministry reports, WHO reports, laboratory data, clinical data	Blogs, discussion forums, mailing lists, media outlets, social networks, Internet articles, eyewitness reports
Reliability of information	More reliable because of confirmation	Less reliable due to false reports
Timeliness	Reports may be delayed because of need for official confirmation or approval	Often earlier reporting
Case definition	Often based on laboratory confirmation	Not necessarily laboratory confirmed, occasionally based on uninformed or misleading information
Outbreak investigation	Useful for serious diseases, such as reportable diseases or diseases of significant socioeconomic impact	Useful for emerging infectious diseases or diseases not reported by official sources
Limitations	Labor-intensive, requires passing through multiple levels of health professionals, underreporting of cases, may not include diseases that are not reportable, may be more costly to obtain formal information	Higher risk of false reports (mis- or disinformation), reporting bias

WHO, and the U.K. Public Health Laboratory Service (3). Traditional sources may include data from hospital/clinical records, questionnaires/surveys, diagnostic lab tests, or health ministry reports. Different collection methods are used to gather formal sources of information. For example, active surveillance may be conducted by interviewing people by telephone or mailing questionnaires for information on animal, plant, and human health. Retrospective studies may also be conducted by using past medical and laboratory records that hold details about specific infectious disease outbreaks. In addition, biological samples suspected of containing pathogens can be collected and submitted to public health, academic, or military labs for testing. More detailed information can further be sought in regards to these samples to determine clues about their origin. Samples may be genotyped and phenotyped and the information then stored in a reference databank. Developed countries often access these databanks to compare past genotypes and phenotypes of diseases to current strains to determine where the outbreak originated. The CDC's PulseNet is an example of this system and focuses on surveillance of food-borne and waterborne bacterial diseases using DNA electrophoretic fingerprints of pathogens, which are stored in the system (2).

In contrast, informal sources of data may provide up-to-date, local information for early recognition of disease outbreaks, even in locations that are resource limited and lack a traditional public health infrastructure. Informal channels of information include news reports, blogs, discussion rooms, social networks, and mailing lists (3, 4). Nongovernmental organizations can also contribute to disease reporting. Examples include the Red Cross and Red Crescent, Médecins Sans Frontières, Medical Emergency Relief International (Merlin), and religious organizations (3). Although informal sources can overload a surveillance system and may result in an increase in reporting bias or greater numbers of false reports, history has proven that informal sources are advantageous in detecting disease outbreaks earlier than with traditional sources. Informal reports have also discouraged countries from hiding outbreak information and encouraged surveillance systems to utilize different forms of data (4).

Today, many Web-based surveillance systems use informal sources of data to gain early knowledge on disease outbreaks. An example is the WHO's GOARN, which currently detects its verified outbreaks mostly through nontraditional information sources (9). The use of informal sources of information is further supported by the WHO's updated International Health Regulations of 2005 (became effective in 2007), which stipulate that the WHO is permitted to take preventative actions in response to these types of data (11). Surveillance systems that currently utilize nontraditional sources of epidemiological data include HealthMap, ProMED-mail, Emergency Prevention System Global Animal Disease Information System (EMPRES-i), and GPHIN, among others.

WEB-BASED SURVEILLANCE SYSTEMS

A number of Web-based surveillance systems have been developed for surveillance of infectious diseases of humans, animals, and plants (Table 2).

Table 2. Examples of digital surveillance systems[a]

Surveillance system	Website	Animal cases	Human cases	Plant cases
BioCaster Global Health Monitor	http://biocaster.nii.ac.jp	X	X	X
Emergency Prevention System Global Animal Disease Information System (EMPRES-i)	http://empres-i.fao.org	X	X	
EpiSPIDER	http://www.epispider.org/	X	X	X
European and Mediterranean Plant Protection Organization (EPPO)	http://www.eppo.int/ QUARANTINE/Alert_List/ alert_list.htm			X
GeoSentinel	http://www.istm.org/geosentinel/ main.html	X		
GermTraX	http://www.germtrax.com/	X		
Google Flu Trends	http://www.google.org/flutrends/	X		
Global Public Health Intelligence Network (GPHIN)	https://www.gphin3.net/	X	X	X
HealthMap	http://www.healthmap.org/en/	X	X	X
International Plant Protection Convention (IPCC)	https://www.ippc.int/			X
MedISys	http://medusa.jrc.it	X	X	X
North American Plant Protection Organization (NAPPO)	http://www.pestalert.org/main.cfm			X
ProMED-mail	http://www.promedmail.org/	X	X	X
Wildlife Data Integration Network (WDIN)	http://www.wdin.org/	X		
World Animal Health Information Database (WAHID)	http://www.oie.int/wahis_2/public/ wahid.php/Wahidhome/Home	X	X	

[a]Last updated April 2013.

ProMED-mail

ProMED-mail (http://www.promedmail.org/) was founded as an Internet-based early warning system for emerging infectious diseases in 1994, and is now a program of the ISID (Fig. 1). The system was one of the earliest Internet-based reporting systems to be utilized for disseminating information on infectious diseases and acute, toxic exposures that threaten human, animal, and food plant health. It operates 7 days a week, and reports are collected from both official and unofficial sources, including alerts from subscribers. Information is sought, analyzed, and commented upon by subject area experts in order to be posted on the ProMED website and e-mailed directly to subscribers through a freely available and open mailing list. Reports are also available via Facebook and Twitter. As ProMED seeks to promote communication among different health professionals, subscribers can discuss their views and work with others; ProMED has been cited as an early form of social networking. Currently, ProMED-mail is available in multiple

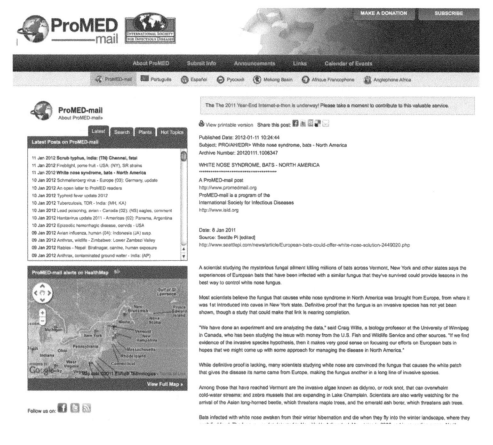

Figure 1. Website of ProMED-mail (http://www.promedmail.org/). ProMED is a service of the ISID and provides reports, moderated by a panel of experts, on outbreaks of emerging diseases in humans, animals, and plants.
doi:10.1128/microbiolspec.OH-0015-2012.f1

languages and has a total of more than 60,000 subscribers from at least 185 countries. Regional networks in the Mekong area of Southeast Asia, the former Soviet Union (in Russian), Latin America (in Spanish and Portuguese), and Africa (in French and English) help less information-rich countries benefit from informal information exchange, and also enhance detection of diseases in areas that are potential hot spots of disease emergence. ProMED is unusual among disease surveillance systems in its coverage of plant diseases affecting food crops and includes a plant pathologist on its staff. These reports are picked up and monitored by some other systems such as HealthMap.

GPHIN

In 1997, the GPHIN (home page, https://gphin3.net/; description at http://biosurveillance. typepad.com/files/gphin-manuscript.pdf) was developed by the Public Health Agency of Canada in collaboration with the WHO. It is managed by the Agency's Centre for Emergency Preparedness and Response. GPHIN pioneered the use of automated Web crawling and serves as an important early warning system for human, animal, and plant disease outbreaks; contaminated food and water; bioterrorist agents; chemical and radionuclear agent exposures; and natural disasters. It also covers drug and medical device safety problems. As one of the earliest digital surveillance networks, GPHIN, along with ProMED-mail, has been credited with detecting severe acute respiratory syndrome before official reports were published. The Microsoft/Java application runs 24/7 real-time in seven languages (Arabic, English, French, Russian, Farsi, Chinese, and Spanish), and data are interpreted by a team of GPHIN analysts based at the Public Health Agency of Canada. A subscription fee is required to access the secure website, with the cost depending on the type of organization.

HealthMap

HealthMap (http://www.healthmap.org/en) is a nonprofit organization based at Children's Hospital Boston and Harvard Medical School. Founded in 2006 (Fig. 2), this digital surveillance system monitors human, animal, and plant diseases and is freely available online without a subscription fee. The automated system operates 24/7 to monitor, organize, integrate, filter, visualize, and disseminate information in near real time. Disparate sources include both informal and formal resources in nine languages. The Linux/Apache/MySQL/PHP application searches from more than 50,000 sources, including news aggregators, eyewitness reports, and verified official reports, for disease names, symptoms, and key words and phrases. Alert sources are organized and filtered using Fisher-Robinson Bayesian filtering and then analyzed by trained personnel to ensure the proper organization of collected data. Users may browse and search for outbreaks by specific location or disease. The original source of information is also linked and available for users to peruse online. A new addition to the website is "The Disease Daily," which highlights outbreak news for the general public. Individual users may also participate in submitting their own outbreak alert online or through a mobile application, "Outbreaks Near Me." This smartphone application allows users to view and search for reports on an interactive map, with the option to receive alerts of local outbreaks.

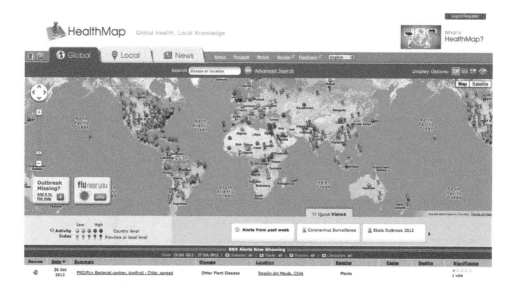

Figure 2. Website of HealthMap (http://www.healthmap.org/en/), based at Children's Hospital Boston, which shows, on an interactive map, infectious disease outbreaks automatically derived from numerous sources and curated by a human team. doi:10.1128/microbiolspec.OH-0015-2012.f2

EMPRES-i

The United Nations FAO created EMPRES-i (http://empres-i.fao.org) to monitor transboundary animal diseases and animal diseases of high impact (Fig. 3). This Web-based application provides an early warning system by utilizing both formal and informal resources, including project and field mission reports, institutions, nongovernmental organizations, government ministries of agriculture and health, FAO or United Nations representatives, public domains, media, and other Web-based surveillance systems. It provides advanced technology to collect sources, analyze animal disease information, and provide information to users. Information is displayed on outbreak maps with the option of viewing additional geospatial layers on livestock populations, biophysical characteristics, socioeconomics of an area, etc., which are provided by the Global Livestock Production and Health Atlas (GLiPHA). Data and graphs can also be created in different formats (e.g., PDF, CSV, or Excel) to be exported for personal use.

World Animal Health Information System (WAHIS)

The OIE, established in 1924, consists of member countries and territories that are legally obliged to report exceptional disease events of OIE-listed animal diseases, including zoonotic diseases and emerging animal diseases. Information is freely available to the general public through the World Animal Health Information Database (WAHID), which provides data from the WAHIS (http://www.oie.int/wahis_2/public/wahid.php/Wahidhome/Home). A more secure site is also available to authorized users, primarily OIE delegates and authorized focal points, that are obligated to notify the OIE within

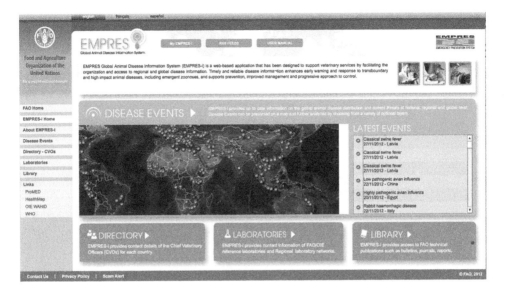

Figure 3. The EMPRES-i website (http://empres-i.fao.org), maintained by the FAO of the United Nations, which reports animal and zoonotic disease outbreaks.
doi:10.1128/microbiolspec.OH-0015-2012.f3

24 hours of confirming a significant animal disease. Information that is collected is verified and validated by the OIE before being published in English, French, and Spanish and sent through the OIE-Info list to delegates. WAHID differs from EMPRES-i by publishing only confirmed disease reports (formal sources of information) to the general public and sharing unconfirmed information (informal sources) to OIE members. The system allows users to search for outbreaks by specific animal diseases or countries/regions. The website provides information on disease characteristics and timelines, veterinary and laboratory services, animal populations, human cases of zoonoses, sanitary conditions of countries, and control measures. The interface also displays maps of disease outbreaks to view disease distribution within a specific country or the world. Older data from 1996 to 2004 may also be sought online from the former system, HandiStatus II, which was replaced by WAHID in 2005. However, a newer version of WAHIS was released in August 2012, with improved reports of wildlife diseases. In addition to routine monitoring of OIE-listed wildlife diseases, the updated system allows voluntary reporting of wildlife diseases that are not officially OIE notifiable.

SEARCH TERM SURVEILLANCE

Syndromic surveillance is another method used for early detection of diseases before they are diagnostically confirmed. By detecting individual and population health indicators, one can potentially recognize an outbreak before traditional reports. Examples of indicators may include an abnormal increase in over-the-counter medication purchases, school and work absenteeism, emergency hospital visits, or data aggregated from Web-based clickstream and key word searching (12).

Online search engines are commonly used by the general public to seek health information. During large-scale outbreaks, an increase in searches for specific diseases may mirror or predict disease outbreaks. For instance, past studies using search queries from Google and Yahoo have shown patterns mimicking disease activity during the H1N1 pandemic (13, 14). Other studies have also used key terms aggregated from social networks, such as Twitter, to show real-time estimates of disease activity (15).

Google Trends

Google Trends (http://www.google.com/trends/) is an automated tool used to monitor search queries in near real time. Although it is available to be used by all Internet users including those seeking non-health-related information, search queries for specific diseases may be aggregated and analyzed to estimate disease activity and geospatial patterns. The more widely studied version is Google Flu Trends (www.google.com/flutrends/), which monitors health-seeking behavior by users who potentially show influenza symptoms. Data on their search queries for influenza-like illnesses may be viewed through a search volume index graph, which is updated on a daily basis. Past studies have shown a strong correlation between Google Flu Trends and the U.S. CDC data from 2003 to 2008. The study also suggests earlier detection by 1 to 2 weeks before the CDC influenza-like illness surveillance reports, which could potentially be followed by an earlier public health response. Although a freely available tool, Google Trends is best used only for highly prevalent diseases, such as influenza, and in developed countries, where a larger population of Internet users are located (13).

TWITTER

Social networks are also powerful tools in connecting people in ways that allow them to share information. Twitter is an example of a free social network that can be used to track health information. The microblog has millions of users who "tweet" or submit messages of up to 140 characters. Most tweets embedded within the Twitter stream contain general conversations, sharing of information, and additional links to items of interest. In one study, researchers used Twitter's streaming application programmer's interface to collect a subset of Twitter messages that contained key words related to influenza-like illness. Using machine learning methods, they were able to aggregate information to measure H1N1 activity and public interest/concern in the United States. However, there is still difficulty with using this type of information because of the lack of specificity, as some tweets may be due to an interest in H1N1 while others may be tweeted because of an onset of symptoms (15).

CONCLUSION

Digital, Internet-based surveillance systems have changed the way we detect disease outbreaks and have created opportunities to conduct surveillance globally at the local, regional, and international level. Automated systems that use machine learning technology function 24/7 and are capable of early monitoring, early warning, and promoting early responses to diseases of public health significance. In addition, information can instantly be displayed on websites or disseminated to subscribers of Web-based surveillance systems.

Currently, Internet-based surveillance systems are better able to detect outbreak information in countries with high levels of Internet access. However, developing countries, while often facing the greatest burden of diseases (10), often lack the public health infrastructure to detect and prevent the spread of infection. Unlike industrialized countries, which may seek to prevent pathogens from entering and reemerging, resource-limited countries are challenged with a more serious problem. Infectious diseases are often endemic to these countries, which must concentrate their efforts on detecting outbreaks to decrease fatalities, reduce spread, and prevent harm to trade and tourism (3). One method of improving disease surveillance in areas that lack resources and Internet penetration is through the use of mobile phones and other hand-held devices that can be used for reporting cases through Short Message Services. The use of such technology has already been rising in resource-limited settings (16) and is likely to continue in the near future to help with disease reporting.

Other challenges for Internet-based disease detection include the obligation to respect privacy. For example, search queries can contain specific geographic information, such as a patient's address. Therefore, care must be taken to use appropriate spatial aggregation according to the public health need, such as mapping administrative units or using spatial skewing (17).

More research will also be needed to solve the problem of overload of information that is often unstructured and difficult to understand. Because the sensitivity and specificity of Internet-based surveillance is often unclear (5), information should be verified by trained personnel, who should also utilize advanced techniques such as machine learning to help organize data. False reports and reporting bias may occur with nontraditional sources of information (4), and media tend to focus their reports on those that can make headlines but fail to accurately communicate risks. An example of this phenomenon occurred in 2011 when Spanish cucumbers were initially and mistakenly blamed for an *Escherichia coli* O104:H4 outbreak causing gastrointestinal disease and hemolytic-uremic syndrome in Europe. These false reports dominated the media, causing a scare that resulted in a drop in cucumber sales. Political and economic tensions grew within the Spanish government, and the culprit was later confirmed as fenugreek sprouts that came from seeds imported from Egypt (18). This example shows that although digital surveillance can help speed the detection of outbreaks, it can only be as good as its data.

Another challenge is harmonizing data from parallel surveillance programs that overlap in function. Systems are currently differentiated by their functions, such as concentrating on specific regions, species types, and types and sources of data. The situation is further complicated by diseases that cross national borders and/or affect more than one species. For instance, FAO's EMPRES-i and OIE's WAHID focus their surveillance efforts on animal health, but many of these infectious agents also affect humans. Although these sources provide information on zoonotic diseases, the direct surveillance of human cases is typically found in other epidemiological systems. Collaborative efforts, therefore, need to be made to bring together resources to build integrated applications that fulfill a variety of needs and communicate disease risks to different populations.

We live in a highly globalized world, where international travel and trade of food, biological products, and live species can serve as potential sources of infectious disease outbreaks and the emergence and reemergence of pathogens (3). By bringing together different types of professionals, including epidemiologists, computer scientists, physicians, veterinarians, and public health professionals from both the private and public sectors, better surveillance systems can be developed to represent animal, human, and plant infections. Furthermore, an integrated system could provide insight into antimicrobial resistance, water quality, animal reservoirs, and insect vectors (8). The need for a One Health approach is evident in the 21st century, as emerging diseases continue to cross species barriers as well as geographic ones.

Acknowledgments. We thank our colleagues at ProMED and HealthMap for their dedication. Dagmar Hanold, ProMED plant disease moderator, provided information on plant disease resources on the Web.

The authors have no commercial affiliations, consultancies, stock or equity interests, or patent-licensing arrangements that could be considered to pose a conflict of interest regarding the manuscript.

Citation. Madoff LC, Li A. 2014. Web-based surveillance systems for human, animal, and plant diseases. Microbiol Spectrum 2(1):OH-0015-2012. doi:10.1128/microbiolspec.OH-0015-2012.

REFERENCES

1. **Taylor LH, Latham SM, Woolhouse ME.** 2001. Risk factors for human disease emergence. *Philos Trans R Soc Lond B Biol Sci* **356:**983–989.

2. **Keusch GT, Pappaioanou M, Gonzalez MC, Scott KA, Tsai P (ed).** 2009. Achieving an effective zoonotic disease surveillance system, p 115–164. *In Global Surveillance and Response to Emerging Zoonotic Diseases.* National Academies Press, Washington, DC.

3. **Heymann DL, Rodier GR.** 1998. Global surveillance of communicable diseases. *Emerg Infect Dis* **4:** 362–365.

4. **Brownstein JS, Freifeld CC, Madoff LC.** 2009. Digital disease detection—harnessing the Web for public health surveillance. *N Engl J Med* **360:**2153–2155, 2157.

5. **Wilson K, Brownstein JS.** 2009. Early detection of disease outbreaks using the Internet. *CMAJ* **180:** 829–831.

6. **Madoff LC.** 2004. ProMED-mail: an early warning system for emerging diseases. *Clin Infect Dis* **39:** 227–232.

7. **Mykhalovskiy E, Weir L.** 2006. The Global Public Health Intelligence Network and early warning outbreak detection: a Canadian contribution to global public health. *Can J Public Health* **97:**42–44.

8. **Heymann DL, Rodier G.** 2004. Global surveillance, national surveillance, and SARS. *Emerg Infect Dis* **10:**173–175.

9. **Heymann DL, Rodier GR, WHO Operational Support Team to the Global Outbreak Alert and Response Network.** 2001. Hot spots in a wired world: WHO surveillance of emerging and re-emerging infectious diseases. *Lancet Infect Dis* **1:**345–355.

10. **Jones KE, Patel NG, Levy MA, Storeygard A, Balk D, Gittleman JL, Daszak P.** 2008. Global trends in emerging infectious diseases. *Nature* **451:**990–993.

11. **Wilson K, von Tigerstrom B, McDougall C.** 2008. Protecting global health security through the International Health Regulations: requirements and challenges. *CMAJ* **179:**44–48.

12. **Mandl KD, Overhage JM, Wagner MM, Lober WB, Sebastiani P, Mostashari F, Pavlin JA, Gesteland PH, Treadwell T, Koski E, Hutwagner L, Buckeridge DL, Aller RD, Grannis S.** 2004. Implementing syndromic surveillance: a practical guide informed by the early experience. *J Am Med Inform Assoc* **11:** 141–150.

13. **Ginsberg J, Mohebbi MH, Patel RS, Brammer L, Smolinski MS, Brilliant L.** 2009. Detecting influenza epidemics using search engine query data. *Nature* **457:**1012–1014.

14. **Polgreen PM, Chen Y, Pennock DM, Nelson FD.** 2008. Using Internet searches for influenza surveillance. *Clin Infect Dis* **47:**1443–1448.

15. **Signorini A, Segre AM, Polgreen PM.** 2011. The use of Twitter to track levels of disease activity and public concern in the U.S. during the influenza A H1N1 pandemic. *PLoS One* **6:**e19467. doi:10.1371/journal.pone.0019467.

16. **Chretien JP, Burkom HS, Sedyaningsih ER, Larasati RP, Lescano AG, Mundaca CC, Blazes DL, Munayco CV, Coberly JS, Ashar RJ, Lewis SH.** 2008. Syndromic surveillance: adapting innovations to developing settings. *PLoS Med* **5:**e72. doi:10.1371/journal.pmed.0050072.

17. **Brownstein JS, Cassa CA, Mandl KD.** 2006. No place to hide—reverse identification of patients from published maps. *N Engl J Med* **355:**1741–1742.

18. **Lebiebicioglu H.** 2012. Enterohemorrhagic *Escherichia coli* epidemic: the sensitive role of the media in the handling of epidemics. *Clin Infect Dis* **54:**450–451.

One Health: People, Animals, and the Environment
Edited by Ronald M. Atlas and Stanley Maloy
© 2014 American Society for Microbiology, Washington, DC
doi:10.1128/microbiolspec.OH-0019-2013

Chapter 15

Genomic and Metagenomic Approaches for Predicting Pathogen Evolution

Veronica Casas[1] and Stanley Maloy[1]

OVERVIEW

Emerging infectious diseases have been defined as microbial infections "whose incidence in humans has increased in the past 2 decades or threatens to increase in the near future" (1). Microbial causes of emerging infectious diseases generally fall into two groups: (i) new pathogens that arise following environmental disturbance or acquisition of novel virulence traits and (ii) existing and known pathogens that have spread to new geographic areas or populations. In both cases, human activities play a key role in the evolution and transmission of these diseases. Human disruption of the natural environment alters not only the physical landscape but also the invisible microbial landscape. This process can facilitate transfer of virulence genes to new hosts or exposure of naïve hosts to previously unidentified pathogens. Due to the tremendous impact of emerging diseases on human and animal populations, we need a better understanding of how new diseases evolve and how to detect emerging diseases in order to develop more effective ways to predict outbreaks before they happen.

GLOBAL CLIMATE CHANGE

One example of the broad impact of human activities is global climate change induced by the extensive use of fossil fuels. Global warming promotes climate change that results in more frequent and damaging extreme weather conditions such as hurricanes and other tropical storms and also affects the ecology and physiology of marine and terrestrial plants and animals (2, 3). In addition to larger organisms, climate change also affects the microbes that determine the health and disease of animals, humans, and the environment (4). Climate change influences the emergence and spread of many infectious diseases by providing new environments for pathogens and expanding the range of disease vectors. Acquisition or enhancement of virulence traits is facilitated by the presence of environmental reservoirs of virulence genes. For example, metagenomics has revealed that a reservoir of exotoxin-encoding genes exists in the environment (5–7). As the temperature increases, there is increased stress on ecosystems such as coral reefs, and this stress makes

---

[1]Center for Microbial Sciences, San Diego State University, San Diego, CA 92182.

organisms more susceptible to infectious disease. A change in the average temperature by as little as 1 to 2°C can have a profound effect on the population of some organisms, reducing the survival of some beneficial microbes while increasing the survival of insect vectors that spread disease and microbes that cause disease (8, 9). Flooding and drought can increase the spread of waterborne pathogens like *Vibrio cholerae* and *Salmonella*, and an increase in temperature allows mosquitoes to thrive at higher elevations, promoting the spread of diseases transmitted by mosquitoes, including malaria, dengue, and yellow fever. Several examples demonstrate these concepts.

The emergence of hantavirus was precipitated by a particularly wet season in the southwestern United States in 1993. The elevated rainfall led to increased plant growth in this typically dry desert region. The resulting verdant vegetation provided an abundant food supply for rodents as well as protection from predators; thus the rodent population surged. Hantaviruses are shed in the urine and feces of infected rodents, but they do not make the animal carrier sick. The deer mouse (*Peromyscus maniculatus*) is the host for Sin Nombre virus, the causative agent of hantavirus pulmonary syndrome in the Four Corners outbreak. The deer mouse is common and widespread in this region, and approximately 10% of deer mice tested show evidence of infection with Sin Nombre virus. When the population of deer mice burgeoned in response to the unusually wet season, the mice moved into new niches that included the living quarters of the local human population, exposing humans to a previously unrecognized disease from wild animals (10). Humans become infected from contaminated dust containing virus in the urine or feces of mice, resulting in high mortality for the infected people. Thus, the Four Corners hantavirus outbreak serves as an example of a disease whose etiologic agent is widespread in the environment but whose transmission to humans was precipitated by environmental change (11).

In many areas of the developing world, fresh water is a scarce resource, and flooding destroys access to uncontaminated water supplies. This is clear from the recent epidemic of cholera in Haiti (12). Since 2005, the reemergence of cholera has paralleled the growing population of vulnerable humans living in regions subject to frequent, extensive flooding. The increased flooding in Southeast Asia has expanded the distribution of *V. cholerae* in its natural estuarine habitats and led to an increase in the incidence of cholera in human water supplies. The pattern of disease suggests that cholera outbreaks begin in coastal regions prior to spreading to inland water supplies. The El Niño-Southern Oscillation, a major source of climate variability from year to year, influences periodic outbreaks of cholera. The incidence of cholera increases after warm cycles and decreases after cold cycles, while in the intervening years the climate-cholera connection breaks down. The outbreaks of cholera are closely correlated with an increase in the abundance of plankton that occurs when the ocean water temperature increases, events that can be tracked by satellite imaging of the marine chlorophyll (13).

There is also a strong correlation between extreme weather events and diarrheal diseases caused by *Salmonella* and other pathogens that are spread by food and water contaminated with animal or human waste. This correlation between certain climate conditions and disease can be used to develop computational models that predict when and where major epidemics are likely to occur, project the severity of disease outbreaks, and provide insight into how we can develop upstream interventions (14, 15).

An outbreak of plague that began in Central Africa in 2004 and abruptly ended in 2009 also shows a strong correlation with El Niño cycles. From 2004 to 2009, eight countries were impacted with more than 12,000 cases and more than 800 deaths attributable to plague. In 2009, there was a sudden decrease in the incidence in plague. The decrease coincided with the worst El Niño cycle since 1998. The wet season in Africa started late, and this might have had a significant impact on the fecundity of the reservoir and movement of wild animals and the associated abundance of fleas that transmit the pathogens (16). Outbreaks of plague are not restricted to developing countries: changes in precipitation also lead to an increase in plague in rodent populations in the southwestern United States.

These examples focus on global climate change. However, the important point is that in each of these examples the emergence of infectious diseases followed an environmental disruption that provided a new niche for microbes, exposing animals to pathogens they had previously not experienced, with subsequent transmission of disease from animals to humans.

DETECTION OF VIRULENCE FACTORS IN THE ENVIRONMENT

Rapid detection of pathogens in the environment will allow the development of approaches to predict disease outbreaks before they happen, thereby facilitating public health approaches to prevent the spread of these emerging infectious diseases instead of treating diseases after they occur. Society often experiences considerable fear and hysteria when there is an outbreak of a new disease, while scientists are trying to identify the cause, find an appropriate drug or vaccine, and distribute the therapy to the exposed population. A One Health approach will allow development of upstream approaches to predict outbreaks and build upstream barriers to transmission. This approach will demand close collaboration among environmental scientists, veterinarians, and physicians coupled with computational scientists and mathematicians who can build powerful predictive models of disease transmission.

Metagenomics has provided insights into the impact of environmental change on the distribution and transmission of pathogens in the environment, in domestic and wild animal populations, and in humans. Given these insights, it is possible to design molecular assays that provide simple, exquisitely sensitive methods for sampling any environment using DNA signatures that probe the biology of that environment and the impact of environmental disturbances. For example, our work has demonstrated that bacterial exotoxin genes are widespread in the environment (5–7). These gene pools of virulence factors exist in diverse habitats and can undergo genetic exchange between microbes, leading to the emergence of new animal and human pathogens. Detection of these genes in the environment provides a sensitive test for new emerging infectious diseases.

MICROBIAL METAGENOMICS

While microbial genomics is the study of the genomes of individual microbes, microbial *metagenomics* is the culture-independent functional and sequence-based analysis of the heterogeneous microbial genomes from a particular environment (17–20). Metagenomics has revolutionized the way researchers investigate the community structure, composition, and distribution of populations of bacteria and bacteriophages (phages) from a multitude of environments, from the mundane to the extreme—including the microbiomes normally associated with animals or humans (21–24). The improvements in the technology for sequencing microbes directly from their habitats have made metagenomics research less expensive and more accessible and also generated an abundance of data that has expanded and transformed our understanding of the microbes that surround us (25).

Sequencing of phages from some of the same environments from which bacterial metagenomes have been constructed has provided invaluable insight into the dynamic interactions and genetic exchange occurring between bacteria and their viruses (26–32). Phages play an important role in determining the types and numbers of bacteria present in a particular population and in the transfer of genetic material between bacteria (19, 33). Many of the novel genes present in bacteria are of phage origin. When the phage genes transferred to the bacterial genome encode virulence factors, such as exotoxin genes, they can serve to confer or enhance the pathogenesis of that bacterial host. Moreover, if these genes are found in alternative, noncognate environmental hosts, they serve as the genetic "raw material" for evolution of novel animal and human pathogens. As described below, the phage-encoded genes for Shiga toxin and staphylococcal enterotoxin A have been found in alternative hosts cultivated from environmental samples (5, 6).

Exotoxins are proteins secreted by certain bacteria that can quickly and effectively cause damage to eukaryotic cells by targeting essential functions (34). Very minute amounts of some exotoxins are sufficient to kill a cell and ultimately cause death. For example, 1 mg of botulinum or tetanus exotoxin can be fatal to an adult human (35), and as little as 100 to 150 ng/kg of body weight of diphtheria toxin is lethal (36). In many cases, exotoxins are responsible for most or all aspects of their associated diseases. As the bacteria grow within the infected individual, the secreted exotoxins exert their deleterious effects at the cellular level, causing damage that leads to symptoms associated with the disease (34). Due to their tremendous potency and the ability of the genes that code for these exotoxins to be horizontally transferred between bacteria and phages, exotoxins are critical virulence factors in a number of emerging infectious diseases of significance to public health.

Recently food-borne illnesses caused by exotoxin-producing pathogens such as *Escherichia coli* O157:H7 have been on the rise worldwide (37–44). The origin of many of these outbreaks has been linked to contaminated food originating from our complex agricultural system; however, the specific source of a pathogen is often difficult to identify definitively. The inability to quickly and precisely identify pathogens in our food sources poses a clear threat to public health. This is exacerbated when the pathogens we encounter contain a novel combination of virulence traits, such as the *E. coli* O104:H4 strain responsible for the 2011 outbreak in Germany (45–47). In the case of *E. coli* O104:H4, genome sequencing provided the necessary clues for the rapid development of diagnostic tests that led to the source of this pathogen. In addition, the genome sequence led to insight into the evolution of *E. coli* O104:H4 by the sequential acquisition of chromosomal mutations, antibiotic resistance plasmids, and Shiga toxin-producing phages.

Survival in the environment is an essential step for the transmission of many pathogens. Recent evidence suggests that the exotoxin genes may enhance the ecological fitness of the bacteria (5, 6). In addition, the phages themselves survive harsh environmental conditions much better than bacteria, allowing transfer of virulence genes to a new bacterial host when the appropriate conditions prevail.

Thus, it has become clear that phages are common elements of our ecosystem and have a major impact on the ecosystem—influencing the population dynamics of bacteria and playing a direct role in bacterial growth and physiology. Phage-encoded genes may increase a bacterium's fitness by providing new metabolic capabilities, allowing evasion of predators, or increasing virulence. Phages may also facilitate the movement of exotoxin genes between microbial hosts, thereby converting avirulent bacteria into toxigenic pathogens. The phage-mediated transfer of virulence traits between bacteria occurs in a variety of environments and facilitates evolution of bacterial pathogens (48–54).

The properties of phages that make them particularly effective vehicles for gene transfer are their abundance and prevalence in natural environments, in animals, and in humans. There are roughly 10-fold more phages than bacteria in each of these environments. Phages are also hardier than their bacterial hosts and can persist without bacteria in harsh environments (55, 56). Phages can survive chlorination and heat treatments, are resistant to inactivation by sunlight, and have been shown to escape sewage/water treatment processes (56–62). Since phages are more impervious to extreme environmental conditions, they can maintain a pool of virulence genes in natural environments, thereby increasing the potential for exchange. Furthermore, the ability of many phages to fluctuate between lysogenic and lytic lifestyles also increases their fitness and the pool of associated virulence genes.

HOW ENVIRONMENTAL DISRUPTION SELECTS FOR NEW PATHOGENS

What happens to the structure, composition, and dynamics of microbial communities upon deforestation, irrigation, coastal zone degradation, wetland modification, expansion of urban areas, global climate change, or other human interventions that disrupt the environment (63)? Reduction of the relative biodiversity of an environment provides an opportunity for invasive plant and animal species that can wreak havoc with the ecosystem. The microbial ecosystem responds similarly, facilitating the evolution and transmission of infectious diseases that affect plants, animals, and humans. For example, the reduced biodiversity associated with the reduction in natural forests and their inhabitants was an important factor in the spread of Lyme disease in the northeastern United States (64). Global expansion of the human population and the growing proximity of humans to wild and domesticated animals have been linked to emergence of Nipah virus in Malaysia (65, 66), as well as the global increase in foodborne illnesses (67).

Use of metagenomics to survey the microbial landscape before and after human activities provides an approach to examine the impact of such changes. The microbial communities associated with humans, animals, and their environment must be investigated concurrently in order to be able to draw a clearer picture of the microbial landscape and the interplay between the microbiomes from these interdependent niches. Prior to the metagenomics era, identification and modeling of the uncultivable microorganisms from a given environment were nearly impossible. Metagenomics has provided novel insights into the structure of the microbial communities in the environment, including the abundance, diversity, and composition of the microbes and viruses. Metagenomics also reveals the distribution of particular genes, including virulence genes, within an environment. Once we know the microbes and potential virulence genes in these environments, it becomes important to better understand what they are doing in these environments, the interactions between organisms and the physical environment, how they interact, and how these dynamics could lead to selection or transmission of organisms that can cause disease. Thus, with some vision and creativity, metagenomics can be used to survey the changing environmental microbial landscape to generate data for models that can predict, and in turn help prevent, impending outbreaks.

ONE HEALTH

Human disruption of the environment promotes alterations in the patterns of infectious disease. For example, global climate change increases food- and waterborne diseases by contamination of fresh water supplies, increases vector-borne diseases by changing the rate and distribution of insect vectors, and alters the vulnerability of organisms to infectious disease by changing the dynamics of the ecosystem. Understanding these factors will demand the integration of a variety of types of data that probe the health of the environment, animals, and humans. The approaches needed extend from the molecular approaches of genomics and metagenomics to geographic information systems, satellite imaging, and mathematical models that can model and predict future outbreaks (68). Bringing together scientists with a broad understanding of computer sciences, mathematics, and the ecology of microbes in humans, animals, and diverse environments can generate predictions that will allow us to anticipate when and where a disease outbreak may occur and provide upstream interventions that protect the health of humans, animals, and the environment.

Acknowledgments. The authors of this manuscript do not have any commercial affiliations, consultancies, stock or equity interests, or patent-licensing arrangements that could be considered to pose a conflict of interest regarding the manuscript.

Citation. Casas V, Maloy S. 2014. Genomic and metagenomic approaches for predicting pathogen evolution. Microbiol Spectrum 2(1):OH-0019-2013. doi:10.1128/microbiolspec.OH-0019-2013.

REFERENCES

1. **Centers for Disease Control and Prevention.** 2010. *Emerging Infectious Diseases* journal background and goals. Centers for Disease Control and Prevention, Atlanta, GA. http://wwwnc.cdc.gov/eid/pages /background-goals.htm (last accessed April 2, 2013).
2. **Parmesan C.** 2006. Ecological and evolutionary responses to recent climate change. *Annu Rev Ecol Evol Syst* **37:**637–669.
3. **Cione JJ, Uhlhorn EW.** 2003. Sea surface temperature variability in hurricanes: implications with respect to intensity change. *Mon Weather Rev* **131:**1783–1796.
4. **Rohwer F, Youle M, Vosten D.** 2010. *Coral Reefs in the Microbial Seas.* Plaid Press, Basalt, CO.
5. **Casas V, Sobrepeña G, Rodriguez-Mueller B, Ahtye J, Maloy SR.** 2011. Bacteriophage-encoded shiga toxin gene in atypical bacterial host. *Gut Pathog* **3:**10. doi:10.1186/1757-4749-3-10.
6. **Casas V, Magbanua J, Sobrepeña G, Kelley ST, Maloy SR.** 2010. Reservoir of bacterial exotoxin genes in the environment. *Int J Microbiol* **2010:**754368. doi:10.1155/2010/754368.
7. **Casas V, Miyake J, Balsley H, Roark J, Telles S, Leeds S, Zurita I, Breitbart M, Azam F, Bartlett D, Rohwer F.** 2006. Widespread occurrence of phage-encoded exotoxin genes in terrestrial and aquatic environments in Southern California. *FEMS Microbiol Lett* **261:**141–149.
8. **Harvell CD, Mitchell CE, Ward JR, Altizer S, Dobson AP, Ostfeld RS, Samuel MD.** 2002. Climate warming and disease risks for terrestrial and marine biota. *Science* **296:**2158–2162.

9. **Harvell CD, Kim K, Burkholder JM, Colwell RR, Epstein PR, Grimes DJ, Hofmann EE, Lipp EK, Osterhaus AD, Overstreet RM, Porter JW, Smith GW, Vasta GR.** 1999. Emerging marine diseases—climate links and anthropogenic factors. *Science* **285:**1505–1510.

10. **Dearing MD, Dizney L.** 2010. Ecology of hantavirus in a changing world. *Ann N Y Acad Sci* **1195:**99–112.

11. **Le Guenno B.** 1997. Haemorrhagic fevers and ecological perturbations. *Arch Virol Suppl* **13:**191–199.

12. **Weil AA, Ivers LC, Harris JB.** 2012. Cholera: lessons from Haiti and beyond. *Curr Infect Dis Rep* **14:**1–8.

13. **Jutla AS, Akanda AS, Islam S.** 2010. Tracking cholera in coastal regions using satellite observations. *J Am Water Resour Assoc* **46:**651–662.

14. **Khasnis AA, Nettleman MD.** 2005. Global warming and infectious disease. *Arch Med Res* **36:**689–696.

15. **Shuman EK.** 2010. Global climate change and infectious diseases. *N Engl J Med* **362:**1061–1063.

16. **Neerinckx S, Bertherat E, Leirs H.** 2010. Human plague occurrences in Africa: an overview from 1877 to 2008. *Trans R Soc Trop Med Hyg* **104:**97–103.

17. **Riesenfeld CS, Schloss PD, Handelsman J.** 2004. Metagenomics: genomic analysis of microbial communities. *Annu Rev Genet* **38:**525–552.

18. **Handelsman J, Rondon MR, Brady SF, Clardy J, Goodman RM.** 1998. Molecular biological access to the chemistry of unknown soil microbes: a new frontier for natural products. *Chem Biol* **5:**R245–R249.

19. **Casas V, Rohwer F.** 2007. Phage metagenomics. *Methods Enzymol* **421:**259–268.

20. **Gilbert JA, Dupont CL.** 2011. Microbial metagenomics: beyond the genome. *Annu Rev Mar Sci* **3:**347–371.

21. **Conlan S, Kong HH, Segre JA.** 2012. Species-level analysis of DNA sequence data from the NIH Human Microbiome Project. *PLoS One* **7:**e47075. doi:10.1371/journal.pone.0047075.

22. **Gevers D, Knight R, Petrosino JF, Huang K, McGuire AL, Birren BW, Nelson KE, White O, Methé BA, Huttenhower C.** 2012. The Human Microbiome Project: a community resource for the healthy human microbiome. *PLoS Biol* **10:**e1001377. doi:10.1371/journal.pbio.1001377.

23. **Ursell LK, Metcalf JL, Parfrey LW, Knight R.** 2012. Defining the human microbiome. *Nutr Rev* **70** (Suppl 1):S38–S44.

24. **Wylie KM, Truty RM, Sharpton TJ, Mihindukulasuriya KA, Zhou Y, Gao H, Sodergren E, Weinstock GM, Pollard KS.** 2012. Novel bacterial taxa in the human microbiome. *PLoS One* **7:**e35294. doi:10.1371/journal.pone.0035294.

25. **Wooley JC, Godzik A, Friedberg I.** 2010. A primer on metagenomics. *PLoS Comput Biol* **6:**e1000667. doi:10.1371/journal.pcbi.1000667.

26. **Breitbart M, Salamon P, Andresen B, Mahaffy JM, Segall AM, Mead D, Azam F, Rohwer F.** 2002. Genomic analysis of uncultured marine viral communities. *Proc Natl Acad Sci USA* **99:**14250–14255.

27. **Breitbart M, Felts B, Kelley S, Mahaffy JM, Nulton J, Salamon P, Rohwer F.** 2004. Diversity and population structure of a near-shore marine-sediment viral community. *Proc Biol Sci* **271:**565–574.

28. **Breitbart M, Hewson I, Felts B, Mahaffy JM, Nulton J, Salamon P, Rohwer F.** 2003. Metagenomic analyses of an uncultured viral community from human feces. *J Bacteriol* **85:**6220–6223.

29. **Cann AJ, Fandrich SE, Heaphy S.** 2005. Analysis of the virus population present in equine faeces indicates the presence of hundreds of uncharacterized virus genomes. *Virus Genes* **30:**151–156.

30. **Culley AI, Lang AS, Suttle CA.** 2006. Metagenomic analysis of coastal RNA virus communities. *Science* **312:**1795–1798.

31. **Zhang T, Breitbart M, Lee WH, Run JQ, Wei CL, Soh SW, Hibberd ML, Liu ET, Rohwer F, Ruan Y.** 2006. RNA viral community in human feces: prevalence of plant pathogenic viruses. *PLoS Biol* **4:**e3. doi:10.1371/journal.pbio.0040003.

32. **Willner D, Furlan M, Haynes M, Schmieder R, Angly FE, Silva J, Tammadoni S, Nosrat B, Conrad D, Rohwer F.** 2009. Metagenomic analysis of respiratory tract DNA viral communities in cystic fibrosis and non-cystic fibrosis individuals. *PLoS One* **4:**e7370. doi:10.1371/journal.pone.0007370.

33. **Edwards RA, Rohwer F.** 2005. Viral metagenomics. *Nat Rev Microbiol* **3:**504–510.

34. **Deng Q, Barbieri JT.** 2008. Molecular mechanisms of the cytotoxicity of ADP-ribosylating toxins. *Annu Rev Microbiol* **62:**271–288.

35. **Dayhoff MO, Schwartz RM, Orcutt BC.** 1978. A model of evolutionary change in proteins, p 345–352. *In* Dayhoff MO (ed), *Atlas of Protein Sequence and Structure*, vol. **5**. National Biomedical Research Foundation, Washington, DC.

36. **Murphy JR.** 1996. Chapter 32, *Corynebacterium diphtheriae*. *In* Baron S (ed), *Medical Microbiology*, 4th ed. University of Texas Medical Branch at Galveston, Galveston, TX. Available from http://www.ncbi.nlm .nih.gov/books/NBK7971/.

37. **Pakalniskiene J, Falkenhorst G, Lisby M, Madsen SB, Olsen KE, Nielsen EM, Mygh A, Boel J, Mølbak K.** 2009. A foodborne outbreak of enterotoxigenic *E. coli* and *Salmonella anatum* infection after a high-school dinner in Denmark, November 2006. *Epidemiol Infect* **137:**396–401.

38. **Sekse C, Muniesa M, Wasteson Y.** 2008. Conserved Stx2 phages from *Escherichia coli* O103:H25 isolated from patients suffering from hemolytic uremic syndrome. *Foodborne Pathog Dis* **5:**801–810.

39. **Vojdani JD, Beuchat LR, Tauxe RV.** 2008. Juice-associated outbreaks of human illness in the United States, 1995 through 2005. *J Food Prot* **71:**356–364.

40. **Franz E, van Bruggen AH.** 2008. Ecology of *E. coli* O157:H7 and *Salmonella enterica* in the primary vegetable production chain. *Crit Rev Microbiol* **34:**143–161.

41. **Charatan F.** 2006. FDA warns US consumers not to eat spinach after *E. coli* outbreak. *BMJ* **333:**673.

42. **Lynch M, Painter J, Woodruff R, Braden C, Centers for Disease Control and Prevention.** 2006. Surveillance for foodborne-disease outbreaks—United States, 1998–2002. *MMWR Surveill Summ* **55:**1–42.

43. **Centers for Disease Control and Prevention (CDC).** 2006. Ongoing multistate outbreak of *Escherichia coli* serotype O157:H7 infections associated with consumption of fresh spinach—United States, September 2006. *MMWR Morb Mortal Wkly Rep* **55:**1045–1046.

44. **Devasia RA, Jones TF, Ward J, Stafford L, Hardin H, Bopp C, Beatty M, Mintz E, Schaffner W.** 2006. Endemically acquired foodborne outbreak of enterotoxin-producing *Escherichia coli* serotype O169:H41. *Am J Med* **119:**168.e7–168.e10.

45. **Scheutz F, Nielsen EM, Frimodt-Møller J, Boisen N, Morabito S, Tozzoli R, Nataro JP, Caprioli A.** 2011. Characteristics of the enteroaggregative Shiga toxin/verotoxin-producing *Escherichia coli* O104:H4 strain causing the outbreak of haemolytic uraemic syndrome in Germany, May to June 2011. *Euro Surveill* **16:**pii=19889. http://www.eurosurveillance.org/ViewArticle.aspx?ArticleId=19889.

46. **Mellmann A, Harmsen D, Cummings CA, Zentz EB, Leopold SR, Rico A, Prior K, Szczepanowski R, Ji Y, Zhang W, McLaughlin SF, Henkhaus JK, Leopold B, Bielaszewska M, Prager R, Brzoska PM, Moore RL, Guenther S, Rothberg JM, Karch H.** 2011. Prospective genomic characterization of the German enterohemorrhagic *Escherichia coli* O104:H4 outbreak by rapid next generation sequencing technology. *PLoS One* **6:**e22751. doi:10.1371/journal.pone.0022751.

47. **Brzuszkiewicz E, Thürmer A, Schuldes J, Leimbach A, Liesegang H, Meyer FD, Boelter J, Petersen H, Gottschalk G, Daniel R.** 2011. Genome sequence analyses of two isolates from the recent *Escherichia coli* outbreak in Germany reveal the emergence of a new pathotype: Entero-Aggregative-Haemorrhagic *Escherichia coli* (EAHEC). *Arch Microbiol* **193:**883–891.

48. **Freeman BJ.** 1951. Studies on the virulence of bacteriophage-infected strains of *Corynebacterium diphtheriae*. *J Bacteriol* **61:**675–688.

49. **Groman NB.** 1953. The relation of bacteriophage to the change of *Corynebacterium diphtheriae* from avirulence to virulence. *Science* **117:**297–299.

50. **Lenski RE, Levin BR.** 1985. Constraints on the coevolution of bacteria and virulent phage: a model, some experiments, and predictions for natural communties. *Am Nat* **125:**585–602.

51. **Waldor MK, Mekalanos JJ.** 1996. Lysogenic conversion by a filamentous phage encoding cholera toxin. *Science* **272:**1910–1914.

52. **Davis BM, Moyer KE, Boyd EF, Waldor MK.** 2000. CTX prophages in classical biotype *Vibrio cholerae*: functional phage genes but dysfunctional phage genomes. *J Bacteriol* **182:**6992–6998.

53. **Ochman H, Lawrence JG, Groisman EA.** 2000. Lateral gene transfer and the nature of bacterial innovation. *Nature* **405:**299–304.

54. **Boyd EF, Davis BM, Hochhut B.** 2001. Bacteriophage-bacteriophage interactions in the evolution of pathogenic bacteria. *Trends Microbiol* **9:**137–144.

55. **Muniesa M, Lucena F, Jofre J.** 1999. Study of the potential relationship between the morphology of infectious somatic coliphages and their persistence in the environment. *J Appl Microbiol* **87:**402–409.

56. **Muniesa M, Lucena F, Jofre J.** 1999. Comparative survival of free Shiga toxin 2-encoding phages and *Escherichia coli* strains outside the gut. *Appl Environ Microbiol* **65:**5615–5618.

57. **Sinton LW, Hall CH, Lynch PA, Davies-Colley RJ.** 2002. Sunlight inactivation of fecal indicator bacteria and bacteriophages from waste stabilization pond effluent in fresh and saline waters. *Appl Environ Microbiol* **68:**1122–1131.

58. **Mocé-Llivina L, Muniesa M, Pimenta-Vale H, Lucena F, Jofre J.** 2003. Survival of bacterial indicator species and bacteriophages after thermal treatment of sludge and sewage. *Appl Environ Microbiol* **69:**1452–1456.

59. **Tanji Y, Mizoguchi K, Yoichi M, Morita M, Kijima N, Kator H, Unno H.** 2003. Seasonal change and fate of coliphages infected to *Escherichia coli* O157:H7 in a wastewater treatment plant. *Water Res* **37:** 1136–1142.

60. **Dumke R, Schröter-Bobsin U, Jacobs E, Röske I.** 2006. Detection of phages carrying the Shiga toxin 1 and 2 genes in waste water and river water samples. *Lett Appl Microbiol* **42:**48–53.

61. **Masago Y, Katayama H, Watanabe T, Haramoto E, Hashimoto A, Omura T, Hirata T, Ohgaki S.** 2006. Quantitative risk assessment of noroviruses in drinking water based on qualitative data in Japan. *Environ Sci Technol* **40:**7428–7433.

62. **McLaughlin MR, Rose JB.** 2006. Application of *Bacteroides fragilis* phage as an alternative indicator of sewage pollution in Tampa Bay, Florida. *Estuar Coast* **29:**246–256.

63. **Patz JA, Daszak P, Tabor GM, Aguirre AA, Pearl M, Epstein J, Wolfe ND, Kilpatrick AM, Foufopoulos J, Molyneux D, Bradley DJ, Working Group on Land Use Change and Disease Emergence.** 2004. Unhealthy landscapes: policy recommendations on land use change and infectious disease emergence. *Environ Health Perspect* **112:**1092–1098.

64. **Schmidt KA, Ostfeld RS.** 2001. Biodiversity and the dilution effect in disease ecology. *Ecology* **82:** 609–619.

65. **Chua KB, Goh KJ, Wong KT, Kamarulzaman A, Tan PS, Ksiazek TG, Zaki SR, Paul G, Lam SK, Tan CT.** 1999. Fatal encephalitis due to Nipah virus among pig-farmers in Malaysia. *Lancet* **354:** 1257–1259.

66. **Lam SK, Chua KB.** 2002. Nipah virus encephalitis outbreak in Malaysia. *Clin Infect Dis* **34**(Suppl 2): S48–S51.

67. **Rose JB, Epstein PR, Lipp EK, Sherman BH, Bernard SM, Patz JA.** 2001. Climate variability and change in the United States: potential impacts on water- and foodborne diseases caused by microbiologic agents. *Environ Health Perspect* **109:**211–221.

68. **Ford TE, Colwell RR, Rose JB, Morse SS, Rogers DJ, Yates TL.** 2009. Using satellite images of environmental changes to predict infectious disease outbreaks. *Emerg Infect Dis* **15:**1341–1346.

One Health: People, Animals, and the Environment
Edited by Ronald M. Atlas and Stanley Maloy
© 2014 American Society for Microbiology, Washington, DC
doi:10.1128/microbiolspec.OH-0014-2012

Chapter 16

Surveillance of Wildlife Diseases: Lessons from the West Nile Virus Outbreak

*Tracey S. McNamara,[1] Robert G. McLean,[2] Emi K. Saito,[3]
Peregrine L. Wolff,[4] Colin M. Gillin,[5] John R. Fischer,[6] Julie C. Ellis,[7]
Richard French,[8] Patrick P. Martin,[9] Krysten L. Schuler,[10]
Dave McRuer,[11] Edward E. Clark,[11] Megan K. Hines,[12] Cris Marsh,[12]
Victoria Szewczyk,[12] Kurt Sladky,[12] Lisa Yon,[13] Duncan Hannant,[14]
and William F. Siemer[15]*

INTRODUCTION

In 1998, before the West Nile virus (WNV), monkeypox, and severe acute respiratory syndrome outbreaks, Childs et al. (1) made the prescient observation that "multidisciplinary teams of ecologists, mammalogists, ornithologists, and entomologists, as well as physicians and epidemiologists, may be required for successful investigations of zoonoses." This was proven to be true in 1999 when the lack of a One Health approach significantly delayed recognition of WNV. This was due to a number of factors including:

* Poor communication across the human and animal sectors
* Weak diagnostic capacity at a state department of natural resources
* Exclusion of captive wildlife from any surveillance efforts

[1]Western University of Health Sciences, Pomona, CA 91766; [2]Division of Biology, Kansas State University, Manhattan, KS 66506; [3]National Surveillance Unit, Centers for Epidemiology and Animal Health, USDA APHIS Veterinary Services, Fort Collins, CO 80526; [4]Nevada Department of Wildlife, Reno, NV 89512; [5]Wildlife Health and Population Lab, Oregon Department of Fish and Wildlife, Corvallis, OR 97330; [6]Southeastern Cooperative Wildlife Disease Study, College of Veterinary Medicine, University of Georgia, Athens, GA 30602; [7]Tufts University, Cummings School of Veterinary Medicine, North Grafton, MA 01536; [8]University of New Hampshire, New Hampshire Veterinary Diagnostic Laboratory, Durham, NH 03824; [9]New York State Department of Environmental Conservation Wildlife Health Unit, Albany, NY 12233-4752; [10]Animal Health Diagnostic Center, Ithaca, NY 14850; [11]Wildlife Center of Virginia, Waynesboro, VA 22980; [12]Wildlife Data Integration Network, Department of Surgical Sciences, University of Wisconsin School of Veterinary Medicine, Madison, WI 53706; [13]School of Veterinary Medicine and Science, University of Nottingham Sutton Bonington Campus, Nottingham LE12 5RD, United Kingdom, and Twycross Zoo-East Midland Zoological Society, Twycross CV9 3PX, United Kingdom; [14]Department of Applied Immunology, School of Veterinary Medicine and Science, University of Nottingham Sutton Bonington Campus, Nottingham LE12 5RD, United Kingdom; [15]Human Dimensions Research Unit, Department of Natural Resources, Cornell University, Ithaca, NY 14853.

- Lack of timely recognition of the geospatial link between the bird and human outbreaks

Given that "60.3% of emerging infectious disease (EID) events are caused by zoonotic pathogens" (2), that "the number of EID events caused by pathogens originating in wildlife has increased significantly with time" (2), and that "wild animals seem to be involved in the epidemiology of most zoonoses and serve as major reservoirs for transmission of zoonotic agents to domestic animals and humans" (2), there is a certain urgency to taking a more integrated approach to zoonotic threats, especially regarding wildlife. Wildlife EIDs not only pose a threat to human health but pose "a substantial threat to the conservation of global biodiversity" (3). But if another WNV-like event were to occur tomorrow, would the recognition and response time differ from that of 14 years ago? The question is, have the issues that caused us to miss early warning of WNV been addressed? Have the lessons of WNV been learned?

Certainly progress has been made. Communication across sectors has improved since 1999. There is increased awareness of "the need for closer collaboration between the veterinary profession, wildlife specialists, and public health personnel" (4). There is now recognition of the role that "veterinarians and other wildlife specialists can play in surveillance, control, and prevention of emerging zoonoses" (6) and that cooperation between human and animal health professionals is "imperative to strengthen the evidence base that will allow for rational use of animal data in public health decision-making" (7). Great strides in cooperation and collaboration were made between the Centers for Disease Control and Prevention (CDC), U.S. Department of Agriculture (USDA), and U.S. Geological Survey (USGS) once WNV was diagnosed. The USGS National Wildlife Health Center (NWHC) established strong ties with CDC's Division of Vector-Borne Infectious Diseases (now the Division of Vector-Borne Diseases in the National Center for Emerging and Zoonotic Infectious Diseases). The CDC developed a remarkable integrated database called ArboNET that included data on people, horses, mosquitoes, and zoo species and included data from the USDA and maps provided by USGS. The CDC even funded a novel public-private partnership with the zoo community that resulted in a national surveillance program of captive wildlife.

Has similar progress been made in the free-ranging wildlife component of the equation? What is the status of wildlife disease surveillance in the United States? If wildlife can serve as sentinels for emerging zoonoses, what guarantees do we have that future sentinels will be diagnosed in a timely manner? In early June 1999, hundreds of crows died and were submitted to the New York State Department of Environmental Conservation (NYSDEC) for evaluation. This was almost 2.5 months in advance of any human morbidity or mortality associated with WNV. Why did it take so long to get a diagnosis in the wild birds? There are two reasons. First, high case fatalities are not unusual in wild populations and often do not trigger the same sense of alarm as they would in human or domestic animal populations. Wildlife personnel manage populations of animals and are not necessarily sensitive to emerging events in individual animals. Second, while "human and domestic animal health are agency mandates at most major levels of government (i.e., municipal, state, federal, provincial) and have direct budget allocations for disease program development and operations, and often are able to obtain supplemental funding when disease emergencies arise," until recently "wildlife disease was not a mandated activity of natural resources agencies and decisions to allocate funds and develop capabilities for this type of activity are internal administrative decisions" (8). As a result, not all states have well-equipped laboratories that deal with wildlife on a regular basis, and many animal facilities that see wildlife specimens may not be prepared to effectively diagnose disease. The NYSDEC was limited in its diagnostic capabilities. The combination of these factors resulted in significant delay in recognition of a sentinel event.

If "efficient surveillance is dependent upon a laboratory system that is capable of identifying and characterizing the pathogens in question" (9), what is the status of diagnostic capabilities for free-ranging wildlife in the United States today? Has anything changed since the WNV outbreak of 1999? Are state wildlife labs better prepared to respond to emerging zoonotic threats? If not, where can they turn? "To increase the capability of recognizing zoonoses with a wildlife reservoir, better national surveillance systems for humans and animals are needed, as well as better national and international integration and sharing of information from such systems" (10). This implies that there must be equal diagnostic and surveillance capabilities across species, and such is not the case.

In his 2006 book *Disease Emergence and Resurgence*, Milton Friend, former director of the USGS NWHC in Madison, WI, comprehensively detailed the associations between wildlife and emerging diseases. Unfortunately, he also noted that although this association is evident, "the true integration of the wildlife component in approaches towards disease emergence remains elusive" and that "the broader community of disease investigators and health care professionals has largely pursued a separatist approach for human, domestic animal, and wildlife rather than embracing the periodically proposed concept of 'one medicine'" (8).

Dr. Friend further analyzed the similarities and disparities of disease programs and found that

> in general, response to disease in humans and domestic animals is guided by well-defined areas of responsibility, established regulations and protocols, existing organizational structures, pre-established communication processes, and other components that provide a reasonably cohesive infrastructure for carrying out this important activity. The situation for wildlife is quite often different. Responses are generally ad hoc and are guided by biologists within the agency managing the site with the disease event (8)

and funding for disease diagnosis is usually limited. Unfortunately, this is because the

> collective resources allocated for wildlife disease investigations within North America by natural resources agencies are only a small percentage of the total resources allocated for the Centers for Disease Control and Prevention (CDC) of the U.S. Department of Health and Human Services (HHS) to combat human disease and those allocated to the U.S. Department of Agriculture (USDA) to combat domestic animal disease. Only a few wildlife disease programs have adequate facilities and are insufficiently staffed or integrated with other programs to provide analyses and the spectrum of expertise

required to meet the demands of rapid, accurate diagnoses for guiding disease response efforts. This is especially true and important when unfamiliar diseases are encountered. (8)

If a One Health approach to zoonotic disease surveillance is to be made a reality, these inequities and coverage gaps will need to be addressed.

WILDLIFE DISEASE SURVEILLANCE AT THE STATE LEVEL

Responsibility for most wildlife rests with the state fish and wildlife agencies that are entrusted to conserve and manage native wildlife within their geographic boundaries. Recently, more states have taken an increasing interest in implementing programs and have integrated fish and wildlife health as part of basic management and research programs.

In 2007, recognizing the need for greater capacity within state agencies throughout the United States to better respond to wildlife disease threats, the Association of Fish and Wildlife Agencies, Fish and Wildlife Health Committee, published the *National Fish and Wildlife Health Initiative Toolkit*. This toolkit provides the framework upon which state and federal fish and wildlife agencies can define current capabilities for disease surveillance, monitoring, and response within their respective agencies, and further build capacity within the agency or through collaborative efforts with partner agencies. The National Fish and Wildlife Health Initiative recognized that state fish and wildlife agencies are responsible for "managing diseases in free-ranging fish and wildlife" (10). In a move toward One Health, it also recognized that there is a need to "foster collaboration, coordination, and communication among fish and wildlife health jurisdictions, as well as with animal health and public health agencies at the state and national level" (10). Several states (Wyoming, Colorado, Michigan, and California) have had long-standing management and research wildlife health programs that serve as models for succeeding state programs. But according to a recent survey (11), most states will need to hire more specialized staff and/or take novel approaches to disease surveillance if the initiative is to be a success. Funding and staffing issues continue to be major hindrances to implementing the initiative nationwide.

In 2012, Siemer et al. (11) conducted a survey that identified factors that affect agency capacity to address disease issues. The survey explored perceptions of how nine factors contribute to agency capacity, including interagency agreements related to staff sharing, interagency coordination, funding sources, regulatory authority, funding level, staffing, diagnostic facilities, funding, and response plans (program management). One terrestrial and one aquatic wildlife health representative was contacted in each state. Response to the terrestrial wildlife survey was 94% (47 states); the only states not represented were Hawaii, Kentucky, and Delaware. Response to the aquatic wildlife survey was 84% (42 states); the states not represented were Connecticut, Hawaii, Oklahoma, Massachusetts, Nevada, Texas, Vermont, and Virginia.

Agency capacity to assist with collection of surveillance data is limited by availability of staff. About 75% of agencies reported that they had adequately sized field staffs to provide a short-term response to a terrestrial disease outbreak, but only 25% had adequate staff to provide a long-term response. About 80% of agencies reportedly had adequate staff for a short-term response to an aquatic disease outbreak, but only 46% had the staff capacity to provide a long-term response. Though many agencies offered limited staff training related to collecting and submitting samples as part of surveillance activities, substantial minorities of agencies reported that training on those topics was less than adequate.

The survey found that the ability to design surveillance programs or collect or interpret surveillance data may also be affected by access to specialized staff. Wildlife veterinarians and wildlife biologists normally conduct investigation, surveillance, monitoring, and research of wildlife diseases and manage the health of free-ranging wildlife primarily in agencies, but also as part of university programs and through the work of nongovernmental organizations and individuals. Wildlife veterinarians and biologists also frequently work with state and federal veterinarians on disease issues that affect livestock and with public health officials if there are zoonotic disease concerns. State emergency management planning activities increasingly include wildlife disease specialists to assist responders and emergency managers with minimizing negative impacts on wildlife populations while safeguarding domestic animal and human health. In 2011, a majority of agencies surveyed did not have veterinarians or pathologists on staff. To date, only half of states have one or more wildlife veterinarians or other staff (wildlife health specialists) dedicated to a wildlife health program for terrestrial and/or aquatic species. Access to veterinarians or pathologists was perceived as an impediment to disease detection and response in about 15% of states.

Another goal of the National Fish and Wildlife Health Initiative is to "establish an integrated surveillance and diagnostic laboratory network" (10). Access to diagnostic testing is variable across states. Using data from the 2011 agency survey, Siemer et al. (12) compared self-identified high-capacity ($n = 7$) and low-capacity ($n = 12$) agencies on multiple traits, including access to diagnostic facilities. Most representatives reported that their agency had access to diagnostic laboratories in other states, National Animal Health Laboratory Network (NAHLN)-accredited facilities to test for chronic wasting disease and highly pathogenic avian influenza (HPAI), and an in-state diagnostic laboratory operated by another agency or a university. But representatives of high-capacity agencies were more likely than those in low-capacity agencies to have access to their own diagnostic facilities (71 vs. 17%), other in-state laboratories (100 vs. 75%), and NAHLN-accredited facilities for HPAI testing (100 vs. 67%). Survey findings suggest that having one's own facilities for routine monitoring and surveillance tasks is not essential to agencies but is more likely to be a trait of high-capacity agencies. Federal funding for WNV and HPAI surveillance within states and within federal agencies has disappeared during the last few years and is unlikely to be replaced. Both of those national surveillance programs provided relatively good national and state surveillance and good training and experience for participants. This trained national workforce will be lost without future support.

Where does the funding for state wildlife agencies come from? State wildlife agencies have a narrow range of funding mechanisms. A major source of funding for state wildlife programs, including many wildlife health programs, is generated from federal funds administered by the U.S. Fish and Wildlife Service under the Pittman-Robertson and Dingle-Johnson Acts. These bills, passed in the mid-20th century, levied federal excise taxes on all firearms and ammunition (Pittman-Robertson) or fishing equipment and boat fuel and motors (Dingle-Johnson). The funds generated are distributed to states for the restoration of wildlife. The money is distributed to the state fish and wildlife management agencies based on a formula derived from the size of the state and the number of hunting and fishing licenses sold in each state. States match 25% of the funding they receive, often through the sale of hunting and fishing licenses. Other funding sources often include the state's general fund, other federally administered grants (U.S. Fish and Wildlife Service, Section 6 and State Wildlife Grants), local or national sportsmen's organizations, mining and energy companies (mitigation funds), and state tax or earmark sources (vehicle license fees). Federal funds earmarked for surveillance for specific diseases of national concern (e.g., chronic wasting disease, HPAI, white-nose syndrome, viral hemorrhagic septicemia, and cold water disease of fish) are also available through competitive and noncompetitive grant sources. These funds are subject to congressional budget approval and are limited in their availability as long-term funding sources. Because disease surveillance levels are dependent on a narrow range of funding sources, surveillance efforts can decline markedly when those sources of funding expire, leaving us vulnerable to disease threats.

About 40% of agency representatives reported that funding for detection and response to disease threats had declined over the past 5 years (20% reported that funding had increased). Representatives in the majority of states reported that funding levels were "adequate" or "partially adequate" to conduct disease monitoring, surveillance, and response activities; about 25% said current funding levels were "not at all adequate" for response to disease outbreaks in terrestrial and aquatic wildlife. Only 24% of wildlife (and 35% of aquatic) representatives reported that the funding level in their agency in 2011 was adequate for purposes of diagnostic testing. So, although state wildlife agencies may now be interested in performing disease surveillance, they do not have sufficient funds to do so.

THE SUMMER OF 1999

During the WNV outbreak, it was fortunate that states were able to turn to a federal wildlife diagnostic laboratory. The USGS NWHC is unique in its breadth of in-house technical disciplines and physical facilities devoted to wildlife disease investigations. These capabilities enabled the NWHC to quickly become a partner in the One Health type of response to this unique outbreak, representing the wildlife health part in collaboration with the public health and domestic animal health parts of the response triad. The NWHC was an active participant in collaborative planning and investigative efforts throughout the early WNV epidemic period and beyond. A federal working group among CDC's Division of Vector-Borne Infectious Diseases, the USGS NWHC, and the USDA Animal and Plant Health Inspection Service (APHIS) Veterinary Services and Wildlife Services was established, and they cooperated closely, in conjunction with relevant state agencies, to conduct WNV surveillance in a One Health manner.

Since its establishment in 1975, the federal NWHC has (i) monitored wildlife diseases and assessed the impact of diseases on wildlife populations; (ii) defined ecological relationships leading to the occurrence of disease in free-ranging wildlife; (iii) provided on-site investigations and control for wildlife disease emergencies; and (iv) provided guidance, training, and technical information for reducing wildlife losses when outbreaks occur. The NWHC provides technical support, knowledgeable guidance, and timely intervention to wildlife managers who are regularly confronted with sick and dead wild animals, frequently on a large scale. The expertise and resources of the NWHC disease diagnostic laboratory are crucial in providing a rapid response to wildlife mortality events.

The USGS NWHC is a high-security biosafety level 3 (BSL3) infectious disease facility in Madison, WI, designed to meet all of the criteria set down by the National Institutes of Health and CDC for BSL3 research. It is the only federal facility devoted exclusively to the diagnosis, prevention, and control of diseases of wildlife.

Another federal program is the National Wildlife Disease Program (NWDP) of the National Wildlife Research Center, Wildlife Services, APHIS, which is located on a 43-acre master facility located on the Colorado State University campus in Fort Collins. The National Wildlife Research Center mission is consistent with lending emergency diagnostic support for specific pathogens, especially those whose reservoirs are in wildlife. Within the context of normal endemic disease emergencies, support for wildlife disease surveillance for foreign animal diseases and support for emergency laboratory testing as a result of a bioterrorism event are within the technical and infrastructure capacity for specific agents and protocols. Wildlife disease biologists conduct surveillance activities in all 50 states and act as Wildlife Services' first responders in cases of emergency, as part of the NWDP's Surveillance and Emergency Response System. As part of their everyday duties, wildlife disease biologists participate in avian influenza surveillance, as well as other disease monitoring and control activities that are of particular interest and concern in their designated regions. Additionally, the NWDP collaborates with nongovernmental organizations and officials from other countries to promote and assist in the development of wildlife disease monitoring programs worldwide.

The NWHC became involved in the WNV outbreak when on September 2, 1999, the Field Investigations Team received a call from the NYSDEC reporting morbidity and mortality in American crows in the Bronx and Queens boroughs in New York City. During early stages of the surveillance, the NWHC was one of only a few BSL3 facilities capable and available to test birds for WNV after it was declared a BSL3 agent. This initial involvement to help NYSDEC with the first group of dead crows was part of the routine service the NWHC provides to state wildlife agencies. It set in motion an intense investigation of these events that would culminate in the examination for WNV of 142 specimens (47 species) from New York in 1999, and 68,578 from 2000 to 2012 (357 species; 50 U.S. states and Canada).

From the investigation of crow mortality in August 1999, the NWHC isolated an unidentified virus in the first week of September that was subsequently confirmed to be WNV. The NWHC then conducted field studies and diagnostic laboratory testing in support of dead bird surveillance in a number of states in the Northeast, especially New York. WNV was isolated and identified from a migratory bird captured in the Bronx; this was the first isolate of WNV from a live, free-ranging wild bird (13) and an early indication that migratory birds could move the virus out of the epidemic focus. In 2000, WNV research was initiated at the NWHC. These studies demonstrated the lethality of the New York 1999 strain, crow reservoir competency, and direct transmission between inoculated crows and controls, likely from WNV-laden discharge (13).

As robust as the initial response was, due to the increase in specimens received, the NWHC did struggle in 2000 to keep up, and this delayed delivery of results to the states.

NWHC staff during these times were challenged by the limited resources, but continued until the states were capable of managing their own testing. This occurred when funding and training became available directly from the CDC to state public health agencies.

The CDC received $4 million for WNV control in the FY2001 budget, and the NWHC received about $200,000 per year for a few years. This significant contrast in funding levels suggests less support for wildlife diagnostics and research even when the country was in full crisis mode.

CREATIVE APPROACHES TO ACHIEVING STATE WILDLIFE DIAGNOSTIC CAPABILITIES

How do states without their own diagnostic labs do disease surveillance? States utilize a number of diagnostic sampling strategies. Carcasses may be sent to a veterinary diagnostic lab for necropsy or examined in the field by a veterinarian or a biologist trained in sample collection, preparation, and shipment. A number of states in the Southeast, East, and Midwest utilize the diagnostic and disease investigation services of the Southeastern Cooperative Wildlife Disease Study (SCWDS) located in Athens, GA, as part of a state contractual agreement. This cooperative approach was the first effort to link state wildlife agencies with a dedicated and specialized wildlife disease diagnostic center.

The SCWDS story began in 1949 when there was a major die-off of deer. Facilities were not available to investigate widespread deer mortality, and conservationists and the general public wanted action. However, it was too costly for any single state to establish and maintain an organization with the expertise to cope with future deer mortality crises.

After careful deliberation, a multistate organization was established for the Southeast, and on July 1, 1957, the Southeastern Cooperative Deer Disease Study (SCDDS) was founded at the University of Georgia's College of Veterinary Medicine. The initial annual SCDDS budget of $18,000 was provided by the 11 southeastern state wildlife management agencies that were the original cooperative members. Membership grew to 13, then to 15, and now numbers 19, including states outside the Southeast. Current members are the wildlife resource agencies of Alabama, Arkansas, Florida, Georgia, Kansas, Kentucky, Louisiana, Maryland, Mississippi, Missouri, New Jersey, North Carolina, Ohio, Oklahoma, Pennsylvania, South Carolina, Tennessee, Virginia, and West Virginia.

In 1960, in recognition of the increasing demand for wildlife health information, the SCDDS expanded its mission to encompass all game and nongame species and changed its name to the SCWDS, as it is known today. SCWDS objectives are to (i) detect causes of morbidity and mortality in wildlife, (ii) define the impacts of diseases and parasites on wildlife populations, (iii) delineate disease relationships between wild and domestic animals, and (iv) determine the role of wildlife in the epidemiology of human diseases.

In 1963, the U.S. Congress enacted a recurring annual appropriation, administered through the U.S. Department of the Interior, to support basic wildlife disease research conducted by the SCWDS. In 1967, a vital alliance between wildlife and domestic animal interests was established when the USDA and SCWDS sponsored a 3-day Foreign and Emergency Disease Surveillance Training Program for wildlife biologists at the University of Georgia. The USDA and SCWDS continue to conduct the annual Wildlife Seminar for Emergency Animal Disease Preparedness every year.

Since its inception, the SCWDS has conducted surveillance and research on zoonotic diseases. The diseases diagnosed run the gamut from those that affect only wild animals to those with significant human or domestic animal health implications, such as rabies, tularemia, plague, WNV, eastern equine encephalitis, and others.

Since its establishment in 1957 as the first regional diagnostic and research center specifically for wildlife diseases, the SCWDS has provided untold benefits to this country's natural resources, wildlife managers, domestic animal and public health officials, and citizens and visitors. With its cooperative approach and pooling of resources, the SCWDS has grown and evolved by leveraging funds from individual supporters with those of the other states, federal agencies, and granting organizations to develop and distribute wildlife health information and services of value to everyone.

In 1970, states in the Northeast took a similar approach and the Northeast Research Center for Wildlife Diseases was established in the Department of Pathobiology, College of Agriculture and Natural Resources, University of Connecticut, Storrs. This cooperative center was established to conduct large-scale projects that would have been difficult to conduct on an individual state basis.

The center consisted of a multidisciplinary team of four pathologists, a microbiologist, a virologist, an immunologist, a toxicologist, an electron microscopist, a hematologist, and veterinarians and PhDs with specialties in clinical medicine and reptilian diseases. The center also engaged extramural consultants from regional affiliated states and universities, including pathologists in human medicine from both Harvard University and Yale University.

The primary functions were identified as (i) research on new and poorly understood diseases of wildlife; (ii) diagnosis of diseases of wildlife; and (iii) dissemination of information and education through teaching of undergraduate students, graduate students, and wildlife biologists about the recognition, control, and prevention of diseases of wildlife. The center was also identified as a participant in the Regional Emergency Animal Disease Eradication Organization established by the USDA. Staff members of the center were on call and assisted as wildlife disease specialists in the early diagnosis and eradication of any infectious foreign and native diseases of animals that might be introduced to the northeastern United States. The activities of the Northeast Research Center for Wildlife Diseases slowly decreased in 1995 after the retirement of its chief pathologist, Svend Nielsen. The center was officially closed in 2007. In 2011, however, another Northeast regional initiative was launched, the Northeast Wildlife Disease Cooperative (NEWDC).

WILDLIFE DISEASE SURVEILLANCE INITIATIVES

Regional coordination of wildlife disease diagnostics and reporting is essential to detect, respond to, and ultimately control disease outbreaks. Successful models of wildlife disease diagnostic and research laboratories exist in California, the southeastern United States, and throughout Canada, but the Northeast has no dedicated wildlife health facility to survey for, detect, or aid in the response to wildlife diseases, even those with potentially severe impacts on the human population. Unlike most western states, many states in the Northeast do not have their own wildlife health specialist. Moreover, the region consists of several small states with many shared borders, necessitating good communication among agencies. Yet there is no coordinated regional disease-reporting system, so information about wildlife health events is not rapidly or effectively disseminated to key stakeholders; as a result, the regional response to disease outbreaks is often sluggish and reactive rather than nimble and proactive. Scientists, veterinarians, and wildlife managers currently submit case material through the same channels used by companion animal veterinary clinics, or submit samples from large-scale die-offs to the USGS NWHC. This approach precludes a holistic, population-level understanding of wildlife and ecosystem health.

In 2010, staff from the Cummings School of Veterinary Medicine at Tufts University, Connecticut Veterinary Medical Diagnostic Laboratory at University of Connecticut, and New Hampshire Veterinary Diagnostic Lab met to discuss the idea of reviving a regional diagnostic program. The Animal Health Diagnostic Center at Cornell University and the University of Maine Animal Health Lab joined the effort soon thereafter. Collectively, these laboratories have considerable expertise in diseases of domestic animals and wildlife in the Northeast. And with multiple laboratories cooperating to provide diagnostics, both the diagnosticians and the "clients" benefit. This new project was named the NEWDC. The overarching goal of the NEWDC is to preserve and protect biodiversity and ecosystem health in the Northeast by offering wildlife diagnostic services, expertise, and cutting-edge research on the interplay of wildlife, domestic animal, and human health. The NEWDC will support and augment the services of the USGS NWHC and the Association of Fish and Wildlife Agencies in a collaborative but regionally focused effort that engages regional expertise and allows for timely and effective response to wildlife diseases. A key contact from each participating state wildlife agency, a regional representative from each of the USDA APHIS Wildlife Services and USDA APHIS Veterinary Services, and a public health veterinarian will be included on the advisory board to ensure a One Health approach.

The specific objectives of the NEWDC are to provide (i) timely diagnoses of wildlife disease outbreaks and mortality events; (ii) surveillance of diseases in live and dead wildlife; (iii) health assessments of live wildlife; (iv) expertise in wildlife-domestic animal and wildlife-human disease transmission; (v) educational opportunities for veterinarians, scientists, and wildlife managers; (vi) an accessible database of regional wildlife disease for use by human and animal health professionals; and (vii) streamlined communication regarding disease outbreaks across state lines and between agencies.

SURVEILLANCE OF WILDLIFE OUTSIDE OF FEDERAL OR STATE AGENCIES

State and federal wildlife agencies are not the only ones handling wildlife in the United States, and there are several new initiatives in the private sector that should be recognized.

Wildlife care centers manned by wildlife rehabilitators represent an untapped source of health data on a diverse array of wild animals, providing a unique "window" into wildlife health. More than 5,000 organizations and individuals in the United States alone hold permits to provide veterinary care and rehabilitation to native wildlife. Current estimates suggest that these rehabilitation programs receive 500,000 birds, mammals, reptiles, and amphibians each year. In the United States, wildlife rehabilitation generally requires state and/or federal permits in addition to filing of annual reports documenting the inventory of species and health issues encountered. However, since the several federal agencies and 44 state agencies that require such reports do not use standardized datasets or terminology or an electronic format, it is nearly impossible to access, let alone compile and analyze, the wildlife health information collected by wildlife care facilities.

The Wildlife Center of Virginia has created a program to establish the validity of data originating from wildlife care facilities. WILD-ONe (Wildlife Incident Log/Database and Online Network) is a system designed to capture admission and health data from wild animals entering rehabilitation facilities. This database provides incentives to encourage timely, standardized data entry, making it a novel source of wildlife health information. WILD-ONe is a free online database created to assist wildlife care facilities in the collection and use of data about their patients. WILD-ONe includes (i) standardized terminology and incident descriptions; (ii) standardized admission documentation; (iii) GPS coordinates for rescue-and-release sites (Google Maps with transferable coordinates); (iv) ability to assess wildlife health trends in wildlife care facilities across states/provinces, regions, and countries; (v) state, federal, and organization report generation; (vi) incentives for the rehabilitators; (vii) scheduled prescription generation; (viii) data fields for entering patient weights, meals, medical notes, etc.; (ix) contact management tools for recording patient history and for use in fund-raising; and (x) annual report generation.

Presently 80 organizations are using WILD-ONe for all patient admissions, and there are more than 25,000 patients currently in the database. It is hoped that in time WILD-ONe will be adopted by most rehabilitation organizations and result in a nationwide searchable database. While it is acknowledged that the successful rehabilitation and release of individual animals is unlikely to have significant impacts on populations or species, the data collected from these individual animals could provide unprecedented insights related to natural and anthropogenic threats to wildlife and aid in the establishment of critical baseline data.

NEW EFFORTS TO ENGAGE THE PUBLIC IN WILDLIFE DISEASE SURVEILLANCE

One of the reasons early recognition of WNV was missed is that there was no way to see the geospatial relationships between the avian and human outbreaks. Although the public was the first to notice the crow die-off, those reports were not captured and could not be visualized. In 2004, a study concluded that "reporting systems for wildlife professionals and the public should be created, and their use should be encouraged to document unusual disease events and die-offs" (7). One effort to do so is a project called the Wildlife Health Event Reporter (WHER). This easy-to-use Web application was created to record wildlife observations by the public concerned about dead or sick wildlife. After being recorded, these observations are connected with other wildlife event sightings and are viewable in tabular reports or in map form, enabling anyone to see where similar events are happening. To keep track of what is being reported to WHER, anyone can sign up for an e-mail alert for a certain area of interest or subscribe to one or more GeoRSS feed options that will connect them with the latest reports as they are shared.

With the help of the public, this system can collect timely and useful information about wildlife mortality events (e.g., date, location, and affected species). The data are integrated and summarized by the system to provide essential information for better understanding of wildlife disease patterns and their potential impact on wildlife, human, and domestic animal health, as well as to provide knowledge about baseline mortality levels. This information is being used by natural resource managers, researchers, and public health officials in an effort to protect the well-being of all living things and promote a healthy ecosystem by (i) assisting in detection of common disease events and biosecurity concerns; (ii) exploring the interconnections between human, domestic animal, and wildlife diseases; and (iii) helping to design and coordinate disease control and prevention strategies.

To build a more robust set of observations, WHER can be configured to import data from external systems and translate the information to match the data and standards used in WHER. In true One Health mode, the WHER application currently ingests mortality or morbidity reports from several other efforts, including HealthMap's mobile application for human outbreaks ("Outbreaks Near Me"). Another volunteer monitoring effort, the Seabird Ecological Assessment Network (SEANET), feeds GIS data directly to WHER about beached bird mortalities observed during periodic monitoring activities along the East Coast from Maine to Florida.

Technical development of the WHER application and framework was performed by the Wildlife Data Integration Network (WDIN) in collaboration with the University of Wisconsin-Madison's Division of Information Technology's Academic Technology group. WDIN is a collaborative research project currently located at the University of Wisconsin School of Veterinary Medicine, the aim of which is to tackle data and information integration, standardization, visualization, and dissemination challenges to increase decision makers' access to information on the health of wildlife. The WDIN project and WHER online application are currently maintained by the University of Wisconsin School of Veterinary Medicine and the WDIN project team.

ZOO SURVEILLANCE

The WNV outbreak showed how "domestic, wild, and zoo animals can be considered 'sentinels,' providing an early warning device for diseases that can harm people" (11). However, "several persons involved in the outbreak commented that the zoo community is currently left out of the animal and public health paradigm" (11). Officials indicated that "because zoo animals are not considered to be wildlife or domestic animals, they do not fall within the jurisdiction of animal health agencies such as the USGS, which tracks wildlife issues, or the USDA, which tracks concerns related to domestic animals" (11). The utility of animals as sentinels for disease has long been recognized, but the power of zoological animals as sentinels for diseases of public health concern remains underrecognized. Inherent characteristics of zoological institutions and their collections make them ideal partners in sentinel surveillance programs.

Zoological institutions manage hundreds of species of animals, both North American native and nonnative species. This represents a vast array of wildlife from many continents, maintained in relatively small footprints. Populations in accredited zoos are closely managed. Unlike most free-ranging wildlife, these animals are relatively stationary and are observed daily by trained professionals. If animals are transferred to another institution, meticulous records detail these movements between zoos. Extensive medical records are kept, and serum and other biomaterials are collected and banked during physical examinations. These biological materials can serve as a historical time-line of disease exposure that is crucial for epidemiological investigation. Most importantly, all animals that die or are euthanized while in the care of an accredited zoo must undergo a complete necropsy. This step can be critical for "early warning" and was paramount in the identification of the unusual pathology that accompanied the emergence of WNV in the Bronx Zoo in 1999.

The location of accredited zoos is also significant. There are 235 Association of Zoos and Aquariums-accredited institutions, located in urban, suburban, and rural locations. Many are situated along flyways with exhibits that allow for interaction with migrating species. Zoos are therefore potential intersections of wildlife, managed animal collections, staff, and visitors.

A national-level database for zoonotic disease surveillance that includes all animal compartments including zoological data still does not exist. An early One Health diagnostic and data integration effort was the Surveillance for West Nile Virus in Zoological Institutions program, which was funded by the CDC and ran from 2001 to 2006. This program, facilitated by Lincoln Park Zoo in Chicago, was a successful effort to integrate outcomes from WNV surveillance in zoos with a national public health database for arboviral diseases (ArboNET). A more modern database has since been developed for HPAI data that is now adaptable for any disease of concern to the zoological community. The data from this pilot project showed how data from zoo cases will automatically be provided to the USDA via the NAHLN. This ensures that the data will be in the hands of animal health officials in a timely manner.

NEW APPROACHES TO WILDLIFE DISEASE SURVEILLANCE OUTSIDE THE UNITED STATES

Researchers at the University of Nottingham are leading a project aimed at developing a state-of-the-art pan-European surveillance system to monitor emerging and reemerging infections in wildlife. Novel Technologies for Surveillance of Emerging and Re-emerging Infections of Wildlife (WildTech) is a proactive attempt to predict and manage disease threats from wildlife and assess the risk to domestic animals and humans. The project has brought together a network of wildlife specialists across 24 countries and combines (i) technological development to enable high-throughput nucleic acid- and peptide-based array screening of samples from a wide variety of wild animals, (ii) surveillance of wild animal species in Europe and from countries that may act as portals of disease entry into the European Union, (iii) epidemiological analysis and risk assessment using data generated during the project and from other sources, and (iv) development and proposal of a model framework for disease surveillance in Europe. The ultimate goal of this huge effort among multiple European countries is to develop analytical tools for multiple diseases. The aim is to prevent and/or limit disease spread among animals of the same and different species as well as from animals to humans. WildTech is working closely with the World Organisation for Animal Health and government bodies to develop an effective pan-European surveillance system with a potential global impact.

CONCLUDING REMARKS

The introduction of WNV into the eastern United States and its subsequent dissemination throughout the North American continent was an unprecedented event that challenged the infrastructure of local, state, and federal public health, domestic animal health, and wildlife health agencies to monitor viral occurrence and spread, to understand the transmission dynamics and ecology, and to try to control it and protect human and animal populations. It exposed significant deficiencies in the abilities of state natural resource and public health agencies to react similarly. In subsequent years, there have been additional high-profile emerging diseases of significance to wildlife, livestock, and public health, exemplified by monkeypox, avian influenza, and white-nose syndrome in bats. While the story of WNV provided the momentum to build additional infrastructure for wildlife disease surveillance and response, it still falls far short of similar capacities for human and domestic animal populations. The contrasts are striking: there are no mandatory reportable diseases of wildlife, there is no integrated national reporting or information system for wildlife morbidity and mortality, many states have minimal or no professional staff dedicated to wildlife disease surveillance, and there is inconsistent communication between health agencies at both the state and federal level. In short, "current measures for the detection and control of human and livestock EIDs are inadequate for the identification of similar threats in wildlife" (8). "We have good earth-monitoring systems, good public health disease-monitoring systems, but we don't have that same proactive systematic collection of data for wildlife health. Until we do that, it's going to be very hard to get a handle on what's driving these diseases" (14).

Many of these deficiencies are resource based, with orders-of-magnitude differences between funding for wildlife health compared with that available for public and livestock health. "There is no real economic incentive to proactively deal with wildlife disease. It gets dealt with during a crisis because of public pressure, but ultimately, there is no highly integrated infrastructure for dealing with disease, period" (14). Some issues may be related to the confusing array of species stewardship responsibilities assigned to state and federal agencies. The prospect of instituting a One Health approach gives some hope for improvement of this situation. When human and animal health agencies accept the concept that there are cross-population shared risks associated with emerging diseases, then the integration of knowledge, capacity, and response will provide a superior platform to address the health threats to all of the nation's inhabitants.

Citation. McNamara TS, McLean RG, Saito EK, Wolff PL, Gillin CM, Fischer JR, Ellis JC, French R, Martin PP, Schuler KL, McRuer D, Clark EE, Hines MK, Marsh C, Szewczyk V, Sladky K, Yon L, Hannant D, Siemer WF, 2013. Surveillance of wildlife diseases: lessons from the West Nile virus outbreak. Microbiol Spectrum 1(1):OH-0014-2012. doi:10.1128/microbiolspec.OH-0014-2012.

REFERENCES

1. **Childs J, Shope RE, Fish D, Meslin FX, Peters CJ, Johnson K, Debess E, Dennis G, Jenkins S.** 1998. Emerging zoonoses. *Emerg Infect Dis* **4:**453–454.
2. **Jones KE, Patel NG, Levy MA, Storeygard A, Balk D, Gittleman JL, Daszak P.** 2008. Global trends in emerging infectious diseases. *Nature* **451:**990–993.
3. **Daszak P, Cunningham AA, Hyatt AD.** 2000. Emerging infectious diseases of wildlife—threats to biodiversity and human health. *Science* **287:**443–449.

4. **Daszak P, Tabor GM, Kilpatrick AM, Epstein J, Plowright R.** 2004. Conservation medicine and a new agenda for emerging diseases. *Ann N Y Acad Sci* **1026:**1–11.

5. **Centers for Disease Control and Prevention.** 2003. Update: multistate outbreak of monkeypox—Illinois, Indiana, Kansas, Missouri, Ohio, and Wisconsin, 2003. *MMRW Morb Mortal Wkly Rep* **52:**642–646.

6. **Chomel BB, Belotto A, Meslin FX.** 2007. Wildlife, exotic pets, and emerging zoonoses. *Emerg Infect Dis* **13:**6–11.

7. **Rabinowitz P, Gordon Z, Chudnov D, Wilcox M, Odofin L, Liu A, Dein J.** 2004. Animals as sentinels of bioterrorism agents. *Emerg Infect Dis* **12:**647–652.

8. **Friend M.** 2006. *Disease Emergence and Resurgence: the Wildlife-Human Connection. Circular 1285.* U.S. Geological Survey, Reston, VA.

9. **Kruse H, Kirkemo AM, Handeland K.** 2004. Wildlife as source of zoonotic infections. *Emerg Infect Dis* **10:**2067–2072.

10. **Association of Fish and Wildlife Agencies.** 2008. *National Fish and Wildlife Health Initiative Toolkit.* Association of Fish and Wildlife Agencies, Washington, DC. http://www.fishwildlife.org/files/Fish-Wildlife-Health-Initiative-Toolkit_rev5-09.pdf (last accessed May 20, 2013).

11. **Siemer WF, Lauber TB, Decker DJ, Riley SJ.** 2012. *Agency Capacities To Detect and Respond to Disease Events: 2011 National Survey Results.* Human Dimensions Research Unit Series Publication 12-1. Department of Natural Resources, Cornell University, Ithaca, NY.

12. **Siemer WF, Lauber TB, Decker DJ, Riley SJ.** 2012. Building capacity to address disease threats: Clues from a study of state wildlife agencies. *North American Wildlife & Natural Resources Conference 77*: In press.

13. **McLean RG, Ubico SR, Docherty DE, Hansen WR, Sileo L, McNamara TS.** 2001. West Nile virus transmission and ecology in birds. *Ann N Y Acad Sci* **951:**54–57.

14. **Nolen RS.** 2012. The CDC for wildlife. *JAVMA News* **241:**1393–1399.

Making One Health a Reality

One Health: People, Animals, and the Environment
Edited by Ronald M. Atlas and Stanley Maloy
© 2014 American Society for Microbiology, Washington, DC
doi:10.1128/microbiolspec.OH-0007-2012

Chapter 17

Defining the Future of One Health

Martyn Jeggo[1] and John S. Mackenzie[2]

INTRODUCTION

During the past few decades, about 75% of newly identified emerging infectious diseases (EIDs) of humans have emerged from animals (1, 2). Microbes naturally cross over between humans, animals, and the environment—we need to adopt a One Health approach that embraces this reality. Diseases in both wildlife and production animals are posing increasingly significant risks to human health as well as the economy (3) and the environment. Good examples of this include Hendra and Nipah viruses, severe acute respiratory syndrome (SARS) coronavirus, bovine spongiform encephalopathy (BSE), avian and swine influenza, drug-resistant tuberculosis and the generation of antibiotic resistance in enterococci and other pathogenic bacteria, and finally and most significantly, HIV/AIDS. In addition, long-established diseases such as rabies, dengue, West Nile virus, and plague are also continuing to reemerge, presenting ongoing challenges and problems (4).

The importance of the role of animals in disease emergence cannot be overemphasized and has led to recognition of the need for an integrated approach to the detection and control of those diseases that affect both animals and man (zoonoses). This One Health approach recognizes not only the importance of integrating human health with animal health and with environmental ecology (5) but, given the transboundary nature of EIDs, the need for widespread surveillance of continental and global dimensions. As the value of this approach has been realized and supported, the concept has been broadened by many to include all aspects of human, animal, and environmental health, even without a causal link among the three and well beyond the linking element of infectious disease. For example, it is clear that current issues of antibiotic resistance in many cases have their origin in direct misuse in treating animals or as a consequence of antibiotics' use as growth promoters in the intensive livestock industries. More broadly, issues of food safety have as much to do with managing food production on the farm as with product preparation postfarm. In this context, of course, infectious disease poses a particular challenge in terms of the impact not just on food production on the farm but on the risks such diseases may pose to humans on the farm, during postfarm production, or through

[1]Geelong Centre for Emerging Infectious Diseases, Deakin University, Waurn Ponds Campus, Geelong, Victoria VIC 3220, Australia; [2]Curtin University, Perth, Western Australia WA 6012, Australia, and Burnet Institute, Melbourne, Victoria VIC 3004, Australia.

the final product (6). To fully and effectively address the issues, it is necessary for practitioners of a number of disciplines (veterinarians, livestock producers, product processors, and producers) to work together in ways that have not occurred in the past.

One Health was first conceptualized in the modern era by the physician Rudolf Virchow in the late 19th century—a time during which Pasteur and Koch were pioneering the field of microbiology (7). Virchow stated that "between animal and human medicine there are no dividing lines—nor should there be" (Virchow was also the first to use the term "zoonosis"), but it was not until recently that this concept has begun to be fully appreciated. In the 1960s, Calvin Schwabe coined the term "One Medicine," which brought the same concept to veterinarians (7). However, it is only during the past decade that there has been a concerted effort to explore and develop the One Health approach with respect to understanding and responding to infectious diseases at the animal-human-environment interfaces, and especially their evolution and transmission (also referred to as One Medicine and One World, One Health at various times).

Today we recognize this fundamental link between human, domestic animal, and wildlife health and the environment and the threat disease poses to people, their food supplies, and their economies. In today's globalized world, no one sector of society or single professional discipline has sufficient knowledge or resources to effectively manage risks of emergence or resurgence of infectious diseases. No one nation could reverse the patterns of habitat loss and extinction that undermine the health of the world's people and animals. Only by breaking down the barriers between agencies, individuals, specialties, and sectors can we utilize the collective expertise and spark the innovation needed to anticipate and combat such challenges to the health of people, domestic animals, and wildlife and to the integrity of ecosystems. We cannot manage today's threats of EIDs and tomorrow's problems of new pandemics and ineffective antibiotics with yesterday's solutions. Instead, there must be an adaptive, forward-looking, and multidisciplinary approach to the challenges that lie ahead, i.e., a One Health approach.

The meaning of One Health is perhaps most eloquently described by the Manhattan Principles developed in 2004 at the Wildlife Conservation Society's meeting on "One World, One Health: Building Interdisciplinary Bridges to Health in a Globalized World" (Table 1). The One Health concept represents a global paradigm shift in the "way we do business." It encourages collaboration and cooperation among clinicians, veterinarians, dentists, and other scientific-health and environmentally related disciplines. (See http://www.onehealthinitiative.com for dialogue on the efforts to advance the One Health concept and the continuing efforts to remove bureaucratic impediments to cooperation across human, animal, and environmental health.)

Traditionally, human health has been managed for the most part separately from animal health, with environment placed in its own silo. The vast majority of countries have ministries of health as large government entities providing a range of public health and clinical services, including that of infectious disease management. Major human health facilities, such as hospitals, diagnostic laboratories, and research institutes, fall for the most part within the remit of these ministries and have distinct funding resources allocated to them. Animal health, on the other hand, which for many years was managed at the government level through ministries of agriculture, has now changed or is changing in most countries. Agriculture has become integrated into environmental management, including that of wildlife, with a focus on ecosystem development and sustainability.

Table 1. The Manhattan Principles defining One Health[a]

1. To recognize the link between human, domestic animal, and wildlife health and the threat disease poses to people, their food supplies and economies, and the biodiversity essential to maintaining the healthy environments and functioning ecosystems we all require
2. To recognize that decisions regarding land and water use have real implications for health. Alterations in the resilience of ecosystems and shifts in patterns of disease emergence and spread manifest themselves when we fail to recognize this relationship
3. To include wildlife health science as an essential component of global disease prevention, surveillance, monitoring, control, and mitigation
4. To recognize that human health programs can greatly contribute to conservation efforts
5. To devise adaptive, holistic, and forward-looking approaches to the prevention, surveillance, monitoring, control, and mitigation of emerging and resurging diseases that fully account for the complex interconnections among species
6. To seek opportunities to fully integrate biodiversity conservation perspectives and human needs (including those related to domestic animal health) when developing solutions to infectious disease threats
7. To reduce demand for and better regulate the international live wildlife and bush meat trade, not only to protect wildlife populations but to lessen the risks of disease movement, cross-species transmission, and the development of novel pathogen-host relationships. The costs of this worldwide trade in terms of impacts on public health, agriculture, and conservation are enormous, and the global community must address this trade as the real threat it is to global socioeconomic security
8. To restrict the mass culling of free-ranging wildlife species for disease control to situations where there is a multidisciplinary, international scientific consensus that a wildlife population poses an urgent, significant threat to human health, food security, or wildlife health more broadly
9. To increase investment in the global human and animal health infrastructure commensurate with the serious nature of emerging and resurging disease threats to people, domestic animals, and wildlife. Enhanced capacity for global human and animal health surveillance and for clear, timely information sharing (that takes language barriers into account) can only help improve coordination of responses among governmental and nongovernmental agencies, public and animal health institutions, vaccine/pharmaceutical manufacturers, and other stakeholders
10. To form collaborative relationships among governments, local people, and the private and public (i.e., nonprofit) sectors to meet the challenges of global health and biodiversity conservation
11. To provide adequate resources and support for global wildlife health surveillance networks that exchange disease information with the public health and agricultural animal health communities as part of early warning systems for the emergence and resurgence of disease threats
12. To invest in educating and raising awareness among the world's people and in influencing the policy process to increase recognition that we must better understand the relationships between health and ecosystem integrity to succeed in improving prospects for a healthier planet

[a]From APEC 2011 (28).

Thus, livestock and agriculture in general are decreasing priority areas for governments, with environmental management becoming significantly more important.

THE ROLE OF INFECTIOUS DISEASE AS A COMPONENT OF ONE HEALTH

Infectious disease has a pivotal role in One Health. Global health security, particularly the emergence and spread of epidemic-prone EIDs, has become a major international concern, not least because of the significant economic impact of outbreaks (Table 2). The term "EID" has become synonymous with new (newly recognized, previously unknown) infectious diseases (such as SARS, which appeared suddenly and unexpectedly in 2003) or with known infections that are increasing in incidence, increasing in geographic scope

Table 2. Economic costs of recent disease outbreaks[a]

Disease	Economic impact
SARS (2003)	Cost to East Asia in excess of US$40 billion
	Global cost approximately US$60 billion
Avian influenza	Direct economic cost currently more than US$20 billion
Nipah (1999)	Cost to Malaysia estimated to be US$500 million
BSE	Cost to the United Kingdom estimated to be US$7.5 billion
Bluetongue virus	France (2007): US$1.4 billion
	The Netherlands: US$85 million
	United States: US$130 million annually
Foot-and-mouth disease (2001)	United Kingdom: US$355 billion
Equine influenza	Australia (2007): A$1 billion

[a]1st International One Health Congress, Melbourne, Australia (24).

(such as the dengue viruses causing dengue fever and dengue hemorrhagic fever), or expanding their host range (such as H5N1 avian influenza). Evidence clearly indicates an increase in the risks from EIDs to humans, to animals, and to the environment. The vast majority of such diseases are transboundary in nature (not respecting state or national borders) and require both national and international approaches for their effective management (8).

The risks from food contaminated with pathogenic microorganisms have been known for many years, and the early approaches dealt with managing these post-farm gate. By applying detection processes for infectious agents as well as chemical contamination linked to food production processes, these risks were seen to have been managed. However, the increasing impact of food-borne pathogens such as *Escherichia coli* or *Salmonella* spp. along with the risk management challenges posed by BSE have led to a whole-of-production-chain approach. Appreciating the risks of these food-borne pathogens to humans and the need to manage them in the animals (or plants) has, by definition, required a One Health approach. In one particular instance, that of antibiotic resistance, it has created more polarization rather than unity. For a number of years, considerable debate took place between human and animal health experts as to the underlying cause of the growing microbial resistance. Driven by the significant value of antibiotics as growth promoters in intensive livestock production systems, it took time for the underlying issues to be recognized. Had a One Health attitude been around at this time, the problem could well have been addressed much earlier.

Many factors (mostly associated with human activities) contribute to disease emergence. Such factors include increased travel and movement of people (particularly by air), increased international trade in live animals and fresh animal products, changes in land use and agricultural production, new developments in technology that provide greater sensitivity in detecting novel diseases, and the spread of exotic vectors to colonize new habitats and thus make new areas receptive to the spread of exotic infections. The greatest challenges for the 21st century may well be climate change, which will have effects on disease patterns and disease emergence as yet uncharacterized, through its effects on the ecology of hosts, vectors, and pathogens (9); and the need to provide food and safe water to an ever increasing world population.

Three important factors in disease emergence have been recognized over the past 2 decades.

1. With the enormous increases in air travel, the world has really become a vast global village with the potential for rapid intercontinental disease transmission.
2. The consequences of climate change include severe ecological disturbance with attendant movements of, and changed relationships between, people, wildlife, and disease vectors.
3. Most novel emerging diseases are zoonotic and originate in wildlife or domestic animals.

These factors have led to recognition that the most effective way to detect and respond to EIDs is through a One Health approach. One Health as a concept for managing the risks from infectious disease has gained wide acceptance in the United States, the European Community, and the World Health Organization (WHO). It recognized that effective global surveillance is essential for the early detection of EIDs, and that this can best be achieved on a global basis by an alliance of the networks established by the WHO, the Food and Agriculture Organization (FAO), and the World Organisation for Animal Health (Office International des Épizooties, or OIE), which provide early detection of and enable early response to EIDs (10). Nevertheless, there is still a major gap in global surveillance, and that is the surveillance of wildlife diseases; nowhere is this carried out with any depth or detail, and most outbreaks in wildlife are only recognized by occasional widespread die-offs.

This early alliance of international organizations (FAO, OIE, WHO, World Bank, United Nations System Influenza Coordination [UNSIC]], United Nations Children's Fund [UNICEF], and the European Union) has continued to interact to further develop the One Health concept. At the national level, a number of countries have undertaken detailed studies to better understand and develop more effective response processes to EIDs. As an example, to help to define EID threats to Australia, an expert working group of the Australian Prime Minister's Science, Engineering and Innovation Council (PMSEIC) on the topic of epidemics was established in April 2009 and reported in June 2009 (11). This report concluded that "it is a matter of when, not if, a lethally catastrophic epidemic will happen." The report recommended that "the Government establish cross-portfolio arrangements essential for effective implementation" of its recommendations "as a matter of immediate priority" (11).

The specific recommendations to which this conclusion referred were:

1. To underpin preparedness to deal with EIDs, that Australia should possess the human capacity to deal with such epidemics
2. To provide early warning of the emergence of EIDs, that Australia should possess a long-term biosecurity information collection, analysis, and interpretation capability

    3. To enhance the wider ability to deal with EIDs, that Australia should develop forward regional engagement to mitigate potential epidemics

Many countries have now embarked on managing the risks from EIDs through a One Health approach (e.g., the United States, Canada, the United Kingdom, Denmark, India, Laos, Cambodia, Mongolia, Philippines, and Thailand), but the approach varies enormously and the level of commitment within national entities is highly variable (12). Examples of One Health approaches for combating infectious diseases include the recent management of the risks from Hendra virus (13) and avian influenza (14), responses to canine rabies (15), and the management of the West Nile virus outbreak in the United States (16). The Australian response to Hendra virus shows the advantages of taking a One Health approach and is included here in more detail as it illustrates some important aspects of what One Health entails (13).

Hendra is a relatively rare viral disease of horses and humans first identified in 1994 when it caused the deaths of 13 horses and a trainer at a training complex in Hendra, a suburb of Brisbane in Queensland, Australia. The causative agent, Hendra virus, is a novel, previously unrecognized virus belonging to a new genus, *Henipavirus*, in the family *Paramyxoviridae*. Since 1994, outbreaks have occurred annually in Australia (most frequently in animals and seven cases in humans, four of which had a fatal outcome [case mortality of 60%]). All cases in horses have been associated with close contact with a flying fox colony, while all cases in humans link to close contact with clinically infected horses, and there is no evidence of direct bat-to-human transmission.

Since the first occurrence of Hendra in Australia, a program of research has been undertaken. The work on the virus has primarily involved virologists and epidemiologists and has focused on fully characterizing the virus and understanding infection and replication in host cells. The work in bats has involved bat carers, wildlife ecologists, immunologists, epidemiologists, and veterinarians and has included studies on the distribution and translocation of various flying fox species as well as more detailed studies on the bat's immune system. Studies of the disease in horses have involved veterinarians, virologists, pathologists, epidemiologists, and immunologists. Studies of how to manage the disease risk to humans have involved infectious disease clinicians, public health physicians, immunologists, general hospital staff, sociologists, and communication experts. Much effort has concentrated on how to convey the messages on the appropriate biosecurity precautions both to horse owners and to veterinary clinicians treating sick horses. In response to the significant cluster of cases in June and July 2011, a Hendra taskforce was established to identify appropriate risk management strategies in the affected states and ensure a coordinated and effective response. The taskforce activities included identification and resourcing of additional research activities to assist risk mitigation and decision making for Hendra management. Hendra is a perfect example of a disease moving from a nidus in wildlife into a livestock species and subsequently causing infection and disease in humans. It is clear that to effectively understand the disease and develop mitigation strategies, the full range of One Health skills and knowledge is required. Bringing these together and developing a viable approach to managing the risk proved crucial in identifying that farm biosecurity measures, linked to an effective horse vaccine, were viable and workable approaches. An understanding of bat ecology proved crucial in dispelling concepts of bat destruction or dispersal, and an appreciation of the timelines for developing a Hendra vaccine for humans negated the value of this in the short term. But these synergies of understanding and knowledge only occurred with some effort in breaking down cultures, removing silos, and sharing resources and results. Viable solutions have been found for managing the current risks of Hendra to both horses and humans without destruction of bats and the contribution they make to the ecosystem. None of this would have been possible without a shared One Health approach.

Over and above this are the political issues that are addressed in utilizing a One Health approach. Hendra gained significant coverage in the press, leading to further community concern and a greater interest by government. Importantly, this interest involved concerns around bats, the risk to horses, and of course, the risk to humans. At the government level, this involved departments managing the environment, agriculture and livestock, and human health. The creation of the Hendra taskforce from all three areas of government, the development of a single set of messages, and the utilization of skills and knowledge from across all sectors was vital in managing the political as well as technical risks. The fact that the premier of Queensland established the taskforce, with direct accountability to her; the fact that it included representatives from both the New South Wales and Commonwealth governments; and the broad nature of the members of the taskforce were essential in addressing community concerns and demonstrating a "whole of government" response. In the context of this Hendra outbreak, the taskforce has spent valuable time in determining its role, its reporting lines, its ability to access and manage resources, and its overall status. Had such a One Health body been in place, time and effort could have been saved, and more importantly, some of the underlying issues may well have been tackled in a "peacetime" scenario.

EVOLUTION OF THE ONE HEALTH CONCEPT

A key driver for the development of a One Health approach has been the international response to the global threat of an avian influenza pandemic caused by highly pathogenic influenza A virus H5N1 (HPAI H5N1) and the risks and fears such a pandemic would pose to human health. There was a recognized need for a sustained, cross-sectoral approach to policy development and coordination to deal with the serious threats that arise at the animal-human-environment interfaces. A series of International Ministerial Conferences on Avian and Pandemic Influenza (IMCAPI) were held to discuss issues relating to the spread, transmission, and possible containment of HPAI under the auspices of the FAO, the OIE, the WHO, UNSIC, UNICEF, the World Bank, and various other international and national agencies. This One Health approach was addressed by IMCAPI in New Delhi, India, in 2007 and by a conference held in Sharm el-Sheikh, Egypt, in October 2008. The latter developed the "Strategic Framework for Reducing Risks of Infectious Diseases at the Animal-Human-Ecosystems Interface," which clearly spelled out the importance and need for a holistic One Health approach in responding to HPAI. A joint agreement among FAO, OIE, and WHO, "The FAO-OIE-WHO Collaboration: Sharing Responsibilities and Coordinating Global Activities at the Animal-Human-Ecosystems Interfaces," underpins the continued development of an internationally integrated global One Health approach (17).

A number of international and national organizations have also been proactive in supporting the development of One Health approaches to pandemic and emerging zoonotic disease threats. The World Bank, which had through a number of initiatives already supported the One Health concept, turned this into real action in the avian and human influenza arena through its own report *People, Pathogens, and Our Planet* (18). Similarly, the European Community has been active, especially in the Asian area, through the European External Action Service's Asia and Pacific Department. Many individual nations have also been developing their own specific action plans and coordinated approaches, as exemplified in the African continent by the Southern African Centre for Infectious Disease Surveillance (SACIDS) One Health Virtual Centre Model (19) and in the Asian and Western Pacific regions by activities in Mongolia and elsewhere (20–22). France also encourages an integrated, intersectoral, and interdisciplinary approach to One Health and has developed a detailed national One Health strategy (23).

In the United States, a One Health Commission was established with strong initial leadership from the American Veterinary Medical Association and included a number of professional partners including the American Public Health Association and the Infectious Diseases Society of America (https://www.onehealthcommission.org/). The American Society for Microbiology has also embraced the One Health concept and organized several sessions at its annual meeting and those of the American Association for the Advancement of Science to conduct further dialogue about One Health. The 1st International One Health Congress was held in Melbourne, Australia, in February 2011 (24). This meeting provided a forum for scientific discourse on the impact of disease on humans, animals, and the environment. The congress generated a series of important One Health principles and concepts (Table 3).

The Public Health Agency of Canada hosted a consultative meeting on "One World, One Health: from Ideas to Action" in Winnipeg, Manitoba, in March 2009 to develop a series of actions that could be implemented at the national level. The partners included the WHO, FAO, OIE, and other national and international agencies. It concluded that the development of the animal-human-ecosystem aspects of One Health needed a continuing commitment at all levels—international, national, regional, and community—to be successful. A second meeting was held in 2010 in Stone Mountain, GA, and hosted locally by the U.S. Centers for Disease Control and Prevention (CDC) and international partners to discuss the future steps needed to "operationalize" One Health, and was entitled "A Policy Perspective—Taking Stock and Shaping an Implementation Roadmap" (25). A major outcome of the Stone Mountain workshop has been the development of a Web-based One Health Global Network (www.onehealthglobal.net) for

Table 3. One Health concepts and principles[a]

1. There is interdependence between human, animal, and environmental health and a need to improve dialogue.
2. Communication, collaboration, and trust between human and animal health practitioners is a key element to successfully developing a One Health strategy.
3. One Health extends to food safety and food security, economics, and social behavior.
4. There is a need to promote the "doable," such as improving EID surveillance and response.
5. There is a need to ensure community participation and an open, broad-based dialogue.
6. Both "ground-up" and "top-down" action is necessary for the advancement of One Health.

[a]APEC 2011 (28).

disseminating information and providing a useful resource site supporting One Health activities.

An essential aspect of One Health development is the need to improve the education of all professionals—veterinarians, medical practitioners, biomedical scientists, wildlife biologists, and other interested groups—to better understand the need for a One Health approach through communication and cooperation across the disciplines, whether it is responding to known or novel zoonotic diseases or detecting and tracking the origins of antibiotic resistance (26, 27). Edinburgh University has initiated a One Health masters postgraduate course (http://www.ed.ac.uk/schools-departments/vet/news-events/news/january2011), and special One Health masters courses for students in the Asia-Pacific region are being established with World Bank support through Massey University in New Zealand (19). In addition, a One Health Institute has been established at the University of California at Davis. The most important and sustainable training developments will be generational as both medical and veterinary programs begin to introduce One Health concepts into their undergraduate and postgraduate degree courses, but the effects of this may not be visible until future clinicians and veterinarians enter their respective professional careers.

DEVELOPMENT OF ONE HEALTH IN ASIAN-PACIFIC COUNTRIES

It is instructive to explore how the Asian-Pacific countries are incorporating a One Health approach into their public health planning. One of the best examples has been that developed by the Asia-Pacific Economic Cooperation (APEC) members, many of which have strong and effective One Health programs in place. From a regional perspective, in 2011 the APEC One Health Action Plan (20) provided a framework to assist APEC economies in strengthening cross-sectoral networks and functioning against the threat of emerging and zoonotic infectious diseases. The plan communicated the current situation in APEC member economies, a common One Health vision and mission (purpose), and six important goals each with a set of actions that can be adopted by member economies to move toward that goal (Table 4). It strongly encouraged a commitment by APEC member economies to progressing implementation of One Health approaches by adopting those actions that are suited to their current capacities and level of One Health engagement. The overall mission is for APEC economies to reduce the risks and impacts of emerging and zoonotic infectious diseases by applying coordinated, collaborative, multidisciplinary, and cross-sectoral approaches at the animal-human-ecosystem

Table 4. One Health goals for Asian-Pacific countries

1. To strengthen cross-sectoral political commitment and government leadership for One Health approaches to emerging and zoonotic infectious disease
2. To strengthen cross-sectoral coordination and collaboration in disease prevention, investigation, response, and control in APEC member economies
3. To increase community awareness and participation in disease prevention and control
4. To incorporate One Health approaches in vocational and university education and training, and expand field-based training in disease prevention, investigation, and control
5. To strengthen international and multilateral cooperation in progressing One Health approaches
6. To ensure that resources are sustainably and efficiently applied in implementing One Health approaches

interface. The APEC goals and associated actions perhaps most clearly define One Health and the underpinning actions that are needed (28).

In the context of political commitment and government leadership, the application of One Health currently varies depending on national economies and between agencies within countries. This is driven by issues of competing priorities, communication between disciplines, and divergences in professional cultures. To be able to compete with these other priorities, the added value of One Health action needs to be demonstrated and communicated widely. This is an ongoing challenge, given that political action is often driven by the need to respond to immediate emergencies and disasters. While a practical commitment to One Health is more common at technical levels, support for One Health approaches at senior government and political levels needs to be strengthened. This will require strengthened cross-sectoral political commitment and government leadership for One Health approaches to emerging and zoonotic infectious disease.

A variety of approaches to cross-sectoral collaboration and coordination are being used in APEC economies. Some economies have formal collaboration agreements for emergencies or for specific diseases such as avian influenza and rabies. In addition, some economies have established One Health units to drive cross-sectoral coordination and collaboration; others have limited or no arrangements in place. The existing focus is generally on improving EID investigation, control, and response, particularly in emergency situations. However, One Health approaches need to be extended to focus on preventing disease emergence, improving ecosystem health, and encouraging collaboration and coordination at all levels. Increased engagement and participation in One Health is required by all, including by universities, businesses, and nongovernment organizations.

In many APEC member economies, disease prevention and control is hampered by lack of essential resources, research, and development to support the prevention and control of EIDs. There is limited application of One Health approaches and a lack of experience in working across disciplines, and in many economies there are shortages of capacity and expertise in relevant disciplines. There also exists minimal capacity for social and economic research and delays or restrictions in sharing research prior to publication. To improve the ability to control the spread of infectious diseases across transnational boundaries, it will be necessary to strengthen cross-sectoral coordination and collaboration in disease prevention, investigation, response, and control in APEC member economies.

Public awareness and participation in disease prevention and control at community levels varies across APEC economies. A number of economies with a limited public health and animal health workforce rely on village animal health and public health workers for implementing disease prevention and control programs. A high-priority need is to strengthen communication and training for workers within communities and for cross-sectoral coordination for the delivery of training. The One Health concept is new to some sections of the public and the media; therefore, effective approaches for engaging with communities and the media need to be identified and shared among APEC economies. Increasing community awareness and participation will help in disease prevention and control.

One Health approaches are beginning to be adopted in universities, and the most notable success has been seen in the field epidemiology training program (FETP). There is generally greater adoption of One Health approaches at the postgraduate level than at the undergraduate and vocational training levels. There is significant potential for promoting One Health approaches through vocational training and undergraduate and postgraduate university education, such as the FETP. Issues to be addressed include determining the number of trainers and mentors required, balancing the demand and supply of graduates, and recognizing the need for opportunities in One Health that support career paths. APEC member economies have variable capacity for delivering education and training. Decisions about investment in emerging and zoonotic infectious disease training programs need to be based on strategic assessment of needs and capacities. APEC economies recognize the importance of learning by doing and the FETP's role in building workforce capacity in human, animal, and ecosystem health. Many economies are implementing FETP in public health, and some training is being undertaken to include veterinarians and wildlife health professionals. However, while there is willingness to adopt FETP in member economies, this is accompanied by a shortage of trainers (particularly epidemiologists) and resources for training. More needs to be done to incorporate One Health approaches in vocational and university education and training and to expand field-based training in disease prevention, investigation, and control.

Fragmentation in planning and implementation of One Health approaches exists at all levels, as the meaning of One Health can apply differently to different member economies. There are also competing priorities among international organizations and member economies. Roles and relationships among APEC member economies also vary in relation to international organizations; for example, some members are donors while others are recipients. Several international organizations such as the WHO, OIE, and FAO are collaborating on the global development of One Health approaches, but strengthening international and multilateral cooperation is critical for progressing One Health approaches is this area.

There is variable capacity for disease prevention, preparedness, and response in and among APEC economies, and there is a need to build capacities across sectors for disease prevention, preparedness, and response. This requires new, cooperative ways of working, including the development of cost-sharing arrangements that lead to more efficient application of resources. There are high costs and consequences for APEC member economies in responding to (rather than preventing) emerging and zoonotic infectious disease incursions and outbreaks. Current systems traditionally focus on responding to emergencies, and the cost and risk to economies of this approach are likely to become unsustainable. There is a need for all APEC members to focus more on priorities for disease prevention and control. One Health approaches require cross-sectoral collaboration, and a major challenge is to develop formal processes for more than one agency to accept joint responsibility for One Health investment, outcomes, and deliverables.

CONCLUDING REMARKS

At the international level, various meetings are being held in low- and middle-income countries under the One Health banner, sponsored and supported by the United Nations agencies (FAO, WHO, and OIE), the European Union, the U.S. Agency for International

Development, and individual countries. For the most part, while these are focused on building capacity to detect and manage zoonotic EIDs, they also strive to bring together animal and human health agencies to foster a collaborative approach in which improved communication and recognition of the roles each can play have been crucial. In Asia, this has been particularly successful and created real change at the national level in a number of countries. There is little doubt that to enable the One Health concept and benefits to be better understood and the current silos to be finally broken down, there need to be improvements in global education at all levels but especially through changes to the curricula for medical and veterinary students. It is also important to stress that the One Health concept is, in reality, a fundamental change in how we do business—the dialogue is an open dialogue and it is inappropriate to discuss terms such as "management" or "governance," or indeed "coordination." Many countries around the globe have now established their own One Health activities, and the tools and support to maintain and sustain these activities are now required.

Acknowledgments. The authors have no conflicts of interest in this manuscript.

Citation. Jeggo M, Mackenzie JS. 2014. Defining the future of One Health. Microbiol Spectrum 2(1):OH-0007-2012. doi:10.1128/microbiolspec.OH-0007-2012.

REFERENCES

1. **Woolhouse ME, Gowtage-Sequeria S.** 2005. Host range and emerging and reemerging pathogens. *Emerg Infect Dis* **11:**1842–1847.
2. **Wolfe ND, Dunavan CP, Diamond J.** 2007. Origins of major human infectious diseases. *Nature* **447:**279–283.
3. **Shaw AM.** 2009. Economics of zoonosis and their control, p 161–167. *In* Rushton J (ed), *The Economics of Animal Health and Production.* CABI, Wallingford, United Kingdom.
4. **Cutler SJ, Fook AR, van der Poel WH.** 2010. Public health threat of new, reemerging, and neglected zoonoses in the industrialized world. *Emerg Infect Dis* **16:**1–7.
5. **Cascio A, Bosilkovski M, Rodriguez-Morales AJ, Pappas G.** 2011. The socio-ecology of zoonotic infections. *Clin Microbiol Infect* **17:**336–342.
6. **de Haan C, Van Veen TS, Brandenburg B, Gauthier J, Le Gall F.** 2001. *Livestock Development: Implications for Rural Poverty, the Environment, and Global Food Security.* World Bank, Washington, DC.
7. **Atlas RM.** 2012. One Health: its origins and future. *Curr Top Microbiol Immunol* [Epub ahead of print.] PMID: 22527177.
8. **Jones KE, Patel NG, Levy MA, Storeygard A, Balk D, Gittleman JL, Daszak P.** 2008. Global trends in emerging infectious diseases. *Nature* **451:**990–993.
9. **Rosenthal J.** 2009. Climate change and the geographical distribution of infectious diseases. *EcoHealth* **6:**489–495.
10. **Vallat B.** 2009. One World, One Health (editorial), p 1–2. *OIE Bulletin* no. 2. OIE (World Organisation for Animal Health), Paris, France. http://www.oie.int/fileadmin/Home/eng/Publications_%26_Documentation/docs/pdf/bulletin/Bull_2009-2-ENG.pdf (last accessed August 19, 2013).
11. **Prime Minister's Science, Engineering and Innovation Council (PMSEIC).** 2009. *Epidemics in a Changing World: Report of the Expert Working Group on Epidemics in a Changing World.* PMSEIC, Canberra, New South Wales, Australia. http://www.innovation.gov.au/Science/PMSEIC/Documents/EpidemicsinaChangingWorld.pdf (last accessed August 19, 2013).
12. **Leboeuf A.** 2011. *Making Sense of One Health: Cooperating at the Human-Animal-Ecosystem Health Interface.* Health and Environment Report no. 7. Institut Français des Relations Internationales, Paris, France. www.ifri.org/downloads/ifrihereport7alineleboeuf.pdf (last accessed August 19, 2013).
13. **Wang LF, Mackenzie JS, Broder CC.** 2013. Henipaviruses, p 286–313. *In* Knipe DM, Howley PM (ed), *Fields Virology,* 6th ed. Lippincott Williams & Wilkins, Philadelphia, PA.

14. **Leong HK, Goh CS, Chew ST, Lim CW, Lin YN, Chang SF, Yap HH, Chua SB.** 2008. Prevention and control of avian influenza in Singapore. *Ann Acad Med Singapore* **37:**504–509.

15. **Drew WL.** 2004. Rabies, p 597–600. *In* Ryan KJ, Ray CG (ed), *Sherris Medical Microbiology*, 4th ed. McGraw-Hill, New York, NY.

16. **Hayes EB, Gubler DJ.** 2006. West Nile virus: epidemiology and clinical features of an emerging epidemic in the United States. *Annu Rev Med* **57:**181–194.

17. **International Ministerial Conference on Animal and Pandemic Influenza.** 2010. *Hanoi Declaration. Animal and pandemic influenza: the way forward*, Hanoi, Vietnam, 19-21 April 2010. International Ministerial Conference on Animal and Pandemic Influenza. http://www.unicef.org/influenzaresources/files/Hanoi_Declaration_21April_IMCAPI_Hanoi_2010.pdf (last accessed August 19, 2013).

18. **World Bank.** 2010. *People, Pathogens, and Our Planet: Volume One—Towards a One Health Approach for Controlling Zoonotic Diseases.* World Bank, Washington, DC. https://openknowledge.worldbank.org/handle/10986/2844 (last accessed June 5, 2013).

19. **Rweyemamu M, Kambarage D, Karimuribo E, Wambura P, Matee M, Kayembe JM, Mweene A, Neves L, Masumu J, Kasanga C, Hang'ombe B, Kayunze K, Misinzo G, Simuunza M, Paweska JT.** 2012. Development of a One Health national capacity in Africa: the Southern African Centre for Infectious Disease Surveillance (SACIDS) One Health Virtual Centre Model. *Curr Top Microbiol Immunol* [Epub ahead of print.] doi:10.1007/82_2012_244.

20. **Gongal G.** 2012. One Health approach in the South East Asia region: opportunities and challenges. *Curr Top Microbiol Immunol* [Epub ahead of print.] doi:10.1007/82_2012_242.

21. **Batsukh Z, Tsolmon B, Otgonbaatar D, Undraa B, Dolgorkhand A, Ariuntuya O.** 2012. One Health in Mongolia. *Curr Top Microbiol Immunol* [Epub ahead of print.] doi:10.1007/82_2012_253.

22. **Coughlan B, Hall D.** 2012. The development of One Health approaches in the Western Pacific. *Curr Top Microbiol Immunol* [Epub ahead of print.] doi:10.1007/82_2012_270.

23. **French Ministry of Foreign and European Affairs.** 2011. *Position française sur le concept "One Health/Une seule santé": pour une approche intégrée de la santé face à la mondialisation des risques sanitaires. Strategic working document.* Ministry of Foreign and European Affairs, Paris, France. http://www.diplomatie.gouv.fr/fr/IMG/pdf/Rapport_One_Health.pdf (last accessed August 19, 2013).

24. **Mackenzie JS, Jeggo MH.** 2011. 1st International One Health Congress (editorial). *EcoHealth* **7:**S1–S2.

25. **One Health Global Network.** 2011. *Expert meeting on One Health Governance and Global Network. Stone Mountain One Health Conference USA. Atlanta report 2011.* One Health Global Network. http://eeas.europa.eu/health/docs/2011_report-experts-atlanta_en.pdf (last accessed August 19, 2013).

26. **Chatham House.** 2010. *Meeting report. Shifting from emergency response to prevention of pandemic disease threats at source.* Chatham House, London, United Kingdom. http://www.chathamhouse.org/sites/default/files/public/Research/Energy,%20Environment%20and%20Development/0410mtg_report.pdf (last accessed August 19, 2013).

27. **Vink WD, McKenzie JS, Cogger N, Muellner P, Boreman B.** 2013. Building a foundation for "One Health": an education strategy for enhancing and sustaining national and regional capacity in endemic and emerging zoonotic disease management. *Curr Top Microbiol Immunol* **366:**in press.

28. **Asia-Pacific Economic Cooperation (APEC).** 2011. *APEC One Health Action Plan.* APEC, Singapore.

One Health: People, Animals, and the Environment
Edited by Ronald M. Atlas and Stanley Maloy
© 2014 American Society for Microbiology, Washington, DC
doi:10.1128/microbiolspec.OH-0016-2012

Chapter 18

Making One Health a Reality—
Crossing Bureaucratic Boundaries

Carol Rubin,[1] Bernadette Dunham,[2] and Jonathan Sleeman[3]

INTRODUCTION

A One Health approach that achieves optimal outcomes requires that nontraditional partners come to a common table to identify solutions that transcend organization-specific mandates. This collaboration requires individuals to go beyond their accustomed comfort zones and function on teams with partners who very likely come from unfamiliar organizational, disciplinary, and even national cultures. Each participant represents a separate mandate and an individual corporate culture and values, and each potentially communicates in agency-specific or industry-prescribed cultural terms that may be foreign to the rest of the team. A recent review paper reports that such interdisciplinary teams are most likely to succeed when they have a unified task and a shared goal and values, and when personal relationships are developed from a foundation of trust and respect (1).

Often, external or imposed forces can actually increase the likelihood of cross-agency collaboration. For example, a One Health approach is more likely to be successful when human, animal, and environmental health entities face a common imminent threat, such as occurred during the 2003 emergence of highly pathogenic avian influenza (HPAI) H5N1. When federal (or other) funding is sufficient and specific enough—as occurred with surveillance for food-borne diseases—interagency activities are likewise streamlined. Sometimes the successful alliances built during periods of imposed necessity form the foundation for trusting relationships that increase the likelihood that subsequent One Health collaborations or alliances will be more easily assembled. However, cross-agency One Health collaborations that are not well focused or compelled by an external exigency are likely to face hurdles that make trust and communication more difficult, especially when fiscal resources are limited and inequitably distributed among agencies and there is a lack of common cause.

Nonetheless, it is not difficult to identify actual cases of cross-sectoral working alliances that reached across bureaucratic boundaries to implement a One Health approach, and thus engendered outcomes of value to all stakeholders.

---

[1]National Center for Emerging and Zoonotic Infectious Diseases, Centers for Disease Control and Prevention, Atlanta, GA 30333; [2]Center for Veterinary Medicine, U.S. Food and Drug Administration, Rockville, MD 20855; [3]National Wildlife Health Center, U.S. Geological Survey, Madison, WI 53711.

CASE STUDY 1: 2003 OUTBREAK OF HPAI H5N1

Background

Beginning in the spring and continuing into the fall of 1997, 18 people in Hong Kong were diagnosed with HPAI H5N1, a newly emerged influenza A virus; 6 of these people died. At the same time, H5N1 was diagnosed in poultry and many of the infected humans were reported to have had contact with sick birds. Although at this early stage transmission appeared to occur from birds to humans rather than from one human to another, the rapid emergence and unusual severity of the disease raised the ominous prospect that the HPAI H5N1 virus could spread globally and cause a pandemic similar to the 1918 "Great Influenza." Concern was intensified because the origin of the infection and exact mode(s) of transmission were unknown (2).

The outbreak was halted by the slaughter of more than 1.5 million chickens at the end of December 1997, along with a ban on the importation of live poultry from mainland China, the only source of live poultry for Hong Kong (3). However, the virus reemerged in Hong Kong in 2003 and since then has spread globally, leading to more than 610 cases and 360 human deaths (4). The threat of human-to-human transmission provoked intense concern and response within the human health community (5). The 2003 outbreaks forced the culling of at least 400 million domestic poultry worldwide. This widespread culling decreased the availability of protein sources, eliminated the livelihood of small farmers, and had a negative impact on poultry export. Ultimately, H5N1 caused an estimated $20 billion in economic damage (6).

Multisectoral Response

Human health and animal health agencies, in-country and globally, were affected by the appearance of HPAI H5N1. Successful response to this pandemic threat demanded international and multiagency response, and fortunately, donor funding was supportive of such collaboration (7). Examples of One Health collaborations established during this crisis included:

- *Coordinated global surveillance.* The Global Early Warning System (GLEWS) is a tripartite undertaking (8). It is an enhanced surveillance and reporting system that builds on existing capabilities of the World Organisation for Animal Health (Office International des Épizooties, or OIE), the United Nations Food and Agriculture Organization (FAO), and the World Health Organization (WHO). Although H5N1 was the tipping point that fostered establishing GLEWS, the system serves a broader, enduring function as it links the international community and stakeholders to assist in prediction, prevention, and control of animal disease threats, including zoonoses. It accomplishes this mission through sharing of information, epidemiological analysis, and joint risk assessment.
- *Coordinated research.* Both the U.S. Centers for Disease Control and Prevention (CDC) and National Institute of Allergy and Infectious Diseases (NIAID) provided research funding that required grantees to form coalitions that included public health and animal health, in order to more

closely examine transmission of H5N1 between animals and humans (9). The NIAID established five Centers of Excellence for Influenza Research and Surveillance (CEIRS). It initiated the CEIRS network as a result of recommendations from the NIAID Blue Ribbon Panel on Influenza Research and as one facet of the overarching Department of Health and Human Services (HHS) pandemic response and preparedness plan.

- *Coordinated response.* The Emergency Center for Transboundary Animal Diseases (ECTAD) was established in 2004 to complement existing FAO systems while strengthening response capabilities for H5N1 and similar emerging pathogens (10). Electronically distributed surveillance maps are promptly shared with human and animal health agencies.
- *New lines of communication.* To enhance effective communication and foster trusted relationships, the CDC has assigned personnel as liaisons to both the OIE and FAO. Although the U.S. Department of Agriculture (USDA) had embedded staff with both international organizations, the CDC assignees represented a new level of partnership with animal health organizations (10).

Case Study Summary

This case study example demonstrates that a One Health outcome is more likely when:

- Agencies with different mandates face an obvious and common external threat.
- International funding is adequate to expand existing systems and form new coordinated alliances.
- Entities are willing to support nontraditional staff secondments.

CASE STUDY 2: COORDINATED SURVEILLANCE TO DETECT AN EMERGING PANDEMIC THREAT

Background

Avian influenza (AI) refers to type A influenza viruses that are naturally found in certain species of waterfowl and shorebirds (11). Wild birds and the virus have become well adapted to each other over time, and infection does not usually cause overt disease in wild birds. AI viruses can be classified as highly pathogenic if they meet certain laboratory-defined criteria and may cause high mortality in domestic birds. Additionally, these viruses could undergo genetic shift and drift and potentially cause human pandemics, with profound and global consequences for human populations. In 2005, a highly pathogenic H5N1 AI virus was found in Asia and Europe (12). This discovery raised concerns regarding the potential impact on wild birds, domestic poultry, and human health—specifically, H5N1's potential introduction into the United States alarmed government health officials. Numerous potential routes for introduction of the virus into the United States were thought to exist, including illegal movement of infected domestic or wild birds, contaminated products, infected travelers, deliberately as a bioterrorism event, and the migration of infected wild birds (13). It was the last possibility that brought public health, agriculture, and wildlife management agencies together to address this urgent issue of mutual concern.

The highly pathogenic H5N1 AI virus first emerged during 1995-1996, when it infected chickens in China (12). Since that time the virus has continued to circulate in Asian poultry and domestic fowl, resulting in significant mortality in these species. The highly pathogenic H5N1 AI virus likely underwent further genetic shift and drift, allowing infection in additional species of domestic birds, mammals, and humans. It then remanifested in wild birds, resulting in significant mortality of several species in China during April 2005.

Coordinated Response

Although the spread of H5N1 AI in Asia had been primarily associated with domestic birds, the presence of this virus in migratory birds raised the possibility that these species could disperse the virus to geographically remote areas. This was thought to be the case in August 2005, when bar-headed geese and whooper swans died on Erkhel Lake, Mongolia, in an area not known to have domestic poultry nearby (14). Concern increased that migrating species could introduce the virus into previously uninfected regions of the world such as North America.

Therefore, at the request of the U.S. Homeland Security Council's Policy Coordinating Committee for Pandemic Influenza Preparedness, the USDA and U.S. Department of the Interior (DOI) were asked to develop a coordinated national strategic plan for early detection of HPAI virus introduced into North America by wild birds (15). To initiate this effort, the USDA Animal and Plant Health Inspection Services (APHIS) Wildlife Services and DOI U.S. Geological Survey (USGS) convened an interagency working group in the fall of 2005 consisting of representatives from the USDA, DOI, HHS, the International Association of Fish and Wildlife Agencies (IAFWA), and other agency and university partners involved in monitoring and managing wild bird populations. This group developed the Interagency Strategic Plan for the Early Detection of H5N1 Highly Pathogenic Avian Influenza in Wild Birds (USDA and DOI, 2006), which was signed by the secretaries of the DOI, USDA, and HHS in March 2006. To detect potential introduction of highly pathogenic H5N1 AI virus by migratory birds, the plan adopted a variety of surveillance techniques, including sampling of live-trapped and hunter-harvested birds as well as testing of wild bird mortality events. During the 6-year period of active surveillance, more than 450,000 birds or environmental samples were tested across the nation, representing one of the largest wildlife disease surveillance projects ever undertaken in North America (16).

This surveillance project represents an example of One Health in action, whereby agencies from different sectors worked together to agree upon and implement a course of action to address an urgent national issue. Factors that contributed to the success of this project included the sense of urgency among all partners and a common mission or purpose to address what was perceived at that time as a serious threat to public health, the economy, and natural resources. Furthermore, the directive from the Coordinating Committee for Pandemic Influenza Preparedness provided the authority to proceed with the work as well as the means to obtain the necessary funding. Thus, we conclude that to implement successful One Health projects, it helps to identify a common mission or purpose, a sense of importance or urgency of the task, agreed-upon core values, and ideally, funding and the authority to conduct the work.

An additional benefit of this AI surveillance was that it allowed diverse agencies to better understand one another's values, cultures, perspectives, and missions and helped build trust and forge common ground among them. These relationships have continued to bear fruit as many of these agencies are seeking ways to work together to conduct wildlife disease surveillance through the formation of a National Fish and Wildlife Health Network (17).

Case Study Summary

This case example demonstrates that a One Health outcome is more likely when:

- There is a sense of urgency and common purpose.
- There is the delegated authority or mandate to conduct the work.
- An interagency steering committee or working group is formed to oversee the work.

CASE STUDY 3: UNIFIED MESSAGING DURING 2009 PANDEMIC H1N1 RESPONSE

Background

In April 2009, several children with respiratory illness presented to health care providers who submitted nasal swabs for influenza testing. These children turned out to be the first reported cases of a newly emerged H1N1 influenza A virus (18). Unfortunately, the media and even scientific agencies quickly began referring to this emergent virus as "swine flu" (19). To a certain extent this moniker was logical because this virus was a unique combination of influenza virus genes never previously identified in either animals or people. Antigenic and genetic characteristics of this virus indicated that it was most closely related to North American swine-lineage H1N1 and Eurasian lineage swine-origin H1N1 influenza viruses (20). However, the term "swine flu" was confusing to many because at that point in time, there was absolutely no evidence that U.S. pigs, or even North American pigs, were infected with the new influenza virus.

The new virus spread rapidly among humans, and the WHO officially declared a pandemic (21). The U.S. public health response was vigorous and transparent, reflected by timely public reporting of human case counts at state and even county levels (18). Rather unexpectedly, some international pork trading partners elected to use the U.S. human case counts as a surrogate for infection among swine herds (22). Several countries that traditionally received U.S. pork products interpreted the human information as a reason to impose state-specific export bans of U.S. swine and pork products. Needless to say, this resulted in an immediate negative economic impact within the swine production community and for the U.S. economy in general. This situation demonstrates how the relationship between human public health and agricultural economic health can become unexpectedly intertwined.

Neither local or federal animal health agencies nor swine producer organizations require that swine influenza virus (SIV) be a reportable disease (23). Although the virus may cause mild clinical illness in animals, infection does not prevent recovered pigs from going to market (24).

The emergence of pandemic H1N1 (pH1N1) among humans inevitably led to some immediate casting of blame. Public health leaders questioned why the USDA was not aware of which SIVs were circulating, why university-based animal diagnostic labs were hesitant to share influenza viral isolates from pigs, and why swine exhibitions and fairs were being held during a human pandemic. At the same time, the animal health community continued to believe that SIV-infected pigs were not a threat to human health and that active surveillance for the virus in pigs and restrictions on exhibitions and sales would create unnecessary market losses. To further inflame this polarization, on August 25, 2009, the *Des Moines Register* carried a story that reported "CDC Selling H1N1 Plush Toys" in a CDC-based (albeit not CDC-controlled) gift shop. Unfortunately, the toy depicted the virus in the shape of a pig's snout (25).

Unified Messaging

The previous interagency collaboration for HPAI H5N1 preparedness (described in Case Study 1) had sown the seeds for a trusting, although tentative, relationship among key governmental leaders in relevant animal and human health communities. To their credit, individuals in the pH1N1 response on both sides built on the previous relationships and communicated honestly, while looking beyond their individual agency perspectives. Public health leaders continued to advocate the importance of sampling and identifying currently circulating SIV. Based on sound science performed by the USDA's National Veterinary Services Laboratories, they were also able to testify to the safety of humans consuming pork from recovered pigs (26). The USDA organized and led 25 separate 1-hour conference calls with a wide variety of key stakeholders, including multiple state and federal agencies, industry representatives, and international organizations and ministries. The goal was to garner agreement for a one-page set of speaking points intended to be released when—inevitably—the pH1N1 virus would be identified in a U.S. swine herd. CDC subject matter experts participated in every call.

This campaign was a key factor in ensuring that the first official 2009 pH1N1 report among U.S. swine did not lead to further embargoes or trade restrictions (27). The potential trade implications associated with 2009 pH1N1 in domestic pork could have led to a loss of approximately $456 million (28). Forward thinking and a cross-boundary One Health approach averted that loss.

Case Study Summary

This case example demonstrates that a One Health outcome is more likely when:

- Agencies with different mandates agree upon a common external threat.
- A foundation of trust exists among key individuals in different agencies, built on a willingness to acknowledge the other agencies' concerns.
- A mutually agreed-upon outcome is science based.

CASE STUDY 4: GOVERNMENTAL MANDATE ENCOURAGES INTERAGENCY COOPERATION—PULSENET AND FOODNET

Background

Between November 1992 and February 1993, an outbreak of *Escherichia coli* O157: H7 was traced back to thousands of pounds of hamburger patties distributed across the western United States, and had public health officials scrambling to prevent additional cases (29, 30). By the time health organizations issued a recall for contaminated meats, the outbreak resulted in more than 700 cases and 4 deaths and led to nationwide panic over the safety of consumer foods. This large-scale incident served as a catalyst, prompting the National Food Safety Initiative to allocate funds to establish enhanced sentinel surveillance systems for preventing and investigating food-borne illnesses (30). Two prominent surveillance systems were established as a result of this legislation: FoodNet and PulseNet (30, 31).

The Foodborne Diseases Active Surveillance Network (FoodNet) is a collaborative, interagency project of the CDC's Emerging Infections Program, multiple state health departments, the USDA, and the Food and Drug Administration (FDA) (30). Since its establishment in 1996, FoodNet has been essential in attributing specific food-borne pathogens to particular foods, as well as in estimating the overall incidence and burden of food-borne illnesses in the United States (32). The system provides active, population-based surveillance for nine bacterial and parasitic infections commonly transmitted through foods. Information generated by the system enables epidemiological studies designed to guide public health officials on how best to control the occurrence of food-borne outbreaks.

Similarly, the National Molecular Subtyping Network for Foodborne Disease Surveillance (PulseNet) is a national system made up of state and local public health laboratories, as well as federal laboratories, all tasked with conducting molecular subtyping of bacterial pathogens associated with food-borne outbreaks (31). This system allows laboratories in all 50 states to compare culture samples from food-related illnesses across multiple outbreaks. While data from FoodNet aids public health officials in conducting epidemiological investigations on food-borne outbreaks, PulseNet uses molecular subtyping to link seemingly unrelated sporadic multistate outbreaks to the same source, resulting in quicker outbreak identification and more rapid outbreak response. Together these two systems have proven vital to timely investigations to identity sources of multistate food-borne outbreaks in the United States (33).

Interagency Cooperation

Cross-sectoral cooperation has been crucial to the development of the FoodNet and PulseNet systems. The two major organizations charged with ensuring food safety in the United States are the USDA Food Safety and Inspection Service (FSIS) and the FDA. Before Congressional backing and financial support was made available for the FSIS and FDA to bring FoodNet and PulseNet to fruition, the U.S. framework for regulating the production of foods for mass consumption consisted of a patchwork of laws and regulations that often lagged far behind current scientific understanding of the risks of food-borne illness (33). In addition, the response of local and state government was often crisis driven and reactive, seldom taking a prophylactic approach to prevent the occurrence of outbreaks. Finally, funding was scarce, making local organizations dependent on third-party agencies to conduct the bulk of their research, thus impeding the potential for the FSIS and FDA to conduct the necessary research to inform their policy decisions. This made for a collection of food safety practices that lacked organizational infrastructure.

During this precollaborative period of food-borne disease control, the varying methods and standards governing the several health and agricultural departments were rarely conducive to sharing information and methodology (33). Although they shared common goals of improving food safety, animal and human health agencies were governed by differing organization-specific cultures that guided and informed their regulatory stance on food safety issues.

Governmental mandates with associated funding not only fostered interagency cooperation, thus prompting the development of FoodNet and PulseNet, but they also promoted cooperating agencies to adopt a One Health approach by creating compatible and collaborating systems to detect related outbreaks in animal and human populations, allowing for a broader understanding of the ways in which pathogens move between the two populations. For instance, by facilitating rapid identification of outbreaks, PulseNet significantly curtails the effects of a food-borne outbreak by helping to inform and mobilize local and state officials early in an epidemic. In addition, epidemiological studies conducted by FoodNet can help inform policy changes, driving health officials to take a preemptive rather than merely reactive approach in the prevention of food-borne illnesses.

With legislative support, PulseNet and FoodNet have also been able to create a standard with which other food laboratories are developing surveillance systems, as is the case with the USDA VetNet, a PulseNet equivalent initiated by the USDA Agricultural Research Service. Similarly, the FDA's National Antimicrobial Resistance Monitoring System (NARMS), which conducts routine surveillance of the retail meat supply, submits results of pulsed-field gel electrophoresis patterns on all *Salmonella* isolates (34). The ability of PulseNet to access the VetNet and NARMS datasets facilitates improvements in the investigation of food-borne outbreaks by making available a greater number of isolates from known sources that can be compared and evaluated for the presence of common pathogens (35).

Finally, the linking of databases between PulseNet and FoodNet, as well as the collaboration with other surveillance systems, creates a gold standard surveillance system that can reliably measure even minute changes in disease incidence and occurrence (36). This sensitivity becomes increasingly important with the emergence and reemergence of food-borne illnesses (i.e., multidrug-resistant pathogens, cholera, etc.). The legislative backing and federal funding available to support these entities is directly linked to their success and expansion, as well as their ability to employ One Health initiatives in their efforts to control the spread and burden of food-borne illnesses.

Case Study Summary

This case example demonstrates that a One Health outcome is more likely when:

- Federal funding and legislative backing mandate collaboration and information sharing.

- Cooperating agencies have clearly defined roles and responsibilities.
- Collaboration between agencies encourages the development of compatible data systems, streamlining the sharing of information and efficiency with which systems help to curtail food-borne outbreaks.

CASE STUDY 5: KENYA ZOONOTIC DISEASE UNIT

Background

In 2005, the International Health Regulations (IHR) were revised by the WHO to explicitly require that each country establish a system for surveillance of zoonoses and potential zoonoses, as well as a mechanism for coordinating all relevant sectors in the implementation of IHR (37). Like most countries, Kenya had not focused on surveillance for zoonotic diseases in either human or animal populations. Human surveillance was under the auspices of the Kenyan Ministry of Public Health and Sanitation (MOPHS) and veterinary surveillance was conducted by the Kenyan Ministry of Livestock Development (MOLD); the two entities did not have formal, established methods of exchanging information.

During 2006-2007, Kenya experienced an outbreak of Rift Valley fever (RVF) that resulted in substantial human and animal morbidity and mortality (38). Cross-sectoral communication was not optimal during the outbreak response, and this led to duplication and redundancy that may have had a negative impact on effective handling of the response (39).

During this same time period, HPAI H5N1 was emerging as a potential global health threat of significant proportion and all countries were being tasked to develop pandemic preparedness plans that encompassed both human and animal health. Although the virus had not yet been reported in Africa, national and international authorities were braced for imminent emergence.

Kenya responded to the threat of H5N1 by forming a National Influenza Task Force (NITF). The NITF assessed lessons learned during the RVF response and recognized the need for a more focused cross-sectoral group dedicated to zoonotic disease response that effectively linked animal and human health experts. To that end, the NITF invited membership from government ministries of public and animal health, military, police, the National Disaster Operation Center, public universities, and research institutions.

In 2008, the NITF expanded its mission to form the Zoonotic Technical Working Group (ZTWG), a multisectoral alliance that includes representatives from public health (MOPHS), animal health (MOLD), and partner organizations including the WHO, FAO, Kenya Medical Research Institute, Kenya Wildlife Services, CDC-Kenya, Kenyan Field Epidemiology and Laboratory Training Program, and National Museum of Kenya. The ZTWG meets quarterly and is chaired on a rotating basis by either the Director of Veterinary Services (representing MOLD) or the Director of Public Health and Sanitation (MOPHS).

Staff working in the ZTWG saw the need to establish a zoonotic disease office that could provide leadership, expertise, and service in laboratory and epidemiological science, bioterrorism preparedness, applied research, surveillance, outbreak response, and policy formation. A memorandum of understanding was signed between directors representing MOPHS and MOLD on August 2, 2011, in support of the formation of the Zoonotic Disease Unit (ZDU) within the government of Kenya. The vision of the ZDU is to provide an effective, efficient, multidisciplinary, and multisectoral surveillance and response system that reduces the burden, risk, and spread of zoonotic diseases in Kenya.

The ZDU is made up of a medical epidemiologist, a veterinary epidemiologist, a data analyst, and administrative staff. Other subject matter experts (such as microbiologists, social economists, and entomologists) are contracted to work with the ZDU as needed. The ZDU serves as the secretariat of the ZTWG, which in turn provides guidance and leadership to the ZDU. Both epidemiologists deployed to the ZDU remain part of their respective ministries and report to their respective heads. The epidemiologists share the leadership of the ZDU equally.

Case Study Summary

This case example demonstrates that a One Health outcome is more likely when:

- A series of external threats or internationally mandated actions imposes cross-sectoral collaboration.
- Leadership rotates rather than being monopolized by one sector.
- Incremental outputs receive favorable responses nationally and by international organizations.

DISCUSSION

The case studies above describe recent events that required cross-sectoral collaboration in order to most effectively respond to global, One Health challenges. The influenza examples, both H5N1 and H1N1, illustrate how a common threat provided the impetus to open lines of communication among partners that have not historically been frequent collaborators. It is to the credit of the various sectors that they recognized the necessity to collaborate with a wide variety of groups in order to respond within their own sector. To a large extent, these collaborations occurred before they were officially mandated, in spite of inequitable funding among the various agencies.

Nonetheless, it can be argued that the actual depth and resiliency of the One Health collaborations were never really tested because H5N1 did not become a pandemic; the transfer of virus remained as bird to human rather than becoming a human-to-human infection. The emergence of pH1N1 in 2009 did, however, challenge the level of trust that had been established among individuals in the separate agencies during H5N1 response planning. Although government agencies were operating under different mandates, U.S. entities were able to build on individual relationships to mount a united One Health collaborative approach that crossed bureaucratic boundaries.

Inequalities among Sectors as a Barrier to Collaboration: Wildlife Agencies

The wildlife health/wildlife management community has struggled with the One Health concept as being focused primarily on human health and secondarily on domestic animal health, while enhanced wildlife and ecological health as a goal appears to be an afterthought (40). The perception in wildlife agencies is that the environment is only considered part of the One Health concept in that environmental changes are threatening human health; i.e., the environment is considered a threat rather than something that can enhance human health or something that has its own inherent value. Nonetheless, several wildlife entities, including the American Association of Wildlife Veterinarians, the Wildlife Conservation Society (40), EcoHealth Alliance (41), and the National Park Service (42), have incorporated the One Health concept into their strategic planning. However, these individual initiatives have yet to move forward in promoting a collective mission in that sector. Furthermore, as we illustrate, agreement on a common set of core values, especially when accompanied by funding, that includes the mutual recognition of the importance of human, animal, and ecosystem health will enable agencies to overcome this apparent impediment to collaboration.

Inequalities among Sectors as a Barrier to Collaboration: Imbalance of D.V.M.'s and M.D.'s

The American Veterinary Medical Association (AVMA) and the Wildlife Conservation Society were early promoters of One Health through publication of the "AVMA Task Force Report on One Health" (43) in 2007 and the wide endorsement of the Wildlife Conservation Society's Manhattan Principles (44) in 2004. Although the human medical community has always been functionally engaged, leadership for One Health continues to be predominantly drawn from the animal health sector. Efforts to overcome this barrier are currently being addressed on several fronts, including (i) the loosely formed One Health Interagency Working Group, where more than a dozen federal agencies, including human health agencies, regularly communicate to exchange information under a One Health banner; (ii) CDC placement of international staff that includes D.V.M.'s, M.D.'s, and Ph.D.'s to work specifically at the interface between animal and human health; and (iii) the inclusion of One Health-focused sessions at meetings and conferences that focus on human health (48).

Team Building as a One Health Core Competency

It may be that cross-agency collaborations referred to as a One Health approach ultimately share the most basic team-building challenges, including building trust, not avoiding the difficult issues or conflicts, commitment to outcome, agency accountability, and attention to results (45). Starting in 2009, several parallel initiatives, including the Rockefeller Foundation project with the University of Minnesota (http://www. rockefellerfoundation.org/grants/grants-and-grantees/384ae11d-d234-4726-ad1b-c647de7ac1e9), the U.S. Agency for International Development Emerging Pandemic Threats RESPOND Program (46), and the Stone Mountain Meeting Training Workgroup (47), have independently tackled the task of defining core competencies for various levels of One Health practitioners. It is of note that each group identified communication and team-building skills as fundamental core competencies. The Stone Mountain Meeting Workgroup took the additional step of aggregating training opportunities that address the core competencies. In the online course listing, a large number of the resources identified as "One Health" focus on leadership, communication, and organizational management skills (47). A successful One Health approach will require that representatives from both animal and human health identify the common mission and goals and form the teams that can achieve these goals.

We also believe that individual leadership of those who participate in One Health work or projects is essential. Specifically, the following individual characteristics are important:

- A commitment and willingness to collaborate
- An ability to think beyond the boundaries of one's agency or organization
- An ability to represent a broad array of interests
- Decision-making authority or influence within one's agency or organization
- Experience in leadership roles and collaborative processes
- The science or knowledge capacity, or active engagement in One Health activities

CONCLUSION

Bureaucratic boundaries are formidable, and they will maintain because each sector has a unique purpose and area of functionality. Nonetheless, the case examples in this review illustrate that bureaucratic boundaries can be overcome and a One Health approach can be viable. Successful operationalizing of One Health is more likely when agencies with different mandates are responding to a common external threat; adequate funding is available to enable each sector to contribute to the outcome; individual entities are willing to accept nontraditional liaisons within their organizations; key individuals have established trusting relationships with counterparts in other agencies; optimal outcomes are mutually agreed upon and are science based; leadership rotates among agencies; and the value of a collaborative One Health approach is visibly demonstrated.

Acknowledgments. None of the authors of this manuscript have any commercial affiliations, consultancies, stock or equity interests, or patent-licensing arrangements that could be considered to pose a conflict of interest regarding this manuscript.

Citation. Rubin C, Dunham B, Sleeman J. 2014. Making One Health a reality—crossing bureaucratic boundaries. Microbiol Spectrum 2(1):OH-0016-2012. doi:10.1128/microbiolspec.OH-0016-2012.

REFERENCES

1. **Anholt RM, Stephen C, Copes R.** 2012. Strategies for collaboration in the interdisciplinary field of emerging zoonotic diseases. *Zoonoses Public Health* **59:**229–240.
2. **Centers for Disease Control and Prevention (CDC).** 1997. Isolation of avian influenza A(H5N1) viruses from humans—Hong Kong, May-December 1997. *MMWR Morb Mortal Wkly Rep* **46:**1204–1207.
3. **Chan PK.** 2002. Outbreak of avian influenza A(H5N1) virus infection in Hong Kong in 1997. *Clin Infect Dis* **34**(Suppl 2):S58–S64.
4. **World Health Organization.** 2013. *Cumulative number of confirmed human cases for avian influenza A (H5N1) reported to WHO, 2003-2013.* World Health Organization, Geneva, Switzerland. http://www.who. int/influenza/human_animal_interface/EN_GIP_20130116CumulativeNumberH5N1cases.pdf (last accessed August 20, 2013).
5. **Peiris JS, de Jong MD, Guan Y.** 2007. Avian influenza virus (H5N1): a threat to human health. *Clin Microbiol Rev* **20:**243–267.

6. **Food and Agriculture Organization, Global Early Warning System (FAO-GLEWS).** 2012. *H5N1 HPAI Global overview: January-March 2012. Bulletin 31.* FAO, Rome, Italy. http://www.fao.org/docrep/015/an388e/an388e.pdf (last accessed August 20, 2013).

7. **Tiensin T, Chaitaweesub P, Songserm T, Chaisingh A, Hoonsuwan W, Buranathai C, Parakamawongsa T, Premashthira S, Amonsin A, Gilbert M, Nielen M, Stegeman A.** 2005. Highly pathogenic avian influenza H5N1, Thailand, 2004. *Emerg Infect Dis* **11:**1664–1672.

8. **Global Early Warning System (GLEWS).** 2013. *Global Early Warning System for Major Animal Diseases Including Zoonoses.* http://www.glews.net/ (last accessed August 20, 2013).

9. **National Institute of Allergy and Infectious Diseases.** 2011. *Centers of Excellence for Influenza Research and Surveillance (CEIRS).* National Institute of Allergy and Infectious Diseases, Bethesda, MD. http://www.niaid.nih.gov/labsandresources/resources/ceirs/Pages/default.aspx (last accessed August 20, 2013).

10. **Food and Agriculture Organization, Emergency Centre for Transboundary Animal Diseases Regional Office for Asia and the Pacific.** 2012. Lessons learned from HPAI. *ECTAD-RAP News*, March-April 2012. http://www.fao.org/docrep/016/an414e/an414e.pdf (last accessed August 20, 2013).

11. **Beigel JH, Farrar J, Han AM, Hayden FG, Hyer R, de Jong MD, Lochindarat S, Nguyen TK, Nguyen TH, Tran TH, Nicoll A, Touch S, Yuen KY; Writing Committee of the World Health Organization (WHO) Consultation on Human Influenza A/H5.** 2005. Avian influenza A (H5N1) infection in humans. *N Engl J Med* **353:**1374–1385.

12. **Kandun IN, Wibisono H, Sedyaningsih ER, Yusharmen, Hadisoedarsuno W, Purba W, Santoso H, Septiawati C, Tresnaningsih E, Heriyanto B, Yuwono D, Harun S, Soeroso S, Giriputra S, Blair PJ, Jeremijenko A, Kosasih H, Putnam SD, Samaan G, Silitonga M, Chan KH, Poon LL, Lim W, Klimov A, Lindstrom S, Guan Y, Donis R, Katz J, Cox N, Peiris M, Uyeki TM.** 2006. Three Indonesian clusters of H5N1 virus infection in 2005. *N Engl J Med* **355:**2186–2194.

13. **Kilpatrick AM, Chmura AA, Gibbons DW, Fleischer RC, Marra PP, Daszak P.** 2006. Predicting the global spread of H5N1 avian influenza. *Proc Natl Acad Sci USA* **103:**19368–19373.

14. **Sakoda Y, Sugar S, Batchluun D, Erdene-Ochir TO, Okamatsu M, Isoda N, Soda K, Takakuwa H, Tsuda Y, Yamamoto N, Kishida N, Matsuno K, Nakayama E, Kajihara M, Yokoyama A, Takada A, Sodnomdarjaa R, Kida H.** 2010. Characterization of H5N1 highly pathogenic avian influenza virus strains isolated from migratory waterfowl in Mongolia on the way back from the southern Asia to their northern territory. *Virology* **406:**88–94.

15. **US Department of Agriculture (USDA), US Department of the Interior, and US Department of Health and Human Services.** 2006. *An Early Detection System for Highly Pathogenic H5N1 Avian Influenza in Wild Migratory Birds: U.S. Interagency Strategic Plan.* USDA, Washington, DC. http://www.usda.gov/documents/wildbirdstrategicplanpdf.pdf (last accessed August 20, 2013).

16. **Deliberto TJ, Swafford SR, Van Why KR.** 2011. Development of a national early detection system for highly pathogenic avian influenza in wild birds in the United States of America, p 156–175. *In* Majumdar SK, Brenner FJ, Huffman JE, McLean RG, Panah AI, Pietrobon PJ, Keeler SP, Shive S (ed), *Pandemic Influenza Viruses: Science, Surveillance and Public Health.* Pennsylvania Academy of Science, Easton, PA.

17. **National Fish and Wildlife Health Initiative for the United States.** 2007. http://www.fishwildlife.org/files/Fish-Wildlife-Health-Initiative-Toolkit_rev5-09.pdf (last accessed August 20, 2013).

18. **Centers for Disease Control and Prevention (CDC).** 2009. Swine influenza A (H1N1) infection in two children—southern California, March–April 2009. *MMWR Morb Mortal Wkly Rep* **58:**400–402.

19. **Rubin GJ, Amlôt R, Page L, Wessely S.** 2009. Public perceptions, anxiety, and behaviour change in relation to the swine flu outbreak: cross sectional telephone survey. *BMJ* **339:**b2651. doi:10.1136/bmj.b2651.

20. **Garten RJ, Davis CT, Russell CA, Shu B, Lindstrom S, Balish A, Sessions WM, Xu X, Skepner E, Deyde V, Okomo-Adhiambo M, Gubareva L, Barnes J, Smith CB, Emery SL, Hillman MJ, Rivailler P, Smagala J, de Graaf M, Burke DF, Fouchier RA, Pappas C, Alpuche-Aranda CM, López-Gatell H, Olivera H, López I, Myers CA, Faix D, Blair PJ, Yu C, Keene KM, Dotson PD Jr, Boxrud D, Sambol AR, Abid SH, St George K, Bannerman T, Moore AL, Stringer DJ, Blevins P, Demmler-Harrison GJ, Ginsberg M, Kriner P, Waterman S, Smole S, Guevara HF, Belongia EA, Clark PA, Beatrice ST, Donis R, Katz J, Finelli L, Bridges CB, Shaw M, Jernigan DB, Uyeki TM, Smith DJ, Klimov AI, Cox NJ.** 2009. Antigenic and genetic characteristics of swine-origin 2009 A(H1N1) influenza viruses circulating in humans. *Science* **325:**197–201.

21. **Chan M.** 2009. *World now at the start of 2009 influenza pandemic. June 11, 2009.* World Health Organization, Geneva Switzerland. http://www.who.int/mediacentre/news/statements/2009/h1n1_pandemic_phase6_20090611/en/ (last accessed August 20, 2013).

22. **Pappaioanou M, Gramer M.** 2010. Lessons from pandemic H1N1 2009 to improve prevention, detection, and response to influenza pandemics from a One Health perspective. *ILAR J* **51**:268–280.

23. **USDA Food Safety and Inspection Service (FSIS).** 2006. *Reportable and foreign animal diseases.* FSIS, Washington, DC. http://www.fsis.usda.gov/wps/wcm/connect/2afa4f5f-e7df-479c-9058-55aecc60d145/PHVt-Reportable ___Foreign_Animal_Diseases.pdf?MOD=AJPERES.

24. **Spronk GD.** 2001. Swine influenza virus. *Adv Pork Prod* **12**:51–54.

25. **Giantmicrobes.** 2013. *Swine flu (influenza A virus H1N1).* Giantmicrobes, Stamford, CT. http://www.giantmicrobes.com/us/products/swineflu.html (last accessed August 20, 2013).

26. **Vincent AL, Lager KM, Harland M, Lorusso A, Zanell E, Ciacci-Zanella JR, Kehrli ME, Klimov A.** 2009. Absence of 2009 pandemic H1N1 influenza A virus in fresh pork. *PLoS One* **4**:e8367. doi:10.1371/journal.pone.0008367.

27. **Gostin LO.** 2009. Influenza A(H1N1) and pandemic preparedness under the rule of international law. *JAMA* **301**:2376–2378.

28. **Zering K.** 2009. Economic disaster in the U.S. pork industry and implications for North Carolina. *NC State University Swine News* **32**:8. http://www.ncsu.edu/project/swine_extension/swine_news/2009/sn_v3209% 20%28september%29.htm (last accessed August 20, 2013).

29. **Tuttle J, Gomez T, Doyle MP, Wells JG, Zhao T, Tauxe RV, Griffin PM.** 1999. Lessons from a large outbreak of *Escherichia coli* O157:H7 infections: insights into the infectious dose and method of widespread contamination of hamburger patties. *Epidemiol Infect* **122**:185–192.

30. **Allos BM, Moore MR, Griffin PM, Tauxe RV.** 2004. Surveillance for sporadic foodborne disease in the 21st century: the FoodNet perspective. *Clin Infect Dis* **38**(Suppl 3):S115–S120.

31. **Swaminathan B, Barrett TJ, Hunter SB, Tauxe RV, CDC PulseNet Task Force.** 2001. PulseNet: the molecular subtyping network for foodborne bacterial disease surveillance, United States. *Emerg Infect Dis* **7**:382–389.

32. **Henao OL, Scallan E, Mahon B, Hoekstra RM.** 2010. Methods for monitoring trends in the incidence of foodborne diseases: Foodborne Diseases Active Surveillance Network 1996–2008. *Foodborne Pathog Dis* **7**:1421–1426.

33. **Woteki CE, Kineman BD.** 2003. Challenges and approaches to reducing foodborne illness. *Ann Rev Nutr* **23**:315–344.

34. **US Food and Drug Administration (FDA).** 2013. *National Antimicrobial Resistance Monitoring System (NARMS).* FDA, Silver Spring, MD. http://www.fda.gov/AnimalVeterinary/SafetyHealth/AntimicrobialResistance/ NationalAntimicrobialResistanceMonitoringSystem/ (last accessed August 20, 2013).

35. **Gerner-Smidt P, Hise K, Kincaid J, Hunter S, Rolando S, Hyytiä-Trees E, Ribot EM, Swaminathan B, Pulsenet Taskforce.** 2006. PulseNet USA: a five-year update. *Foodborne Pathog Dis* **3**:9–19.

36. **Jones TF, Scallan E, Angulo FJ.** 2007. FoodNet: overview of a decade of achievement. *Foodborne Pathog Dis* **4**:60–66.

37. **von Tigerstrom B.** 2005. The revised international health regulations and restraint of national health measures. *Health Law J* **13**:35–76.

38. **Centers for Disease Control and Prevention (CDC).** 2007. Rift Valley fever outbreak—Kenya, November 2006–January 2007. *MMWR Morb Mortal Wkly Rep* **56**:73–76.

39. **Breiman RF, Minjauw B, Sharif SK, Ithondeka P, Njenga MK.** 2010. Rift Valley Fever: scientific pathways toward public health prevention and response. *Am J Trop Med Hyg* **83**(2 Suppl): 1–4.

40. **Wildlife Conservation Society.** 2013. *One World–One Health.* Wildlife Conservation Society, Bronx, NY. http://www.wcs.org/conservation-challenges/wildlife-health/wildlife-humans-and-livestock/one-world-one -health.aspx (last accessed August 20, 2013).

41. **EcoHealth Alliance.** 2010. *One Health for One World. April 13, 2010.* EcoHealth Alliance, New York, NY. http://www.ecohealthalliance.org/news/146-one_health_for_one_world (last accessed August 20, 2013).

42. **National Park Service, US Department of the Interior.** 2013. *Disease detection and response.* National Park Service, Washington, DC. http://www.nps.gov/public_health/di/di.htm (last accessed August 20, 2013).

43. **One Health Commission.** 2013. *Historical background summary of the One Health Commission.* https://www.avma.org/KB/Resources/Reports/Documents/onehealth_final.pdf (last accessed August 20, 2013).

44. **Cook RA, Karesh WB, Osofsky SA.** 2004. *One World, One Health: building interdisciplinary bridges to health in a globalized world. One World, One Health symposium.* http://www.oneworldonehealth.org/sept2004/owoh_sept04.html (last accessed August 20, 2013).

45. **Lencioni PM.** 2006. *The Five Dysfunctions of a Team: a Leadership Fable.* John Wiley & Sons, New York, NY.

46. **US Agency for International Development.** 2013. Emerging Pandemic Threats program. U.S. Agency for International Development, Washington, DC. http://www.usaid.gov/news-information/fact-sheets/emerging-pandemic-threats-program (last accessed August 20, 2013).

47. **Rubin C.** 2011. *Operationalizing One Health: the Stone Mountain meeting.* Presented at 1st International One Health Congress, February 16, 2011. http://www.cdc.gov/onehealth/pdf/atlanta/australia.pdf (last accessed August 20, 2013).

48. **Centers for Disease Control and Prevention.** 2012. *One Health related meetings.* http://www.cdc.gov/onehealth/meetings.html.

One Health: People, Animals, and the Environment
Edited by Ronald M. Atlas and Stanley Maloy
© 2014 American Society for Microbiology, Washington, DC
doi:10.1128/microbiolspec.OH-0017-2012

Chapter 19

One Health: Lessons Learned from East Africa

Dominic A. Travis,[1] David W. Chapman,[2] Meggan E. Craft,[1]
John Deen,[1] Macdonald W. Farnham,[1] Carolyn Garcia,[3]
William D. Hueston,[1] Richard Kock,[4] Michael Mahero,[1]
Lawrence Mugisha,[5] Serge Nzietchueng,[1] Felicia B. Nutter,[6]
Debra Olson,[7] Amy Pekol,[2] Katharine M. Pelican,[1]
Cheryl Robertson,[3] and Innocent B. Rwego[1,8]

INTRODUCTION

Africa is faced with many of the most daunting challenges (food insecurity, poverty, and disease) of our time. With an area of 30 million square kilometers, it is the second-largest continent, covering 6% of the Earth's surface and 20% of its land mass. It currently comprises 54 sovereign countries accounting for roughly 15% of the world's human population. In 2009, 22 of 24 nations identified as having "Low Human Development" on the United Nations' Human Development Index were located in sub-Saharan Africa (http://hdr.undp.org/en/statistics/). Today, 33 of the 48 nations on the United Nations' list of least developed countries are in Africa. On the other hand, Africa also has arguably the largest proportion of intact natural ecosystems, biodiversity, and sociocultural capital and the lowest impact on global warming of any continent, with considerable "carbon credit." Africa's ratio of biocapacity (capacity of an area to provide resources and absorb wastes) to consumption (ecological footprint) (>150%) is much higher than that for the developed world, which is dramatically negative in these indicators. When an area's ecological footprint exceeds its biocapacity, unsustainability occurs (www.footprintnetwork.org).

[1]Department of Veterinary Population Medicine, University of Minnesota College of Veterinary Medicine, St. Paul, MN 55108; [2]Department of Organizational Leadership, Policy, and Development, University of Minnesota-Twin Cities, Minneapolis, MN 55455; [3]School of Nursing, University of Minnesota-Twin Cities, Minneapolis, MN 55455; [4]Department of Pathology & Infectious Diseases, The Royal Veterinary College, North Mymms, Hatfield, Hertfordshire AL9 7TA, United Kingdom; [5]Department of Wildlife and Resource Management, Makerere University College of Veterinary Medicine, Animal Resources and Biosecurity, Kampala, Uganda; [6]Department of Biomedical Sciences, Cummings School of Veterinary Medicine, Tufts University, North Grafton, MA 01536; [7]School of Public Health, University of Minnesota-Twin Cities, Minneapolis, MN 55455; [8]Department of Biological Sciences, Makerere University, Kampala, Uganda.

African leaders are faced with daily competing demands and values among a multitude of complex issues such as high human population growth, extreme poverty, food insecurity, land use policy, climate change, and biodiversity conservation. In this context, building sustainable national systems for human and/or animal health is one of the grand challenges of this generation. Fortunately, the international community has made very large investments in health over a long period of time in Africa. Unfortunately, these investments often come with requirements or priorities that do not reflect those of the local people or government. This donor-recipient mismatch has led to further frustration of local health experts while reinforcing the need for more sustainable solutions aimed at systematically connecting communities with national governments and ministries. Nowhere is this more obvious than in the prevention and control of infectious diseases, including but not limited to malaria (1, 2), tuberculosis (3), HIV (4), and yellow fever (5).

Today's global and complex health and development challenges require long-term commitment (6) and a range of approaches that are too broad for any one discipline, institution, or country to implement on its own (7). The One Health concept recognizes the interconnectedness of global health issues and, as such, promotes the importance of and need for international, interdisciplinary, and cross-sectoral communication and collaboration at local, national, and international levels. This concept, therefore, is a deliberate attempt to move away from the traditional narrow disciplinary approach to a more holistic, integrated approach that requires a new set of skills to implement, including leadership, team building, communication, and multidisciplinary project management on top of the traditional discipline-based training. Thus, the One Health approach is a long-term strategy that requires the development of future global health leaders with the skills, knowledge, and experience in collaborating across disciplines and sectors to solve pressing and complex global health problems.

By taking advantage of natural cultural tendencies for shared leadership, resource allocation, and community values, African leaders are currently proactively demonstrating the principles of One Health, and thus becoming a model for this global vision. And by focusing on partnerships rather than donor-recipient relationships, they are fostering the development of shared priorities and are increasingly driving their own health agenda to fulfill their own needs. Although there is a long way to go, this holistic approach may provide a much needed sustainable platform for saving valuable resources while increasing human health, food security, and the conservation of natural resources. The following are a few initiatives and/or lessons learned from East Africa as experienced by the authors.

UNIVERSITIES IN SUPPORT OF ONE HEALTH

To realize One Health, there is a need for an interprofessional and transdiciplinary educational framework focused on developing a new generation of professional and academic leaders who can create an integrated scientific knowledge base. Universities have long been recognized for their potential to further national economic and social development goals. As centers of knowledge production, innovation, collaboration, and training, universities offer many advantages in this regard. James Coleman used the term "developmental universities" to describe the potential of universities to direct their work and mission toward national and social development goals (8). In recognition of this potential, the 1980s saw universities become indispensible parts of international development partnerships, which up until that point had been limited to a relationship between the donor and recipient governments. After a period of neglect and overshadowing by basic education reforms in the 1990s, there is now a resurgence of interest in investing in higher education for development purposes (7, 9).

When it comes to implementing and institutionalizing the international, interdisciplinary, and cross-sectoral One Health approach in particular, universities offer many advantages. Their strong community and government ties make them ideally situated to promote collaboration between international aid agencies, governments, the private sector, and local communities. In addition, as centers of education, training, and research, they can provide interdisciplinary training for the next generation of One Health professionals.

While universities have great potential, implementing and institutionalizing the One Health approach in Africa requires financial resources that exceed the capacity of African governments and institutions alone. Recognizing these limitations, cross-border university collaborations have become a widely accepted strategy for building institutional capacity to achieve broad development and global health goals (7). Among the different forms of cross-border university collaborations, university networks have recently emerged as a popular development strategy with support from leading international aid agencies and organizations such as the U.S. Agency for International Development (USAID), Asian Development Bank, and UNESCO. University networks typically bring together a group of institutions to collaborate on a broad set of activities or common issue. These university networks, therefore, lend themselves well to One Health initiatives, which promote intersectoral, interinstitutional, and interdisciplinary research collaborations to solve local and global health challenges. This is evidenced by the growing number of One Health networks and consortia in which institutions of higher education and their respective health-related schools play a major role. A number of One Health networks involving universities are already under way in sub-Saharan Africa, and they are supported by a diverse group of donors, which suggests a global trend toward using university networks to address global health challenges (Table 1).

While university networks have a great deal of support and potential in the field of global health and development, systematic evaluation of this approach remains limited. This is partially because university networks are a relatively new development phenomenon, they take considerable time to develop, and their administrative structure and activities can be quite broad and difficult to track. As a result, little is known about the strengths and limitations of university networks as a strategy for development, and even less is known about the role of university networks in implementing a One Health approach to global health issues. In an attempt to fill these gaps, the following section identifies key themes that have emerged during the design and implementation of one particular One Health university network initiative, the One Health Central and Eastern Africa (OHCEA) university network.

The OHCEA university network was founded in 2010 as part of a 5-year USAID-funded project (http://ohcea.org/). It expanded upon a preexisting network of seven schools of public health called the Higher Education Alliance for Leadership through Health (HEALTH), and currently includes 14 public health and veterinary medicine institutions and government ministries in the Democratic Republic of Congo, Ethiopia, Kenya, Tanzania, Rwanda, and Uganda (http://halliance.org/). The OHCEA network

Table 1. One Health networks operating in Africa[a]

One Health-related network/consortium	Participating countries	Primary funder(s)
One Health Initiative-African Research Consortium on Ecosystem and Population Health (Afrique One)	Tanzania, Ghana, Ivory, Uganda, Senegal, Chad	Wellcome Trust
One Health Central and Eastern Africa (OHCEA) university network	Ethiopia, Democratic Republic of Congo, Kenya, Rwanda, Tanzania, Uganda	USAID
One Health National Networks for Enhanced Research in Infectious Diseases (NRN-Biomed)	Tanzania, Ghana, Uganda (with partners in the global North)	European Union
Cysticercosis Working Group in Eastern and Southern Africa (CWGESA)	Tanzania, Kenya, Uganda, Zambia, Zimbabwe, South Africa, Madagascar, Mozambique, Rwanda, Burundi	Principal sources of funding include membership fees, annual subscriptions, grants, donations, and other contributions
Southern African Centre for Infectious Disease Surveillance (SACIDS)	Democratic Republic of Congo, Mozambique, South Africa, Zambia, Tanzania (with research center partners in the global North)	Wellcome Trust, Rockefeller Foundation, Google.org
Southern African Development Community Transboundary Animal Diseases (SADC TADs)	Angola, Botswana, Democratic Republic of Congo, Lesotho, Malawi, Mauritius, Mozambique, Namibia, Seychelles, South Africa, Swaziland, Tanzania, Zambia, Zimbabwe	Member states, through SADC's Regional Development Fund
Training Health Researchers into Vocational Excellence (THRiVE)	African partners: Uganda, Tanzania, Rwanda; Northern partners: United Kingdom	Wellcome Trust
Consortium for Advanced Research Training in Africa (CARTA)	Tanzania, Kenya, Uganda, Rwanda, Malawi, South Africa, Nigeria	Wellcome Trust

[a]Note: This is a sample, rather than an exhaustive list, of One Health networks currently operating in Africa.

embodies a One Health approach to collaboration in the area of emerging and infectious zoonotic diseases, and its long-term strategy is to build the necessary skills, knowledge, and One Health attitudes among health professionals and leaders. While the OHCEA network is still relatively young, there are already a number of very relevant lessons learned with respect to university network development and implementation in Africa (D. W. Chapman, A. Pekol, and L. W. Wilson, unpublished data).

1. A benefit of a university network is that it can draw on and mobilize a wide range of talent and address a large number of issues. They are also widely perceived to achieve more efficient and sustainable development outcomes. Nonetheless, it can be extraordinarily difficult to communicate and coordinate activities across different institutions, countries, languages, legal systems, and operating procedures. Such differences may slow the pace of network activities, hinder cooperation, and cause some partners to feel disenfranchised. A strong communication system and an

administrative structure that accounts for the strengths and limitations of each member institution are important to keep network activities moving at a steady pace and in a mutually agreeable direction.

2. Since university networks can promote collaboration on many issues, narrowing in on a particular issue and approach can require hard decisions and consume a lot of time. Time spent negotiating the organization and governance of the network itself often comes at the expense of making progress on more substantive activities. This can result in the appearance of minimal progress and cause momentum and support to waver. On the other hand, not taking appropriate time for organizational development can limit the strength and sustainability of the network. Emerging university networks must strike a balance between developing a strong administrative structure and implementing a steady stream of network activities early on to keep partners informed and engaged.

3. Network success depends on having champions at each member university as well as one or numerous overall network champions. These people are key players in developing support and enthusiasm for the network and projects. While network champions are key to mobilizing interest and pushing agendas, placing too much decision-making authority within a single entity may heighten the perception that resources are disproportionately allocated or exploited. Thus, network champions are important, but they are in a delicate position; there should be checks and balances embedded into the network to support the development of trust and ensure that network decisions reflect the interests, needs, and capabilities of all partners.

4. External funding is advantageous in that it can contribute needed resources and make new initiatives possible. However, local institutions and external funders have distinct operating procedures, resources, and abilities and are likely to approach university networks with different priorities and timelines. Whereas local institutions must take a long view and focus on capacity building and creating a sustainable network structure, donor agencies typically need to demonstrate progress on short-term goals. Given their different abilities and priorities, local partners and external funders need to work together early on to establish clear and reasonable goals, indicators, and timelines for the network. Ensuring that member institutions have more input at this stage is also advantageous in that it fosters a greater sense of ownership and increases buy-in for the creation of a sustainable long-term platform.

5. Collaboration is most attractive when it is among equals. Each partner wants to benefit from participation in the network, but not all institutions can contribute equally or reap the same benefits. OHCEA partners cite "limited and unequal access to resources" as a major factor for the fair and equitable growth of the network. Reaching an agreement a priori on how each partner can expect to benefit, as well as recognition of individual resources and capabilities, can help reduce competition and improve collaboration efforts across the network.

As outlined above, university networks offer many advantages for governments and universities to collaborate and solve pressing global health challenges. The OHCEA network serves a dual purpose of implementing a One Health approach across Central and Eastern Africa while also strengthening African institutions of higher education. While university networks can expand resources and capabilities, they also increase operational complexity. University partners enter networks with different resources, capacities, and constraints, which in turn shape how they participate in and what they expect from the network. Keeping partners informed, represented in decisions, and engaged in activities is necessary for maintaining network momentum and long-term support. The greatest challenge is getting this structure in place in the short term while also maintaining a steady stream of activities and taking steps to ensure the long-term sustainability of the network once short-term external project funding and technical assistance ends.

ZOONOTIC DISEASE PREVENTION AND CONTROL: A ONE HEALTH GRAND CHALLENGE

Zoonotic and emerging infectious diseases pose a significant threat to animal and human health, food security, the economy, and the environment; they even affect the social stability and well-being of entire communities, countries, and geographic regions (10). More than 75% of emerging infectious diseases are zoonotic, with the majority having their origin in wild animal populations. There also is a significant relationship between socioeconomic, environmental, and ecological factors and emerging infectious disease events. Resources for countering disease emergence are poorly allocated on a global scale, with the majority existing in areas where emerging infectious disease events are least likely to occur (11, 12). Despite the evidence, a major disconnect remains between human, animal, and environmental health in terms of funding, infrastructure, and general capacity to address this common problem. However, recognition of this problem is growing, and numerous global, regional, and local health organizations are now proactively engaged in fostering One Health approaches, many of them in Africa.

At the global level, the intergovernmental agencies are working at a variety of levels to promote a One Health approach to address the threat of emerging zoonotic disease. The World Organisation for Animal Health (Office International des Épizooties, or OIE) is conducting training and sensitization workshops in Africa at both regional and country levels to help reinforce international standards aimed at many zoonotic diseases (http://www.rr-africa.oie.int/en/en_index.html). Specific activities include systematic assessment of national veterinary services' disease surveillance and control methods and capacity; training country focal persons in disease risk analysis, surveillance, and diagnostics; and building laboratory capacity and disease identification knowledge through a tripartite agreement with the World Health Organization (WHO) and Food and Agriculture Organization of the United Nations (FAO) (13). The FAO has long been engaged in Africa and prioritized a number of "pressing needs" for dealing with zoonotic and emerging infectious diseases, including the need for increased veterinary expertise to control zoonoses such as rabies, brucellosis, and echinococcosis; recognition and planning for the utilization of animal disease outbreaks as sentinels for emerging human and environmental health risks; and improvement of the safety of food derived from animals and animal products (14–16). In the past few years, most of the above initiatives have been designed to include public and wildlife health experts—thus increasing their One Health approach to these issues.

The WHO has invested heavily in prevention and control of infectious disease in Africa by supporting implementation of its Integrated Disease Surveillance and Response (IDSR) technical guidelines, which outline reporting recommendations and requirements for diseases of human health concern, many of which are zoonotic. Training is often accompanied by allocation of resources toward diagnostics-based surveillance systems and interventions for high-priority diseases (as defined by WHO member states) (17). Thus, the WHO supports the development of robust disease surveillance systems, connecting local and national governments to regional and global health authorities. Unfortunately, these training and system-strengthening programs rarely include resource allocations for domestic animal and wildlife populations so often fall short as One Health initiatives. As a result, the burden of creating and maintaining such systems typically lies with individual animal producers/farmers (10, 14). This, in turn, results in a significant gap between human and animal disease surveillance systems. The tripartite agreement between the WHO, FAO, and OIE acknowledges this gap, states that these organizations will seek to actively foster One Health efforts globally, and in Africa specifically; and supports linkages, partnerships, and networks to strengthen systems-based thinking and approaches (13).

At the regional level, many One Health initiatives are gaining acceptance after successful proof of concept. For example, the African Union Interafrican Bureau for Animal Resources (AU-IBAR) was founded in 1951 explicitly to control one of the key animal diseases in the world: rinderpest. Since its initial mandate, the goals of AU-IBAR have expanded to address all aspects of animal resources (fish, livestock, and wildlife) throughout Africa. It aims to provide leadership in the development of animal resources for Africa "by supporting and empowering the African Union member states and the Regional Economic Communities (RECs) in a vision of an Africa free from hunger and poverty in which animal resources make a significant contribution within the global arena" (http://www.au-ibar.org/about/vision-mission-and-mandate). AU-IBAR has a strategic plan for One Health, has conducted several One Health outbreak investigations and trainings, and supported advocacy for a One Health approach to ministerial-level health authorities of most member countries. One specific example is support for the "One Health Training on disease investigation in Wildlife, Livestock and Public Health" (http://www.au-ibar.org/component/jdownloads/finish/25/848, where human, domestic animal, and wildlife health regulatory officials from multiple African countries attend 7- to 10-day workshops focused on learning One Health approaches through integrative case studies and field experiences.

At the country level, using Uganda as a case in point, several high-profile, confusing outbreaks of emerging diseases (e.g., Ebola virus, yellow fever, anthrax, trypanosomiasis, Marburg virus, and nodding disease within the past 3 years) have resulted in increased public awareness with increased expectation of effective, proactive government response (18). The yellow fever outbreak in northern Uganda in 2010 did not match expected clinical appearance (lack of marked jaundice in the majority of cases), which prolonged a definitive diagnosis. Nodding disease in northern Uganda has continually frustrated efforts to understand and control the disease. Even in major animal disease outbreaks like the death of hundreds of hippos from anthrax in Queen Elizabeth National Park, submission of samples to the existing laboratories is delayed due to significant challenges with sample collection, cold chain maintenance, and transport from remote locations to laboratories in urban areas that will accept animal samples. As a result, the Ugandan government is promoting multisectoral cross-ministry collaboration in its National Task Force (NTF) for Epidemic Preparedness and Response. Previously called in on an ad hoc basis, and dissolved at the conclusion of an outbreak, the NTF is now a standing entity. The NTF coordinates efforts across ministries and sectors, from local to national levels, and provides a platform to coordinate efforts of intergovernmental and nongovernmental organizations, donors, development partners, and other stakeholders from the central level.

The case study of Uganda is not unique, and every African country is faced with similar problems to a greater or lesser extent. Thus, it is imperative that lessons learned are communicated to the broader scientific community. Some lessons from the efforts above:

- There is a need for better overall coordination and planning within countries and with external strategic partners and donors.
- There is still too much of a focus on short-term issues and needs rather than long-term sustainable solutions.
- There is a disconnect between specialized service laboratories and national/regional/global disease surveillance infrastructure.
- There is an overreliance on passive versus active surveillance and a general lack of appropriate training and continuing education for diagnosticians.
- Marketplace stakeholder demand for services that support surveillance infrastructure is low; incentivizing animal producers, veterinarians, associated industry, local/national/international regulatory authorities, and other key stakeholders to value disease diagnostics and surveillance as good business remains a significant One Health challenge (10).

EAST AFRICAN INFECTIOUS DISEASE ONE HEALTH CASE STUDIES

Great Ape Conservation and Zoonotic Infectious Disease Risk

As our closest phylogenetic relatives, chimpanzees (*Pan troglodytes*), gorillas (western *Gorilla gorilla* and eastern *Gorilla beringei* species), and bonobos (*Pan paniscus*) share genetic similarities that facilitate the spread of infectious pathogens among humans and great apes (19–22). Wild great apes can be reservoirs for pathogens that infect humans, such as the simian immunodeficiency virus (SIVcpz) that evolved into HIV-1 (23); and can be infected with human-origin pathogens, such as metapneumovirus (24–26), polio (27), measles (28), and scabies (29). Great apes and humans can also both be infected with pathogens from other wild or domestic animal hosts, such as Ebola virus (30), *Cryptosporidium* and *Giardia* (31), and anthrax (32). All great apes are endangered and therefore of high conservation value, making the risk associated with pathogens that pass between humans and apes a concern in both directions (33).

Long-term great ape behavioral research sites established in the 1960s and 1970s to study chimpanzees (in Gombe and Mahale Mountains National Parks, Tanzania, and Tai National Park, Côte d'Ivoire) and mountain gorillas (in Volcanoes National Park, Rwanda) provide compelling examples of the need for and benefits of the One Health approach. Behavioral researchers working at each of these field sites independently observed infectious disease epidemics in their study populations, and analysis of historical data showed that disease was the most common cause of great ape death at several sites (27). The potential for disease transmission among great apes, humans (researchers, tourists, and local communities), domestic animals, and other wildlife was recognized (25, 27, 28, 34, 35), and various One Health-consistent responses devised.

One Health medical programs, including syndromic surveillance and response systems in apes (36–38), preventive health programs for conservation and research personnel (39, 40), and domestic animal health programs, have been designed and implemented. The expertise developed and results achieved through these programs have helped inform the development of policy guidelines for the continued protection of great ape health in conjunction with growing human and domestic animal populations and increasing demand for ecotourism access (33). The positive impact that holistic human-animal health care can have on a great ape and local human populations has recently been conclusively demonstrated for the mountain gorilla population (41), and data supporting successful implementation of the One Health concept are currently being collected at many other long-term great ape monitoring sites as well.

The Second Successful Global Eradication: Rinderpest

Rinderpest, a morbillivirus, emerged along with the expanding domestic cattle populations some 2,000 or more years ago in Central Asia. Its impact on other artiodactyls only became apparent when it established in Africa with massive die-off of cattle, antelope, and buffalo during the great pandemic in the 1890s. Its impact was catastrophic, and ultimately whole communities starved or lost livelihoods. Control was achieved in a few areas quite rapidly through quarantine, but it persisted in the great nomadic wildlife and cattle herds of East and West Africa throughout the 20th century (42, 43). The slow road to eradication started with the advent of an efficacious vaccine developed in Kenya in the 1960s (44), which was immediately implemented in a series of vaccination campaigns. Considerable progress was made initially using these conventional vaccination and control measures, and the disease was reduced to cryptic foci and occasional epidemics. This approach alone, however, was not enough to fully eradicate the disease, and it continued to reemerge, to the frustration of the donors and governments alike, through the '70s, '80s, and '90s (45).

Failure to fully understand the disease ecology and epidemiology in Africa was at the root of this eradication failure. There was little time for research, as each event was usually dramatic and the vaccine was applied immediately, preventing understanding of the diversity of pathogen strains and the multihost dynamics that existed. Rinderpest was considered to be exclusively a livestock problem, and the livestock departments jealously guarded the mandate for control, and thereby the resources and strategies. Ironically, it was only when other disciplines became accidentally engaged in the monitoring and management of the disease, first by wildlife managers in places where rinderpest was also causing an impact (but hitherto hardly acknowledged by veterinary services) (46) and second through the use of participatory epidemiology and paraveterinarians (47) to engage farmers and communities. There was little or no control over these sectors by the veterinary departments, and at first they actively discouraged their activities. This may also have been because the results exposed flaws in the surveillance systems and control measures being applied. The disease was diagnosed regularly among wildlife while knowledge of virus circulation in livestock remained rudimentary.

Reluctantly at first but with growing momentum through the 1990s, wildlife personnel and veterinary ecologists were engaged, and in time this became a highly cooperative activity between the veterinary services, wildlife departments, and communities, with the important result of expanding the surveillance systems and networks and allowing more precise and accurate determination of endemic areas (48). As a consequence, through focal vaccination, rinderpest virus was finally suppressed, with the last outbreak recorded globally affecting buffalo in Meru National Park in Kenya in 2001. The last cattle vaccinations were undertaken in 2003, and no further cases were reported until declaration of global freedom from rinderpest was made by the OIE and FAO in 2010-2011 (49). This success showed how sectors with quite different mandates, but common interests and goals, could collaborate and thereby eradicate a major disease of the animal world for the first time. This was probably the first significant achievement from using an intersectoral One Health approach.

Rabies Prevention and Control: the Creation of Science-Based Policy

Rabies is a zoonotic, preventable, neglected tropical disease that, in Africa, has been historically underreported and poorly controlled. One successful model for rabies control has incorporated a One Health approach in the Serengeti ecosystem, Tanzania. In the Serengeti ecosystem, rabies kills humans (mostly children) and domestic animals (dogs, cows) and threatens endangered wildlife species (wild dogs). The Serengeti rabies story is one of hard work from a dedicated multidisciplinary team and can be viewed as a successful example of a One Health project.

In the 1990s, a team of ecologists, veterinarians, public health officials, and wildlife biologists working together in the Serengeti established a ring vaccination program for domestic dogs in the villages around the Serengeti National Park. Before the study, it was thought that rabies was uncontrollable in developing countries due to feral dogs and potential wildlife reservoirs (50). Study results show that rabies spills over from domestic dogs to other wildlife hosts (51) and that each rabid animal on average only affects ~1.2 others; therefore, rabies elimination is feasible through domestic dog vaccination (52). Following ring vaccination of domestic dogs around the park, human bites decreased, as did the incidence of rabid animals in the villages and inside the protected area (53). As a result of data-driven science and long-term commitment and investment from a team of researchers and local health officials, it was acknowledged that it is feasible to eliminate rabies in developing countries. As a result of this study, the WHO, with support from the Bill & Melinda Gates Foundation, chose Tanzania as a rabies eradication demonstration country.

The rabies One Health story in the Serengeti ecosystem can be viewed as a success not only for the impact on rabies control but also for the One Health approach itself. Specifically, (i) the study was strengthened through multi-institutional and cross-sectoral partnerships with local and foreign universities (in the United Kingdom, United States, Canada, and Tanzania), nongovernmental organizations (Lincoln Park Zoo and Frankfurt Zoological Society), government ministries (Tanzania Wildlife Research Institute), and private partnerships (donation of dog vaccines) (54). (ii) Local people were trained at all levels of the research implementation; Tanzanians were employed as staff and Tanzanian masters and Ph.D. students were trained. (iii) Multidisciplinary teams of academics, such as ecologists, veterinarians, modelers, and animal behaviorists, actively engaged in collaborative research. (iv) The research was based on strong surveillance, novel field diagnostics, and integrative information management (55–58). (v) A long-term commitment was created with long-term monitoring and ongoing implementation of rabies control. An added benefit of this long-term surveillance approach is that new pathogens have been discovered (59), and (vi) there is local buy-in due to education of local communities.

Once field data on interventions were collected, another reason this project was successful is because the research was used to inform policy. This was obtained in three ways. (i) Raw data were published (60, 61). (ii) Raw data could be used to statistically and mathematically model cost-effective interventions (62–64). And (iii) information was relayed back to ministries, the Gates Foundation, and global partnerships (54). Thus, this case study represents an effective holistic approach to complex issues.

A Cautionary Tale: Lessons Learned from the Threat of Pandemic Avian Influenza

Avian influenza subtype H5N1 most likely emerged in China around Poyang Lake after massive development of the domestic and semidomestic duck industry. The first outbreaks involved spillover to people from infected chickens in Hong Kong, and over the next decade there were additional outbreaks in poultry as well as severe disease in migrating wild waterfowl—most dramatically in Qinghai Lake (65). At first, wild birds were assumed to be an important source of viral shedding and global spread of the H5N1 virus. Despite this hypothesis, ecologists and wildlife health specialists were noticeably absent from the discussions regarding disease control and prevention in the first few years following emergence of the highly pathogenic avian influenza strain. As a result, wild bird surveillance was poorly managed and lacked sufficient expertise in species identification and wildlife monitoring (66). This in turn compromised the quality of results and led to misinformation about the role of wildlife in the avian influenza pandemic.

Unfortunately, the focus on the risk of spread via migrant birds deterred officials from focusing on the most important threat—the rapidly industrializing poultry sector in China and Southeast Asia—and acted synergistically with public and media panic (67). In the end, global spread was primarily through the poultry trade, not through wild bird epidemics; the latter burned out quite rapidly, with no spillover to people or poultry confirmed in any country (68). After well over 1 million wild birds were sampled, at considerable cost, no reservoir of infection in wildlife could be confirmed. Africa had major programs internationally funded at both regional and national levels in anticipation of the virus's arrival, focused on preparedness and response to this emerging pandemic. However, it was never found in most of the continent, though there is no doubt that other benefits accrued from this effort. It is a shame that the focus of these programs was so specific that other more pressing disease problems were often ignored. Today, the reservoir for the virus remains within the domestic poultry sector of the Far East, and the endemic focus is largely in the region of its origin, as well as in other regions with similar agricultural ecology to the main endemic zone, including South Asia and Egypt (69, 70).

COMMUNITY-BASED ONE HEALTH CAPACITY

The One Health concept is gaining momentum at many levels, partially due to the demonstration of the application of these principles to the control and management of emerging infectious diseases in eastern Africa. The number and depth of networks (Table 1) supported by international agencies and donors to address these issues is testimony to this fact. What remains to be seen is how these efforts translate to the practical implementation of helpful activities at the community level. Many well-funded international nongovernmental organizations are playing a crucial role in implementing One Health principles in Africa. However, a gap still exists in the support for or recognition of local organizations that may lead One Health initiatives at the community level. Local organizations or civil societies at large offer a comparative advantage over others in that they are made up of people from the relevant culture and are in direct contact with local communities faced with the challenges of concern. In addition, they fully understand and are working with local governments that are quite often *not* involved in discussions of One Health at national, regional, and global levels. We believe this is a critical area that needs to be recognized and addressed for any effective implementation and sustainability of One Health activities. For example, response to high-profile disease outbreaks such as Ebola and Marburg viruses is often handled largely by international organizations that fly in with the resources needed (such as personal protective equipment and rapid diagnostic tests) and then leave without having built significant infrastructure (the African Field Epidemiology Network [AFENET] is one caveat to this example). In most cases, this marks the end of all activity in this arena until the next outbreak, which will find the local authorities again underfunded and unprepared. Recent interviews conducted in communities affected by these outbreaks reveal a great deal of posttraumatic stress in recovered individuals and affected communities, yet these issues remain largely unaddressed (71). Local organizations with expertise in both science (health, ecology, conservation, etc.) and community-based approaches are critical. For example, two locally created and run organizations, Conservation & Ecosystem Health Alliance (http://www.ceha.co/) and Conservation through Public Health (http://www.ctph.org/), have a programmatic focus in western Uganda at the interface of wildlife, human, and livestock health and conservation issues. They have built strong research and community engagement pillars in conjunction with local governments and a host of external partners. Examples include understanding contact between great apes and humans in nonconserved areas; improvement of canine and public health in multiple urban centers through public education campaigns, rabies vaccination, population control via spay-and-neuter clinics, and external parasite control; as well as tuberculosis and brucellosis household risk factor surveys, domestic animal health surveys, and wildlife surveillance. AFENET (http://www.afenet.net/new/) has been at the center of epidemiological studies and disease outbreak investigations advocating for a One Health approach, successful outbreak investigation and control studies, as well as training programs such as a Masters of Preventative Veterinary Medicine with Field Epidemiology track, in conjunction with Makerere University, and several short courses in diagnostics and disease outbreak investigation. In the future, these local and regional organizations will be key to a true operationalization of the One Health approach in Africa.

As an example strategy for teaching students to work across disciplines and to encourage appreciation for cross-disciplinary collaboration, a One Health student club was generated and piloted in Rwanda. Students from veterinary medicine, nursing, and agricultural sciences identified the club as a framework they are familiar with, and one in which they could provide leadership and self-driven initiation of activities or projects that not only enhance their learning but also support and provide services to the local community. The students listed numerous ideas for coming together, across their disciplines, to encourage health promotion initiatives in the community. These included outreach exercises, support for community-based health screenings and outbreak response, and even formation of education teams that could go into secondary-level schools and inform students about the One Health principles and strategies. The students see this club as an opportunity to come together, learn from one another, and practice collaboration in ways they have not previously done through their specialized educational programs. Based on the success of this model, One Health student clubs are currently being formed across East and Central Africa.

THE WAY FORWARD

The challenges Africa faces at the interface of humans, animals, and ecosystems are not simple problems. Rather, these issues are complex and present compelling dilemmas with no simple technical solutions. No individual, discipline, sector, or organization can effectively manage these dilemmas alone; they require the transdisciplinary, integrated systems-based approaches promoted by One Health. Precipitating transformational change in behavior requires a long-term, multifaceted strategy; pan-African adoption of the One Health approach requires a conscious effort to catalyze transformational change. While technology advances may spur transformational change—like the development of the cell phone, which revolutionized communications in Africa—this change was an unintended impact. Precipitating transformational change with intention, i.e., with a clear objective in mind, requires a more strategic approach that involves a series of catalysts such as:

- *New heroes and compelling stories*. Throughout human history, compelling stories of heroes conquering daunting challenges have influenced behavior. One Health needs heroes with compelling stories that serve to provide role models and encouragement for the next generation.
- *New reward systems*. Society consciously and unconsciously rewards certain types of behavior. Celebrating One Health successes and recognizing and rewarding people and organizations that are doing it will speed the adoption of One Health.
- *New language*. A shared language is key to effective communications. Developing a language of One Health will facilitate cooperation and potentiate transdisciplinary, multisectoral partnerships and action. Creating this new language means not necessarily the invention of new words but rather the fostering of widespread shared understanding of key terms and concepts such as "ecosystem," "teamwork," and indeed, "One Health."
- *Value systems and norms*. Value systems underpin societal behavioral norms. Valuing of free speech, for example, sets the stage for the norm of candor and open discussion of various perspectives and opinions. Valuing the core competencies of One Health will expedite adoption of One Health

as the new normal. Teamwork is easier to develop within organizational systems when there is clear valuing of the norms of cooperation and interconnectedness. Language should be developed to effectively communicate the norms of One Health to stakeholders and bring relevancy to the concept—One Health can then provide the right language for stakeholders to understand and make it relevant to their systems.

- *New approaches to education.* Education embodies the means for communicating the compelling stories of new heroes, rewarding the desired behavior, teaching the new language, and instilling the value systems and new behavioral norms. Educational institutions committed to training the next generation as change agents require a redesign for "mutual learning and joint solutions offered by global interdependence due to acceleration of flows of knowledge, technologies and financing across borders." Transformed learning will emphasize searching and synthesis rather than fact finding and will manifest itself in achieving core knowledge, skills, and attributes as the primary end point for the learner rather than the credential.

CONCLUDING REMARKS

The One Health approach has special traction in Africa because of the tradition of Ubuntu leadership (72).

> When I share the value of my African upbringing, I proudly share the sociological richness of that otherwise (seemingly) harsh rural background. Those conditions of material lack were rich learning environments in many ways. They laid solid foundations for my understanding the value of human interconnectedness, of humaneness, of valuing collective good over individual interests, of the traction of human goodness found in Ubuntu.

> DUMISANI NDELELE,
> "The value of the African philosophy of Ubuntu in leadership"

The principles of Ubuntu support an African strategy of collaboration. Ubuntu is one of the most resilient African wisdoms, grounded in principles and practices of interconnectedness. "Ubuntu essentially means that each one of us can only effectively exist as fully-functioning human beings when we acknowledge the roles that others play in our lives. Most Nguni languages in Southern Africa describe Ubuntu as 'umuntu ngumuntu ngabantu' (in isiZulu this means: 'a person is a person through other persons', or 'I am because we are')" (73).

> Africans have a thing called 'Ubuntu'; it is about the essence of being human, it is part of the gift that Africa is going to give to the world. It embraces hospitality, caring about others, being willing to go that extra mile for the sake of another. We believe that a person is a person through other persons; that my humanity is caught up and bound up in yours. When I dehumanize

you, I inexorably dehumanize myself. The solitary human being is a contradiction in terms, and therefore you seek to work for the common good because your humanity comes into its own in community, in belonging.

DESMOND TUTU, Archbishop Emeritus of Cape Town

Acknowledgments. The authors of this manuscript have no commercial affiliations, consultancies, stock or equity interests, or patent-licensing arrangements that could be considered to pose a conflict of interest regarding the manuscript.

In addition, we would like to acknowledge collective input from members of the One Health Central and East Africa University Network, and affiliated support from RESPOND, Emerging Pandemic Threats Program, United States Aid in Development (USAID), USG.

Citation. Travis DA, Chapman DW, Craft ME, Deen J, Farnham MW, Garcia C, Hueston WD, Kock R, Mahero M, Mugisha L, Nzietchueng S, Nutter FB, Olson D, Pekol A, Pelican KM, Robertson C, Rwego IB. 2014. One Health: lessons learned from East Africa. Microbiol Spectrum 2(1):OH-0017-2012. doi:10.1128/microbiolspec.OH-0017-2012.

REFERENCES

1. **Donnelly MJ, McCall PJ, Lengeler C, Bates I, D'Alessendro U, Barnish G, Konradsen F, Klinkenberg E, Townson H, Trape JF, Hastings IM, Mutero C.** 2005. Malaria and urbanization in sub-Saharan Africa. *Malar J* **4:**12. doi:10.1186/1475-2875-4-12.

2. **Hay SI, Guerra CA, Tatem AJ, Atkinson PM, Snow RW.** 2005. Urbanization, malaria transmission and disease burden in Africa. *Nat Rev Microbiol* **3:**81–90.

3. **Chaisson RE, Martison NA.** 2008. Tuberculosis in Africa—combating an HIV-driven crisis. *N Engl J Med* **358:**1089–1092.

4. **Dunkle KL, Jewkes RK, Brown HC, Gray GE, McIntyre JA, Harlow SD.** 2004. Gender-based violence, relationship power, and risk of HIV infection in women attending antenatal clinics in South Africa. *Lancet* **363:**1415–1421.

5. **Barnett ED.** 2007. Yellow fever: epidemiology and prevention. *Clin Infect Dis* **44:**850–856.

6. **de Beyer JA, Preker AS, Feachem RG.** 2000. The role of the World Bank in international health: renewed commitment and partnership. *Soc Sci Med* **50:**169–176.

7. **Buse K, Walt G.** 2000. Global public-private partnerships: part I—a new development in health? *Bull World Health Organ* **78:**549–561.

8. **Coleman JS.** 1984. The idea of the developmental university, p 85–104. *In* Hetland A (ed), *Universities and National Development*. Almqvist & Wiksell International, Stockholm, Sweden.

9. **Samoff J, Carrol B.** 2004. The promise of partnership and continuities of dependence: external support to higher education in Africa. *Afr Stud Rev* **47:**67–199.

10. **Conraths FJ, Schwabenbauer K, Vallat B, Meslin FX, Füssel A-E, Slingenbergh J, Mettenleiter TC.** 2011. Animal health in the 21st century—a global challenge. *Prev Vet Med* **102:**93–97.

11. **Jones KE, Patel NG, Levy MA, Storeygard A, Balk D, Gittleman JL, Daszak P.** 2008. Global trends in emerging infectious diseases. *Nature* **451:**990–993.

12. **International Livestock Research Institute.** 2012. *Mapping of Poverty and Likely Zoonoses Hotspots. Zoonoses Project 4: Report to Department for International Development, UK.* International Livestock Research Institute, Nairobi, Kenya. http://cgspace.cgiar.org/bitstream/handle/10568/21161/ZooMap_July2012_final.pdf (last accessed June 5, 2013).

13. **Food and Agriculture Organization/World Organisation for Animal Health (OIE)/World Health Organization.** 2010. *Stakeholders Meeting for Emerging Pandemic Threats: FAO, OIE and WHO IDENTIFY Project.* OIE, Paris, France. http://www.oie.int/doc/ged/D11474.PDF (last accessed August 23, 2013).

14. **Food and Agriculture Organization.** 2003. *Veterinary public health and control of zoonoses in developing countries.* Food and Agriculture Organization, Rome, Italy. http://www.fao.org/docrep/006/y4962t/y4962t01.htm (last accessed August 23, 2013).

15. **Kuzmin IV, Bozick B, Guagliardo SA, Kunkel R, Shak JR, Tong S, Rupprecht CE.** 2011. Bats, emerging infectious diseases, and the rabies paradigm revisited. *Emerg Health Threats J* **4:**7159. doi:10.3402/ehtj.v4i0.7159.

16. **Stephen C, Ribble C.** 2001. Death, disease and deformity—using outbreaks in animals as sentinels for emerging environmental health risk. *Global Change Human Health* **2:**108–117.

17. **World Health Organization (WHO)/Centers for Disease Control and Prevention.** 2010. *Technical Guidelines for Integrated Disease Surveillance and Response in the African Region*, 2nd ed. WHO Regional Office for Africa, Brazzaville, Republic of Congo. http://www.cdc.gov/globalhealth/dphswd/idsr/pdf/ Technical%20Guidelines/IDSR%20Technical%20Guidelines%202nd%20Edition_2010_English.pdf (last accessed August 23, 2013).

18. **Wamala JF, Malimbo M, Okot CL, Atai-Omoruto AD, Tenywa E, Miller JR, Balinandi S, Shoemaker T, Oyoo D, Omonyo EO, Kagirita A, Musenero MM, Makumbi I, Nanyunja M, Lutwama JJ, Downing R, Mbonye AK.** 2012. Epidemiological and laboratory characterization of a yellow fever outbreak in northern Uganda, October 2010–January 2011. *Int J Infect Dis* **16:**e536–e542.

19. **Homsy J.** 1999. *Ape Tourism and Human Diseases: How Close Should We Get? A Critical Review of Rules and Regulations Governing Park Management & Tourism for the Wild Mountain Gorilla, Gorilla gorilla beringei*. International Gorilla Conservation Programme, Nairobi, Kenya. http://www.igcp.org/wp-content/ themes/igcp/docs/pdf/homsy_rev.pdf (last accessed August 23, 2013).

20. **Scally A, Dutheil JY, Hillier LW, Jordan GE, Goodhead I, Herrero J, Hobolth A, Lappalainen T, Mailund T, Marques-Bonet T, McCarthy S, Montgomery SH, Schwalie PC, Tang YA, Ward MC, Xue Y, Yngvadottir B, Alkan C, Andersen LN, Ayub Q, Ball EV, Beal K, Bradley BJ, Chen Y, Clee CM, Fitzgerald S, Graves TA, Gu Y, Heath P, Heger A, Karakoc E, Kolb-Kokocinski A, Laird GK, Lunter G, Meader S, Mort M, Mullilkin JC, Munch K, O'Connor TD, Phillips AD, Prado-Martinez J, Rogers AS, Sajjadian S, Schmidt D, Shaw K, Simpson JT, Stenson PD, Turner DJ, Vigilant L, Vilella AJ, Whitener W, Zhu B, Cooper DN, de Jong P, Dermitzakis ET, Eichler EE, Flicek P, Goldman N, Mundy NI, Ning Z, Odom DT, Ponting CP, Quail MA, Ryder OA, Searle SM, Warren WC, Wilson RK, Schierup MH, Rogers J, Tyler-Smith C, Durbin R.** 2012. Insights into hominid evolution from the gorilla genome sequence. *Nature* **483:**169–175.

21. **Wallis J, Lee DR.** 1999. Primate conservation: the prevention of disease transmission. *Int J Primatol* **20:**803–826.

22. **Woodford MH, Butynski TM, Karesh W.** 2002. Habituating the great apes: the disease risks. *Oryx* **36:**153–160.

23. **Heeney JL, Dalgleish AG, Weiss RA.** 2006. Origins of HIV and the evolution of resistance to AIDS. *Science* **313:**462–466.

24. **Kaur T, Singh J, Tong S, Humphrey C, Clevenger D, Tan W, Szekely B, Wang Y, Li Y, Alex Muse E, Kiyono M, Hanamura S, Inoue E, Nakamura M, Huffman MA, Jiang B, Nishida T.** 2008. Descriptive epidemiology of fatal respiratory outbreaks and detection of a human-related metapneumovirus in wild chimpanzees (*Pan troglodytes*) at Mahale Mountains National Park, Western Tanzania. *Am J Primatol* **70:**755–765.

25. **Köndgen S, Kühl H, N'Goran PK, Walsh PD, Schenk S, Ernst N, Biek R, Formenty P, Mätz-Rensing K, Schweiger B, Junglen S, Ellerbrok H, Nitsche A, Briese T, Lipkin WI, Pauli G, Boesch C, Leendertz FH.** 2008. Pandemic human viruses cause decline of endangered great apes. *Curr Biol* **18:**260–264.

26. **Palacios G, Lowenstine LJ, Cranfield MR, Gilardi KV, Spelman L, Lukasik-Braum M, Kinani JF, Mudakikwa A, Nyirakaragire E, Bussetti AV, Savji N, Hutchison S, Egholm M, Lipkin WI.** 2011. Human metapneumovirus infection in wild mountain gorillas, Rwanda. *Emerg Infect Dis* **17:**711–713.

27. **Williams JM, Lonsdorf EV, Wilson ML, Schumacher-Stankey J, Goodall J, Pusey AE.** 2008. Causes of death in the Kasekela chimpanzees of Gombe National Park, Tanzania. *Am J Primatol* **70:**766–777.

28. **Hastings BE, Kenny D, Lowenstine LJ, Foster JW.** 1991. Mountain gorillas and measles: ontogeny of a wildlife vaccination program, p 198–205. *In* Junge RE (ed), *Proceedings of the Annual Meeting of the American Association of Zoo Veterinarians*. Blackwell, Philadelphia, PA.

29. **Kalema-Zikusoka G, Kock RA, Macfie EJ.** 2002. Scabies in free-ranging mountain gorillas (*Gorilla beringei beringei*) in Bwindi Impenetrable National Park, Uganda. *Vet Rec* **150:**12–15.

30. **Bermejo M, Rodríguez-Teijeiro JD, Illera G, Barroso A, Vilà C, Walsh PD.** 2006. Ebola outbreak killed 5000 gorillas. *Science* **314:**1564.

31. **Nizeyi JB, Cranfield MR, Graczyk TK.** 2002. Cattle near the Bwindi Impenetrable National Park, Uganda, as a reservoir of *Cryptosporidium parvum* and *Giardia duodenalis* for local community and free-ranging gorillas. *Parasitol Res* **88:**380–385.

32. **Leendertz FH, Lankester F, Guislain P, Néel C, Drori O, Dupain J, Speede S, Reed P, Wolfe N, Loul S, Mpoudi-Ngole E, Peeters M, Boesch C, Pauli G, Ellerbrok H, Leroy EM.** 2006. Anthrax in Western and Central African great apes. *Am J Primatol* **68:**928–933.

33. **IUCN.** 2012. *The IUCN Red List of Threatened Species. Version 2012.2.* International Union for Conservation of Nature and Natural Resources, Cambridge, United Kingdom. http://www.iucnredlist.org (downloaded November 30, 2012).

34. **Goodall J.** 1986. *The Chimpanzees of Gombe: Patterns of Behavior.* Harvard University Press, Cambridge, MA.

35. **Nishida T.** 1990. *The Chimpanzees of the Mahale Mountains.* University of Tokyo Press, Tokyo, Japan.

36. **Decision Tree Writing Group.** 2006. Clinical response decision tree for the mountain gorilla (*Gorilla beringeii*) as a model for great apes. *Am J Primatol* **68:**909–927.

37. **Lonsdorf EV, Travis D, Pusey AE, Goodall J.** 2006. Using retrospective health data from the Gombe chimpanzee study to inform future monitoring efforts. *Am J Primatol* **68:**897–908.

38. **Cranfield M, Minnis R.** 2007. An integrated health approach to the conservation of Mountain gorillas (*Gorilla beringei beringei*). *Int Zoo Yb* **41:**110–121.

39. **The Mountain Gorilla Veterinary Project 2002 Employee Health Group.** 2004. Risk of disease transmission between conservation personnel and the mountain gorillas: results from an employee health program in Rwanda. *EcoHealth* **1:**351–361.

40. **Ali R, Cranfield M, Gaffikin L, Mudakikwa T, Ngeruka L, Whittier C.** 2004. Occupational health and gorilla conservation in Rwanda. *Int J Occup Environ Health* **10:**319–325.

41. **Robbins MM, Gray M, Fawcett KA, Nutter FB, Uwingeli P, Mburanumwe I, Kagoda E, Basabose A, Stoinski TS, Cranfield MR, Byamukama J, Spelman LH, Robbins AM.** 2011. Extreme conservation leads to recovery of the Virunga mountain gorillas. *PLoS One* **6:**e19788. doi:10.1371/journal.pone.0019788.

42. **Spinage C.** 2003. *Cattle Plague: a History.* Kluwer/Plenum Press, New York, NY.

43. **Roeder PL, Taylor WP, Rweyemamm MM.** 2006. Rinderpest in the twentieth and twenty-first centuries, p 105–142. *In* Barrett T, Pastoret PP, Taylor WP (ed), *Rinderpest and Peste des Petits Ruminants: Virus Plagues of Large and Small Ruminants.* Academic Press, London, United Kingdom.

44. **Plowright W.** 1968. Rinderpest virus, p 25–110. *In* Gard S, Hallauer C, Meyer KF (ed), *Virology Monographs,* vol **3**. Springer-Verlag, New York, NY.

45. **Rossiter PB, Jessett DM, Wafula JS, Karstad L, Chema S, Taylor WP, Rowe L, Nyange JC, Otaru M, Mumbala M, Scott GR.** 1983. Re-emergence of rinderpest as a threat in East Africa since 1979. *Vet Rec* **113:**459–461.

46. **Kock RA, Wambua JM, Mwanzia J, Wamwayi H, Ndungu EK, Barrett T, Kock ND, Rossiter PB.** 1999. Rinderpest epidemic in wild ruminants in Kenya, 1993-97. *Vet Rec* **145:**275–283.

47. **Mariner JC, Roeder PL.** 2003. Use of participatory epidemiology to study the persistence of lineage 2 rinderpest virus in East Africa. *Vet Rec* **152:**641–647.

48. **Kock RA, Wamwayi HM, Rossiter PB, Libeau G, Wambwa E, Okori J, Shiferaw FS, Mlengeya TD.** 2006. Re-infection of wildlife populations with rinderpest virus on the periphery of the Somali ecosystem in East Africa. *Prev Vet Med* **75:**63–80.

49. **Anderson J, Baron M, Cameron A, Kock R, Jones B, Pfeiffer D, Mariner J, McKeever D, Oura C, Roeder P, Rossiter P, Taylor W.** 2011. Rinderpest eradicated; what next? *Vet Rec* **169:**10–11.

50. **Lembo T, Hampson K, Kaare MT, Ernest E, Knobel D, Kazwala RR, Haydon DT, Cleaveland S.** 2010. The feasibility of canine rabies elimination in Africa: dispelling doubts with data. *PLoS Negl Trop Dis* **4:**e626. doi:10.1371/journal.pntd.0000626.

51. **Lembo T, Hampson K, Haydon DT, Craft M, Dobson A, Dushoff J, Ernest E, Hoare R, Kaare M, Mlengeya T, Mentzel C, Cleaveland S.** 2008. Exploring reservoir dynamics: a case study of rabies in the Serengeti ecosystem. *J Appl Ecol* **45:**1246–1257.

52. **Hampson K, Dushoff J, Cleaveland S, Haydon DT, Kaare M, Packer C, Dobson A.** 2009. Transmission dynamics and prospects for the elimination of canine rabies. *PLoS Biol* **7:**e53. doi:10.1371/journal.pbio.1000053.

53. **Kaare M, Lembo T, Hampson K, Ernest E, Estes A, Mentzel C, Cleaveland S.** 2009. Rabies control in rural Africa: evaluating strategies for effective domestic dog vaccination. *Vaccine* **27:**152–160.

54. **Lembo T, Attlan M, Bourhy H, Cleaveland S, Costa P, de Balogh K, Dodet B, Fooks AR, Hiby E, Leanes F, Meslin FX, Miranda Müller T, Nel LH, Rupprecht CE, Tordo N, Tumpey A, Wandeler A, Briggs DJ.** 2011. Renewed global partnerships and redesigned roadmaps for rabies prevention and control. *Vet Med Int* **2011**:923149. doi:10.4061/2011/923149.

55. **Lembo T, Niezgoda M, Velasco-Villa A, Cleaveland S, Ernest E, Rupprecht CE.** 2006. Evaluation of a direct, rapid immunohistochemical test for rabies diagnosis. *Emerg Infect Dis* **12**:310–313.

56. **Cleaveland S, Packer C, Hampson K, Kaare M, Kock R, Craft M, Lembo T, Mlengeya T, Dobson A.** 2008. The multiple roles of infectious diseases in the Serengeti ecosystem, p 209–239. *In* Sinclair AR, Packer C, Mduma SA, Fryxell JM (ed), *Serengeti III: Human Impacts on Ecosystem Dynamics*. University of Chicago Press, Chicago, IL.

57. **Halliday J, Daborn C, Auty H, Mtema Z, Lembo T, Bronsvoort M, Handel I, Knobel D, Hampson K, Cleaveland S.** 2012. Bringing together emerging and endemic zoonoses surveillance: shared challenges and a common solution. *Philos Trans R Soc Lond B Biol Sci* **367**:2872–2880.

58. **Lembo T, Auty H, Hampson K, Craft ME, Fyumagwa R, Ernest E, Haydon D, Hoare R, Kaare M, Lankester F, Mlengeya T, Travis DA, Cleaveland S.** 2013. Infectious diseases in the Serengeti: what we know and how we know it. *In* Sinclair AR, Metzger K, Mduma SA, Fryxell JM (ed), *Serengeti IV: Sustaining Biodiversity in a Coupled Human-Natural System*. University of Chicago Press, Chicago, IL, in press.

59. **Marston DA, Horton DL, Ngeleja C, Hampson K, McElhinney LM, Banyard AC, Haydon D, Cleaveland S, Rupprecht CE, Bigambo M, Fooks AR, Lembo T.** 2012. Ikoma lyssavirus, highly divergent novel lyssavirus in an African civet. *Emerg Infect Dis* **18**:664–667.

60. **Hampson K, Dushoff J, Cleaveland S, Haydon DT, Kaare M, Packer C, Dobson A.** 2009. Transmission dynamics and prospects for the elimination of canine rabies. *PLoS Biol* **7**:e53. doi:10.1371/journal.pbio.1000053.

61. **Lembo T.** 2007. *An investigation of disease reservoirs in complex ecosystems: rabies and canine distemper in the Serengeti. Ph.D. thesis.* University of Edinburgh, Edinburgh, United Kingdom.

62. **Beyer HL, Hampson K, Lembo T, Cleaveland S, Kaare M, Haydon DT.** 2012. The implications of metapopulation dynamics on the design of vaccination campaigns. *Vaccine* **30**:1014–1022.

63. **Beyer HL, Hampson K, Lembo T, Cleaveland S, Kaare M, Haydon DT.** 2011. Metapopulation dynamics of rabies and the efficacy of vaccination. *Proc Biol Sci* **278**:2182–2190.

64. **Fitzpatrick MC, Hampson K, Cleaveland S, Meyers LA, Townsend JP, Galvani AP.** 2012. Potential for rabies control through dog vaccination in wildlife-abundant communities of Tanzania. *PLoS Negl Trop Dis* **6**:e1796. doi:10.1371/journal.pntd.0001796.

65. **Liu J, Xiao H, Lei F, Zhu Q, Qin K, Zhang XW, Zhang XL, Zhao D, Wang G, Feng Y, Ma J, Liu W, Wang J, Gao GF.** 2005. Highly pathogenic H5N1 influenza virus infection in migratory birds. *Science* **309**:1206. doi:10.1126/science.1115273.

66. **Knight-Jones TJ, Hauser R, Matthes D, Stärk KD.** 2010. Evaluation of effectiveness and efficiency of wild bird surveillance for avian influenza. *Vet Res* **41**:50. doi:10.1051/vetres/2010023.

67. **Alexander DJ.** 2007. An overview of the epidemiology of avian influenza. *Vaccine* **25**:5637–5644.

68. **Hogerwerf L, Wallace RG, Ottaviani D, Slingenbergh J, Prosser D, Bergmann L, Gilbert M.** 2010. Persistence of highly pathogenic avian influenza H5N1 virus defined by agro-ecological niche. *EcoHealth* **7**:213–225.

69. **Lebarbenchon C, Feare CJ, Renaud F, Thomas F, Gauthier-Clerc M.** 2010. Persistence of highly pathogenic avian influenza viruses in natural ecosystems. *Emerg Infect Dis* **16**:1057–1062.

70. **Abdelwhab EM, Hafez HM.** 2011. An overview of the epidemic of highly pathogenic H5N1 avian influenza virus in Egypt: epidemiology and control challenges. *Epidemiol Infect* **139**:647–657.

71. **Hewlett BS, Hewlett BL.** 2008. *Ebola, Culture and Politics: the Anthropology of an Emerging Disease.* Thompson/Wadworth Press, Belmont, CA.

72. **Van der Colff L.** 2003. Leadership lessons from the African tree. *Manage Decision* **41**:257–261.

73. **Ncube LB.** 2010. Ubuntu: a transformative leadership philosophy. *J Leadership Stud* **4**:77–82.

One Health: People, Animals, and the Environment
Edited by Ronald M. Atlas and Stanley Maloy
© 2014 American Society for Microbiology, Washington, DC
doi:10.1128/microbiolspec.OH-0018-2012

Chapter 20

The Future of One Health

Ronald M. Atlas[1] and Stanley Maloy[2]

The recognition that human, animal, and ecological health are integrally interconnected has given rise to a growing recognition of the importance of crossing boundaries that have arisen in education, research, and practice. The value of the One Health approach is obvious to microbiologists who confront the frequent emergence of zoonotic diseases and the ecological factors that bring about changes in the distribution and activities of microorganisms across the globe. Microbes readily cross the boundaries of ecosystems—they have evolved to jump environmental barriers, including those that differentiate humans from other animal species (1).

This is not a new idea: the pioneering microbiologists Louis Pasteur and Robert Koch carried out research on both animal and human diseases and recognized the interconnection between animal and human health (2). Medical and veterinary educators of that era, including Rudolph Virchow and Sir William Osler, also freely crossed the boundaries of human and animal health (3, 4). Virchow is quoted as saying: "Between animal and human medicine there are no dividing lines—nor should there be" (5). Calvin Schwabe, who helped establish the modern One Health movement, shared this perspective when he said: "There is no difference of paradigm between human and veterinary medicine. Both sciences share a common body of knowledge in anatomy, physiology, pathology, on the origins of diseases in all species" (6). Although a major thrust for One Health has emerged from the veterinary community, the value of One Health goes well beyond cooperation between veterinarians and physicians. Importantly, "in the past decade, the concept of One Health has expanded beyond an examination of the human-animal health interface to encompass the health and sustainability of the world's ecosystems" (7).

Although it is an old concept, the need for One Health approaches is more important than ever. The risks of not adopting a One Health approach were clearly evident in 1999 when a lack of coordination between veterinary and human diagnostic labs delayed recognition of the outbreak of West Nile fever in New York City (8). Subsequently this disease has spread across the United States and around the world.

Given that more than 60% of emerging infectious disease events are caused by the transmission of an infectious agent from animals (zoonoses), with 75% of these originating from wildlife, employing a systematic One Health approach has great potential for reducing threats to global health from infectious diseases. In other countries, particularly

[1]Department of Biology, University of Louisville, Louisville, KY 40292; [2]Center for Microbial Sciences, San Diego State University, San Diego, CA 92182.

in the developing world, there is less of a division between the veterinary and human health communities. In fact, many countries now are seeking better ways to ensure early detection of zoonotic diseases. Canadian ministries and major international organizations have initiated consultations entitled "One World, One Health: from Ideas to Action." There also now is a One Health office within the Centers for Disease Control and Prevention (CDC) and increased cooperation between the CDC and the U.S. Department of Agriculture. The One Health approach should advance health care for the 21st century and beyond by accelerating biomedical research, enhancing public health efficacy, expeditiously expanding the scientific knowledge base, and improving medical education and clinical care (6).

Despite the obvious benefits, the barriers to achieving a comprehensive One Health approach are formidable. Education, research, diagnostics, surveillance, and funding for human medicine, veterinary medicine, and environmental health often exist as separate silos with limited exchange. Medical students often are trained only in human diseases. Similarly, veterinarians concentrate on nonhuman animals. Environment is often not even considered in introductory microbiology courses. These barriers must be overcome if the benefits of One Health are to be realized. One critical aspect involves reforming the fundamental system of education in the way Virchow, Osler, and Schwabe envisaged. Fortunately, some academic medical centers are beginning to rise to this challenge, providing the interdisciplinary educational opportunities needed to form the foundation of a One Health approach, including consideration of environment and its health implications (7).

This challenge is both regional and global. Changing demographics, the resulting environmental disruption, and international travel have a major impact on animal and human health (7). Expansion of farms and cities into wilderness areas and ecological disruption of animal habitats have led to new niches for pathogenic microbes and promoted the transmission of new diseases from animals to humans (Fig. 1). Human developments have resulted in global climate change that influences the distribution of animal habitats and disease vectors. Furthermore, the expansion of global travel and food

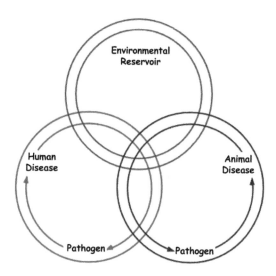

Figure 1. The interrelationship among human disease, animal disease, and the environment. One Health is represented by the region of overlap.
doi:10.1128/microbiolspec.OH-0018-2012.f1

distribution networks has facilitated the rapid transmission of disease between urban and rural regions of the entire world. Hence, it is clear that international cooperation in many areas will be required to thwart these threats.

In addition, solving these problems will demand new tools for rapid identification and response. A variety of new tools such as environmental metagenomics, geospacial modeling, and mobile communication technologies have made it possible to rapidly detect many diseases in the environment, and provide a window of opportunity to develop upstream barriers to transmission before the diseases become a major health risk. This changes the way we deal with infectious disease from responding to an outbreak by treating patients to detecting and intervening in the process upstream (Fig. 2). When this One Health approach is most successful, it prevents disease outbreaks before they are recognized as a problem by the public and funding agencies; thus it will demand constant effort to inform policymakers about the need to support these efforts.

In addition, to foster the necessary research there will need to be cross-agency funding opportunities. Traditionally, funding for human, animal, and environmental health has been supported by different agencies in the United States, limiting the potential for supporting interdisciplinary One Health approaches. One step in the right direction is the interagency program by the U.S. National Institutes of Health (NIH) and the National Science Foundation to support research on the evolution and ecology of infectious diseases. The NIH has also supported work on the emergence of potential human infectious agents in wildlife populations. The work on viral chatter by Nathan Wolfe and his efforts at viral forecasting (9) (http://www.globalviral.org/) as well as work by Peter Daszak are nice examples of the need for such cross-disciplinary research. Recent concerns about the potential jump of H5N1 influenza viruses into a human-transmittable form highlight the extreme need for such molecular surveillance programs in nonhuman animal populations and the environment. Nevertheless, there is tremendous need for more cross-agency support for interdisciplinary research on One Health approaches.

Current paradigm:

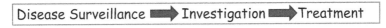

- Human disease

One Health paradigm:

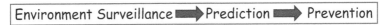

- Environment
- Animals
- Human disease

Figure 2. The current human health versus the One Health paradigm. doi:10.1128/microbiolspec.OH-0018-2012.f2

One Health approaches are likely to have a major impact on public health, with a focus on surveillance and upstream interventions that are likely to reap obvious and rapid benefits for the health of human populations. For that reason public health agencies such as the CDC and the World Health Organization are joining with veterinary organizations and agricultural departments in advancing the One Health agenda. The chapters in the book *One Health: People, Animals, and the Environment* (10) provide compelling examples of the imperatives and opportunities for One Health and the impact of this approach on our future.

Acknowledgments. The authors have no conflicts of interest regarding this manuscript.

Citation. Atlas RM, Maloy S. 2014. The future of One Health. Microbiol Spectrum 2(1):OH-0018-2012. doi:10.1128/microbiolspec.OH-0018-2012.

REFERENCES

1. **Kolter R, Maloy S.** 2012. *Microbes and Evolution: the World That Darwin Never Saw.* ASM Press, Washington, DC.
2. **Atlas RM.** 2013. One Health: its origins and future. *In* Mackenzie JS, Jeggo M, Daszak PS, Richt JA (ed), *One Health: The Human-Animal-Environment Interfaces in Emerging Infectious Diseases. Curr Top Microbiol Immunol* **365**.
3. **Kahn LH, Kaplan B, Steele JH.** 2007. Confronting zoonoses through closer collaboration between medicine and veterinary medicine (as 'One Medicine'). *Vet Ital* **43**:5–19.
4. **Kahn LH, Kaplan B, Monath TP, Steele JH.** 2008. Teaching "One Medicine, One Health." *Am J Med* **121**:169–170.
5. **Saunders LZ.** 2000. Virchow's contributions to veterinary medicine: celebrated then, forgotten now. *Vet Pathol* **37**:199–207.
6. **Atlas R, Rubin C, Maloy S, Daszak P, Colwell R, Hyde B.** 2010. One Health: attaining optimal health for people, animals, and the environment. *Microbe* **5**:383–389.
7. **Shomaker TS, Green EM, Yandow SM.** 2013. One Health: a compelling convergence. *Acad Med* **88**: 49–55.
8. **American Society for Microbiology.** 2011. *Microbeworld Video: One Health and the lessons learned from the 1999 West Nile virus outbreak (MWV46).* American Society for Microbiology, Washington, DC. http://www.microbeworld.org/podcasts/microbeworld-video/898-one-health-and-the-lessons-learned-from-the-1999-west-nile-virus-outbreak-mwv46- (last accessed August 26, 2013).
9. **Wolfe ND, Dunavan CP, Diamond J.** 2007. Origins of major human infectious diseases. *Nature* **447**: 279–283.
10. **Atlas RM, Maloy S.** 2014. *One Health: People, Animals, and the Environment.* ASM Press, Washington, DC.

INDEX